Afflicted

Basic Bioethics
Arthur Caplan, editor

A complete list of the books in the Basic Bioethics series appears at the back of this book.

Afflicted

How Vulnerability Can Heal Medical Education and Practice

Nicole M. Piemonte

The MIT Press
Cambridge, Massachusetts
London, England

© 2018 Massachusetts Institute of Technology

All rights reserved. No part of this book may be reproduced in any form by any electronic or mechanical means (including photocopying, recording, or information storage and retrieval) without permission in writing from the publisher.

This book was set in Stone Serif by Westchester Publishing Services. Printed and bound in the United States of America.

Library of Congress Cataloging-in-Publication Data

Names: Piemonte, Nicole M., author.
Title: Afflicted : how vulnerability can heal medical education and practice / Nicole M. Piemonte.
Description: Cambridge, MA : The MIT Press, [2017] | Series: Basic bioethics | Includes bibliographical references and index.
Identifiers: LCCN 2017021517 | ISBN 9780262037396 (hardcover : alk. paper)
Subjects: LCSH: Medicine—Philosophy. | Medical education—Philosophy. | Medical ethics.
Classification: LCC R723 .P476 2017 | DDC 610.1—dc23
LC record available at https://lccn.loc.gov/2017021517

10 9 8 7 6 5 4 3 2

For my mother, Joy, who always seemed to embody her name

Contents

Prologue   ix
Acknowledgments   xiii
Introduction   xv

1 Exploring the Shortcomings of a "Scientific" Medical Education   1
2 The "Remainder" in Modern Medicine: The Lived Experience of Illness and Existential Anxiety   29
3 Turning toward Suffering Together   63
4 The Formation of Medical "Professionals"   97
5 The Journey Back to Oneself: Reimagining Medical Education   127
   Epilogue   165

Notes   171
Bibliography   227
Index   249

Prologue

The ideas presented in this book are ones I have had for a long time—ideas that were critically important to me before I started my graduate work in the medical humanities, though at the time they were more nebulous and intuitive and, indeed, not yet coherent. I started my doctoral program not long after caring for my mother, a joyful woman filled with a fierce love who was diagnosed at fifty with advanced ovarian cancer and died a little more than two years later. After living alongside her illness and plunging deep into the disorienting world of hospital rooms, anxious sickbed vigils, and isolating suffering, I emerged with something I never asked for: a vivid, embodied understanding of the triumphs and failings of the complex world of medicine.

Looking back, I know that my mother's doctors cared for her, both as a patient and as a person; they were kind, compassionate, professional, and knowledgeable—all of the things we want our doctors to be. But, as she lay dying in a hospital room instead of at home, having been told only twelve hours earlier—by a palliative care doctor whom she had never met—that she was dying, I also knew that, somewhere along the way, something had gone wrong. Her doctors, who genuinely cared about her and also about me, were afraid. They were afraid of telling us that she was dying, though they undoubtedly knew she was, having seen the scans that showed the disease had spread throughout her lungs and abdomen and into her brain. They were afraid—that is the only way I can make sense of their offering her a new chemotherapy treatment the day before she died rather than acknowledging that the end was so near.

It would have been easy for me, and at times it was easy, to blame the doctors for not being candid with us, for not simply addressing my mother's inevitable death. Wasn't it their job to "break bad news," to diagnose and prognosticate, to tell us what was happening inside her body? And, more than that, weren't they, as healers, called to do something more than medically treat her disease? Shouldn't they have acknowledged the reality of her existential suffering, that she was facing the end of her life much earlier than she had ever imagined? Shouldn't they have made sure she was comfortable, that she could say her good-byes to her friends and family and die at home?

It is easy to ask these questions and to become angry that things could have, or should have, been different. But this anger, it seems to me, fails to consider that my mother's doctors were human beings with their own struggles, limitations, and vulnerabilities. If doctors are more than just medical technicians or dispensers of healthcare, if they are, in fact, also human beings, who, like the rest of us, experience sadness and fear and disappointment, then it is understandable that confronting human suffering and mortality might be difficult for them. It is much easier to look at the statistical chances for a patient's living another few months and to offer her more treatment than to tell a scared woman and her scared daughter that they need to confront the one reality they simply can't bear to face.

My research over the past six years and my time spent with patients, doctors, residents, and students, both medical and premedical, has revealed to me that, though our anger and frustration toward doctors can sometimes be justified, they can sometimes be misguided, too. Seeing firsthand how doctors are trained has in many ways transformed my anger and frustration into a kind of empathy for those who are shaped by, and even perpetuate, the systems that fail patients and doctors alike. It is easy to criticize doctors for being unempathetic, uncaring, and self-serving, but doing so often covers over the root of the problem: the educational and institutional cultures that so powerfully (trans)form medical students and doctors; that promote reductionistic understandings of care, illness, and suffering; and that virtually ignore the personal development—the *self*—of students who are becoming doctors.

Not long ago, while attempting to make my thoughts about these issues cohere into some kind of written work, I opened an e-mail that was part of a thread I had been following on a large listserv. It was from a doctor who was writing in response to the topic of physicians who behave badly:

This conversation has resonated deeply with me as a physician who has intended well, and who nearly burned out because of the insidious process of physician formation that left me a mess at the threshold of the suffering of other human beings. I won't begin to tell you the sad things I have seen and done, and it has taken me years to find my way out, and back into compassionate care. . . . We have a deep, deep problem in this country with physician formation. Among other things. I was—pardon the sentiment—loved back into a good medical practice as a form of growing wisdom and care. And believe me, I am still learning.[1]

When I read this doctor's candid and poignant message, I knew right then he had captured the very problem I wanted and needed to explore. Despite all the scholarly work focusing on professionalism, empathy erosion, and the need for holistic care, little has been said about how the process of forming future doctors leaves them ill equipped to handle the realities of medicine—and how it leaves them a mess at the threshold of human suffering. Surprisingly, even less has been said about *why* medical training tends to avoid the cultivation of the self and an authentic confrontation with human suffering and the fear and self-doubt that can come with it. And almost nothing has been said about how medical students and doctors might be "loved back" into compassionate care for themselves and others.

I am well aware that the idea of "loving" someone back into compassionate care sounds effusive and even silly, especially within a medical culture that tends to valorize objectivity and "professional" detachment. Yet this word seems right to me. It is somehow too vague, too profound, too imprecise, and too perfect all at once. In this context, the word is strange; it stops us in our tracks; its incongruity forces us to consider the very humanness of medicine. In Arthur Kleinman's classic text *The Illness Narratives*, a doctor he interviewed asserts that "to care for humans is to be *human* and to see the limits and failures and also successes of our small humanity writ large in the struggle to help someone who hurts and fears and just plain is in need. The moral lesson is that this is what our life is about, too, what we must prepare for."[2] In this sense, being a doctor is about being human, and the medical act is simply a human act—a response to another human who needs help. Although professional codes state that doctors must use their medical knowledge to aid patients, students are rarely told that they are called to simply respond to another human being in need. Perhaps all that medical knowledge obscures this simple fact. Perhaps the preoccupation with scientific and clinical facts, rote memorization, and test scores sends the message that doctors confronting their own limitations and fears and learning to respond to the persons in front of them are not what *really* matters in medicine. Yet, by not preparing students for the suffering they will inevitably encounter time and again, by letting them believe that medicine is just about attending to biological dysfunction, and by ignoring the fact that medical education will change in a significant way *who* they are, we leave these future doctors a mess in the face of suffering patients—patients whose suffering is intensified by doctors who do not know how to respond to it.

Afflicted, then, is not about me, or my mother, or making sense of my experience with her. In some ways, it is not even about medicine—it is about recognizing our own vulnerability and learning how to respond to the vulnerability of others. It is about exploring why, as human beings, we desire to turn away from suffering and death. And it is about cultivating a self who acknowledges this desire and still chooses to face others in their suffering and show them care. Some might say that this topic is too idealistic and emotive for anyone to realistically write about, let alone ask those who practice or teach medicine to take seriously. In some ways, they may be right. But as I spend more time teaching and learning from medical students, residents, and faculty, I have come to see that—not unlike their patients—our caregivers desire authenticity and connection; they, too, want to be seen and known, to engage in meaningful work, and to find their way back to the reasons why they chose their profession in the first place. It is difficult to discuss things like authenticity, meaning, and connection without toeing the line of naïve idealism, and I admittedly take the risk of crossing that line. My hope is that in doing so, I can help reveal our need for one another—a need that so often gets covered over in medicine—so that we might all learn how to more authentically engage with one another and care for each other well.

Acknowledgments

Although it would be hard to acknowledge and express gratitude to all who have made this book possible, there are those without whom it simply would not exist. I am eternally grateful to my family—my father, Ralph, my brother, Chris, my grandma, Rose Marie, and my partner, Shawn Abreu, for their love and their steadfast support. So much of what I have learned about medicine has been through personal experiences we have walked through together as a family.

During my time at the University of Texas Medical Branch, I was fortunate enough to learn from Dr. Michael Malloy, Dr. Susan McCammon, Dr. Steve Lieberman, and Susan Minello, clinical faculty who represent the gleaming bright spots of medical education. I am grateful for the time, energy, and resources they invested in me and so many other students simply because they are passionate about practicing medicine and helping to form future healers. I am also indebted to so many faculty members who have pushed me, throughout my graduate and postgraduate education, to think deeply and critically about our shared world. I want to thank in particular Drs. Michele Carter, Ramsey Eric Ramsey, Kevin Aho, Jason Robert, Carla Fisher, Ronald Carson, Anne Hudson Jones, Jason Glenn, Douglas Kelley, Vincent Waldron, and Jeff Sugimoto. I will always carry with me what I have learned from you, both personally and professionally.

To my friends, from both Phoenix and Texas, whose love has sustained me while writing this: you have, whether you know it or not, lent me your courage when I needed it most. I am especially grateful for one of my truest friends, Erica Fletcher, who kept me alive through it all—the woman who taught me that even when life becomes an existential nightmare, you just have to keep typing. And, finally, I must thank the premeds, medical students, and residents who have taught me so much when I was supposed to be teaching them. I will keep fighting for a healthcare system that supports you in the way you deserve.

Introduction

The question has been posed to me many times, and every so often I ask myself the same thing: how can I possibly say anything about medical practice and education—let alone write a book about it—if I am not a clinician myself? The question is fair enough, and (most of the time) I appreciate when people are direct enough to ask me it. My response usually takes one of two forms. Sometimes I respond by emphasizing my insider knowledge, pointing to my experience taking care of my mom or explaining how I went to graduate school at an academic medical center where I learned from medical ethicists and doctors, rounded in hospitals, and spent time with patients—and where the majority of my peers and closest friends were medical students. These were friends I watched fumble and prevail in a shockingly imperfect educational system and stayed up late with having the conversations they weren't having in school about death and suffering and poverty, about Board scores and career decisions and the pains of being a twenty-something, about whether and how they could possibly survive it all. I then explain that I currently work at a hospital and medical school where my job is to teach, mentor, and support medical students and residents and help establish a culture that reconnects students, residents, and doctors to why they went into medicine in the first place. And I tell how I share my life and my home with a new doctor, whom I try to love and support the best way I can as I watch him struggle to offer compassionate care in a dispassionate healthcare system.

Other times, I respond by simply embracing my role as an outsider. As I discuss later in this book, medical culture does a particularly fine job of enculturating newcomers into its rituals and norms—almost all adopt the values, assume the behaviors, and embrace the ideals of medicine, for better or for worse and without even knowing it. It is hard to see the norms of a culture when one is so entrenched in that culture. Thus, as an outsider with an admittedly privileged view from the nearby margins, I am at times able to recognize and speak to issues that others simply cannot see. Or, as Peter Cahn said in a recent issue of *Academic Medicine*: "Outsiders are particularly well positioned to notice unspoken assumptions because they bring a different set of perceptions against which to contrast the prevailing model. People steeped in the predominant metaphors can rarely articulate the underlying conceptual system because it has become naturalized to them."[1] It is for this reason that I find working in medicine as a nonclinician to be a virtue; offering a different view for my colleagues, friends, and loved ones in medicine is sometimes exactly what is needed. And yet the point that an outsider cannot possibly understand the lived experience of a doctor is not lost on me. I will never know what it is like to stay up all night on a labor and delivery shift, make a life-or-death decision for a stranger, or face the consequences of a serious medical mistake. So, even as I lament the stigma that surrounds the Ph.D. in an M.D.'s world while recognizing the value of my unique standpoint, I also acknowledge and accept the limitations of my perspective.

Outside, inside, or in between, those of us who are concerned about medicine and medical education focus on problems that are, quite honestly, not particularly new. For years, scholars, clinicians, and patients alike have pointed to the ways in which patients' encounters with physicians have left them feeling dehumanized and misunderstood. I have lost count of the times when people I have just met—after I explain to them briefly what it is that people like me "do" in the medical humanities—exclaim, "Well, doctors certainly need that kind of thing, so keep it up!" What I think most people are referring to when they say their doctors "need" something is that, as patients, they feel their illness experiences and an essential part of themselves are overlooked in the clinical encounter—some aspects of their suffering are deemed invalid or simply rendered invisible. As physician Eric Cassell observed over thirty years ago, "Patients and their friends and families do not make a distinction between physical and nonphysical sources of suffering in the same way that doctors do."[2]

The idea that medicine is concerned only with particular kinds of suffering, specifically those physically manifested on or within the corporeal body, helps to explain why even patients who do not appear to be suffering profoundly might feel as though they are not "seen" by their doctors. Because suffering ensues when people perceive a threat to their "intactness"—when they perceive a potential destruction of their identities, routines, futures, relationships, roles, and so forth—the sources of suffering are multifarious and intricate, and the "remedies" usually involve finding, restoring, or making new meaning.[3] It is true that some conditions, like a broken arm or a minor infection, can be treated successfully through technical interventions alone; yet, even patients with minor or straightforward complaints come to the doctor because they are experiencing a perceived disruption in their normal way of life. Thus, the lived experience of patients who are ill or injured—even those who are not acutely vulnerable or suffering profoundly—includes more than biological breakdown. Patients seek the help of the doctor because they desire a restoration of their way of being-in-the-world. And when they are facing serious illness, even if not terminal, the experience can rip them out of their relations of meaning and being, shatter their worlds, and bring on intense *"existential* suffering"[4] as they struggle to find meaning, security, or connectedness.[5]

The failure of medicine to address these complex realities of illness and the kinds of suffering that extend beyond the workings of the biological body is a long-lived and persistent problem, one that has often been traced back to the ways doctors are trained. In the 1960s, philosophers, theologians, and practitioners began to draw attention to how medical care that privileged exactitude and certainty was failing to address the lived experiences of patients. These early medical humanists (though they did not yet refer to themselves as such) expressed concerns about "the way medical students of the rising generation were being trained and, in particular, [about] what was lacking in their education."[6] Daniel Fox, who offers a historical account of the political origins of the medical humanities, observes that groups concerned with medical education during this time focused primarily on three issues: depersonalization in medicine, the centrality of molecular biology in medical education, and the teaching of "mechanistic medicine." They believed that the best way to deal with these issues was to infuse "human values" into formal medical education—even though their presumption that human values could be identified, measured, and judged, and value deficits remedied by a "dose of the humanities" might have been mistaken.[7]

The argument that a simple dose of humanities will never remedy the problems in medical education is not uncommon.[8] Incorporating the humanities post hoc into a curriculum that scholars claim is so deeply entrenched within a culture of detachment and within an epistemology of science and certainty can do very little to change how students engage with patients and how they conceive of what it means to care. Not surprisingly, then, much of the recent scholarship concerning medical education indicates that the problems early medical humanists faced nearly fifty years ago are still present with us today. And not only are they still present, but they are also reinforced and perpetuated both within medical culture and within the contemporary medical school curriculum—a curriculum still preoccupied with identifying and treating biological disease states, potentially encouraging students to see themselves as mere technical problem solvers.[9] Most would agree that, despite efforts to incorporate studies of the humanities, communication workshops, and empathy training into medical schools, we find ourselves not far from where we were five decades ago.

Making Headway: Recent Curricular Changes

Due in part to the persistence of these issues, attention has been paid more recently to professionalism or professional identity formation in medical education—that is, to whether and how medical education fosters values such as compassion, altruism, honesty, integrity, and respect. Although professionalism standards, charters, and credos have become ubiquitous, many scholars have argued that there exists a considerable disconnect between the professional values and ideals espoused within the professionalism movement and the implicit values that are communicated to students on the wards through their interactions with peers and mentors—what they learn from the "hidden curriculum." Unfortunately, with its emphasis on efficiency, compliance, and the acquisition of scientific or technical knowledge and its tendency to focus on biological disease processes and technical cures, this hidden curriculum undermines the espoused values of professionalism and leaves little room to focus on what kind of person the doctor should be.[10]

Over the past decade or so, much scholarship has emerged focusing on the harmful consequences of the hidden curriculum and suggesting remedies. These almost always include quality mentoring of students by their attending physicians and residents, given that these mentors have such a profound effect on students' development.[11] As physician Thomas Inui argues, the hidden curriculum of medical education "constitutes the most powerful influence on students' understanding of professionalism in medicine."[12] Yet, even though discourse about the hidden curriculum has found its way into the literature and suggestions have been offered for addressing it, less attention has been paid to *why* the disconnect between espoused values and the ways students and mentors actually behave on the wards exists and persists. It is unlikely that this disconnect is simply a result of unprofessional physicians who engage in unethical decision making within a morally vacuous profession. Rather, as literary scholar and medical educator Kathryn Montgomery has pointed out, this hidden curriculum is likely a result of the fact that students and physicians are trained within a culture that views medicine as the direct application of science in the clinical setting, rather than a science-using *practice* imbued with uncertainty and ambiguity.[13]

Because of this view, the hidden curriculum of medical education sends a very clear and persistent message to students: medicine is a science concerned with the biological body and the efficient amelioration of disease states; doctors are therefore not required to attend to existential suffering. Claiming that medicine is akin to a kind of "impartial" natural science, Montgomery argues, bolsters clinical detachment and perpetuates what she calls the "the professional façade" that distances clinicians from the reality of illness, pain, and death.[14] Like Montgomery, philosopher and clinician Jeffrey Bishop claims that the education and training future doctors receive obscure how suffering extends beyond the biological body; students are "seduced by the efficient and effective manipulation of bodies and psyches as the most important response to suffering."[15] Thus, as medical students progress through their training, tending to the body becomes paramount, and other sources of suffering fall from view.

To me, the work of scholars like Montgomery and Bishop speaks to a "way of knowing" that German philosopher Martin Heidegger (borrowing from Aristotle) deemed "calculative thinking," a kind of thinking that is associated with the natural sciences and their methodologies, one set over and against the world and its objects in order to discover "correct" answers.[16] Although calculative thinking is appropriate for medicine in many ways and certainly leads to valuable technical knowledge, the danger lies in the propensity of modern medicine to conceive of calculative thinking as the *only* proper way of knowing anything at all. Indeed, Heidegger warns that "calculative thinking may someday come to be accepted and practiced *as the only* way of thinking."[17] Unsurprisingly, it is science and, by extension, medicine that have most tenaciously championed this way of knowing. "Science," argue biologist Linda Wiener and philosopher Ramsey Eric Ramsey, "represents itself not simply as a particular kind of methodology, but as the only method that can produce universally replicable descriptions of the world. It is from this point of view that the objectified body of anatomy and physiology, for example, becomes the only body that we are capable of acknowledging as valid."[18] When scientific methodologies are seen as the best or only way to think through medical problems, addressing the needs of the tangible, physical, measurable body can appear to be the doctor's only task at hand.

Although the scientific methodologies that constitute much of medicine's predominant approach to care are not inherently problematic, the perception that scientific interpretations of the world are more real or reliable than any others can narrow the kind of care that medicine considers within its purview. In other words, the professed telos of medicine—which is often conceived of as the good of the patient and the alleviation of human suffering—is narrowed significantly by a medical practice that is single-mindedly concerned with the physical body.[19] Educated within a system that almost exclusively embraces calculative thinking, which does not, indeed cannot, account for the lived, phenomenological experience of either patients or practitioners, medical students are ill prepared to address the kind of human suffering they will inevitably encounter.

Next Steps: Looking beyond—and before—Epistemology

Some of the scholarly work mentioned above has made the important argument that medicine is grounded within a normalized and rarely acknowledged epistemology that privileges scientific, objective, and verifiable truth, and that this accepted epistemology significantly influences patient care. Less work, however, has focused on why this kind of thinking—especially within medicine where human suffering and death are so prevalent—is so seductive.[20] Therefore, one point of the present work is to draw attention to the taken-for-granted assumptions of medical epistemology and pedagogy and to efforts toward "giving up the science claim," as Montgomery says, which

Introduction

requires us to consider the way medical education and practice personally shapes those who participate in it.[21] But the scope of the present work extends beyond an acknowledgment of the taken-for-granted, normalized culture, epistemology, and pedagogy of medicine and imagining ways of changing it. *Afflicted* aims to understand *why* it is that students, practitioners, educators, and patients so readily subscribe to and perpetuate calculative thinking. With the aid primarily of existential and phenomenological philosophy, I argue that the propensity to ground medicine within a scientific, objective, and anatomo-biological worldview is, in fact, a manifestation of a fundamental and ontological or existential desire to turn away from our shared vulnerability of being human. Rather than encouraging introspection and authentic engagement with others, the pedagogy and epistemology of modern medicine perpetuate this flight from the ontological reality of illness, suffering, loneliness, and death. In other words, I contend that depersonalization in medicine is not primarily an epistemological but an *ontological* problem—that is, it is related to *who we are* as finite, mortal beings and our beliefs about what it means to live and to be. The epistemology of medicine, or rather the privileging of this epistemology and the pedagogy it gives rise to, is a manifestation of our shared ontological or existential struggle to authentically face the realities of death and meaningless suffering. This does not mean that the way medicine is practiced and taught is consciously *intended* to conceal suffering, loss, and vulnerability, but rather that it is imperceptibly, yet substantially, molded by deep existential qualms about the human condition.

It is important to address these issues not only because they affect the kind of care patients receive, but also because they have real consequences for those who are exposed to patients' unacknowledged suffering. The moral conflicts that can and do arise in medicine often point to clinicians' own personal struggles to find some meaning or purpose in the face of death and tragedy.[22] As Michele Carter and Sally Robinson put it, "by submerging and denying these personal conflicts instead of realizing they are part of the human condition, practitioners may find themselves harboring significant negative emotions of anger, despair, or helplessness, which in turn can impede their professional judgments."[23]

Avoiding or trivializing personal responses to human suffering can have significant and tangible consequences in the clinical setting, but, just as important, these personal responses are not unique to those who work in healthcare—they are "part of the human condition." With that clearly in mind, *Afflicted* argues that it is too simple to conclude that doctors simply lack compassion, empathy, or the desire to help. Rather, like their patients, doctors share in the human desire to avoid suffering and the existential anxiety it produces. But this desire poses a particular problem for doctors and other healthcare professionals. Even though the medical profession requires practitioners to extend care to others, medicine's epistemological stance (grounded in calculative thinking) offers them an all-too-easy means of turning away from vulnerability—and thus also from providing care in the fullest sense—by comporting themselves as technicians. That is to say, the primary curative ethos of medicine, which emphasizes a "medical doing something," perpetuates a calculative understanding of care that, however unintentionally, encourages physicians to turn away from the suffering of their patients.

In my view, then, the preoccupation with cure over care, pervasive clinical detachment, poor or nonexistent communication between clinicians and patients, compassion fatigue and burnout, and even "coping strategies" like gallows humor are symptoms of deeper issues underlying medical education and practice—symptoms that will persist until we address the existential issues that give rise to them.[24] As such, readers looking for a "handbook" or "roadmap" for effective communication interventions need read no further, for I believe such interventions fail to address the core of medicine's inability to adequately deal with vulnerability and existential suffering. And though I see the present work as practical and applied, especially in relation to the changes I suggest for premedical and medical education, it offers no specific behavioral or communication interventions. From my own experience researching and developing medical and premedical curricula and teaching medical students and residents, it is clear to me that many communication interventions, as well as research and pedagogy in interpersonal communication in medicine, are grounded in the assumption that communication is transactional in nature. So, rather than teaching future clinicians how to authentically engage with patients, to be present with the dying, or to bear witness to suffering, we have them memorize checklists and mnemonics to assist with difficult clinical interactions and with "delivering" information to patients. To "break bad news," for instance, many medical students are taught the SPIKES (**S**et the stage, **P**erception,

Inform, Knowledge, Empathy, and Summarize) method, memorizing the mnemonic in preparation for giving a patient-actor a terminal diagnosis.[25] Although methods like SPIKES might offer some guidance for novices who have little or no experience addressing existential suffering and mortality, it is unlikely that they will offer much help in navigating a complex, all-too-human situation fraught with uncertainty, fear, and vulnerability.

Yet the appeal of communication and educational interventions in healthcare, even those which are reductionistic and formulaic, remains: they seem practical, relevant, and expedient, thus perfectly suited for the rational, fast-paced culture of medicine. Communication training, though absolutely necessary for future clinicians, is woefully insufficient in and of itself, and any attempt I might make to offer an efficient and practical roadmap to improve clinical communication would require me to engage in the kinds of efforts *Afflicted* intends to critique. Indeed, relying too heavily on such downstream efforts is one of the reasons why medicine has for decades made little progress in encouraging authentic engagement between clinicians and patients.[26] To explain *why* these "how to" efforts continue to fail, I will explore the deeper philosophical and psychological reasons why medical practitioners avoid vulnerability, how this avoidance both influences and is perpetuated by medical epistemology and pedagogy, and why handbooks and checklists regarding competencies and behaviors *will not change* medical culture in any substantive way until we address the deeper issues that manifest in practitioners' poor communication, burnout, and inappropriate coping.

In the chapters that follow, I draw on the ideas of Emmanuel Levinas, Mikhail Bakhtin, and Hans-Georg Gadamer to argue that, in turning away from suffering and vulnerability, practitioners not only diminish the care they offer patients, but also diminish their own being. Through a philosophical analysis of the patient-practitioner encounter as an encounter between two persons each of whose being is constituted by the other's, I emphasize that the doctor, in escaping from authentic engagement with a patient who is profoundly suffering is, in fact, "escap[ing] from herself."[27] I argue that physicians who authentically respond to the call of suffering on the part of their patients approach not only their patients but also *themselves*: their subjectivity is deepened and expanded with the recognition of their own potential for suffering that is always already at hand. It is this understanding of the patient-practitioner relationship—an understanding that highlights the mutual giving and receiving within an encounter between two people who are both struggling to make meaning in the face of vulnerability and mortality—that will begin to orient us toward to a richer understanding of illness and suffering and will cultivate a more capacious understanding of care for healthcare professionals.

Finally, I suggest ways in which future physicians might be "brought back to themselves" through a pedagogy that values the cultivation of the self, openness and humility, and a fuller conception of what it means to be a healer. Following medical humanist Ronald Carson, I argue that the cultivation of new ways of understanding and interpreting the world and the lived experiences of others can be taught—not didactically but "maieutically"—that is, by "indirection," the way we learn from reading literature and poetry, for example.[28] Teaching by indirection helps cultivate the "moral imagination"—emotional and intellectual capacities that allow us to imagine something of what it might be like to be in the situation of someone else.[29] And teaching by indirection, rather than didactically, with literature, art, poetry, and narrative can foster new ways of seeing and thinking and can open up spaces for dialogue and reflection in order to garner personal moral clarity, empathic understanding, and an appreciation for others and their experiences. This approach is similar to the one advocated by the existential philosopher Søren Kierkegaard, who himself adopted the Socratic ideal of "indirect communication," an approach that was in no way dogmatic but rather guided his readers from behind to where they would make decisions for themselves based on interior reflection and introspection.[30]

As might be painfully obvious at this point, much of the present work is informed by a philosophical tradition shaped by a group of thinkers who share many things—including being very white and very male. And though this is true, much of *Afflicted* is also informed by postcolonial and feminist theory—which I hope will become apparent in later chapters. Specifically, my thoughts on pedagogical approaches are informed by a feminist ethics of care and by the ideas of feminist and activist writer bell hooks, who has helped me come to see the classroom and clinic as "radical space[s] of possibility," where both students and educators learn about how to live in the world as "whole human beings."[31] And though I recognize and later discuss the intersections between Levinas's philosophy and feminist approaches to ethics, especially in their shared emphasis on responsibility to others, I also point out that feminist theory is essential to medicine—where power

Introduction

hierarchies reign supreme—for it speaks to issues of oppression and subordination that too often taint the experiences of patients, learners, and nonphysician healthcare professionals alike.[32] Yet, despite the presence of diffuse power, racism, sexism, sanism, ableism, and so forth, I remain cautiously optimistic that Alan Bleakley is right when he says, "Medical education need not act as a handmaiden to normative medicine, but can formulate resistance to, and critique of, the institutional norms of medicine [that are] unproductive to patient care, collaborative, interprofessional teamwork, and doctors' self-care."[33] That is, of course, if we are truly committed to making real changes.

In an attempt to catalyze such changes, *Afflicted* is unabashedly interdisciplinary and draws on different analytical methods and modes of thinking. Much of it involves the close reading of both philosophical works and contemporary scholarly literature in medicine and medical education and brings these works into conversation with one another in order to develop an analysis that is at once philosophically rigorous, practical, and relevant. Chapter 1 begins with a synopsis of the scholarly literature that discusses the epistemology and pedagogy of medicine and the effects these have on physician formation. It then shows how this perspective can be deepened and expanded by an understanding of calculative thinking, as explained by Heidegger, to offer a more comprehensive grounding for the discussion about the inherent problems of medical education and practice. It highlights that calculative thinking—the default and preferred way of thinking not only in medicine, but also in contemporary society more generally—is actually derived from our more primordial (what Heidegger calls "meditative") way of thinking and being in the world. Privileging calculative thinking closes us off from other "truths," truths that are unverifiable, unquantifiable, or intangible. A Heideggerian critique helps to illustrate medicine's tendency toward a calculative understanding of illness that is defined by a hurried curiosity, as opposed to a meditative thinking that is slower, open to wonder, embraces ambiguity, and considers the ineffable and unquantifiable to be just as "true" or valid as things that might be scientifically "proven,"[34] a point more fully explored in later chapters. Recognizing the dominance and seductiveness of calculative thinking within medicine is important, for it speaks to the human tendency to turn away from contingency, vulnerability, and death—a point clarified and expanded in chapter 2.

Because medicine and medical education focus on the "real" and the "scientific" (namely, assessing and treating biological disease), the phenomenological or lived experience of illness—including existential issues such as suffering, fear, and inescapable uncertainty—are left largely unaddressed. Thus practitioners trained within this environment, especially those who view themselves as scientists or technicians, may believe that they are not called to attend to these issues. Chapter 2 examines why calculative or technical thinking is pervasively privileged and particularly problematic in medical practice. It is not enough, however, to say that doctors turn away from answering this call to care simply because they have been trained within a medical culture that fails to acknowledge the lived experiences of patients that fall outside the bounds of calculative thinking and technical rationality.[35] Turning away from the reality of vulnerability and mortality is, I argue, part of the shared condition of being human. Through an exploration of the philosophical work of Søren Kierkegaard, Martin Heidegger, Maurice Merleau-Ponty, and Friedrich Nietzsche, I attempt to show that medicine's preoccupation with science, detachment, and scientific certainty is a manifestation of the basic human desire to turn away from the anxiety that emerges in the face of human suffering and the struggle to make meaning in the face of profound illness and death.

In chapter 3, with philosophical help from Heidegger, Levinas, Charles Taylor, and Bakhtin, I contend that, by turning away from patients' suffering in the name of objectivity and "clinical detachment," physicians not only compromise the care they offer their patients but also diminish both their own practice and their own being. What is more, I argue, only through responding to the call of the face of suffering can physicians become authentic or resolute. For it is through facing the reality of their own mortality and potential for suffering that physicians deepen their subjectivity and begin to recognize and respond to their patients' call for care. In authentically responding to this call from the other, doctors come to see that they *need* their patients, not only to determine how to help them, but in a more fundamental way: they need their patients in order to heal, in order to *be healers*. As Heidegger would say, doctors need patients and their calls outward to them in order to become what they already are.[36]

Chapter 3 ends with a discussion about how clinicians might come to know how to respond to the suffering of their patients. With the help of hermeneutic phenomenology, particularly that of Hans-Georg Gadamer, Frederik Svenaeus, and S. Kay Toombs, I explore how physicians can come to a shared understanding with their patients about "what is the matter." This discussion emphasizes the necessity of reflective discernment and practical wisdom ("phronesis") within the clinical encounter. It is not enough to simply confront suffering; the physician as healer is called to respond to this suffering in a way that is appropriate for and meaningful to a particular patient.

Chapter 4 explores how educators might help cultivate qualities such as humility, openness, and gratitude toward patients among doctors in training. It argues that medicine's preoccupation with calculative thinking will persist until educators can cultivate within clinicians and clinicians in training the capacity to face the reality of existential anxiety through a pedagogy that values and fosters vulnerability and reflection. Although recent trends in the professionalism movement, including those in "professional identity formation," have made progress toward these ends, by focusing on outcomes and assessments, they may actually serve to reinforce calculative thinking. This chapter looks critically at such trends in medical education and contends that ideas concerning professionalism can be enriched and expanded through an understanding of virtue ethics and the Aristotelian concept of phronesis, one that emphasizes personal development, experiential and habitual learning, and quality mentorship.

Chapter 5 discusses specific curricular interventions that can work toward getting students to think critically and to "reflect broadly and deeply on what it means to be human."[37] It highlights pedagogical approaches that allow students to see that the "real" scientific facts of biological disease cannot be separated from the existential reality of illness and that human beings always already dwell within their lived experiences, even before science and medicine inscribe their particular, abstract truths onto the body. Through exposure to patients' stories—whether as narratives or in face-to-face encounters—and through reflective writing, dialogue, and quality mentorship, students may come to appreciate the lived experience of illness, to expand their moral imaginations, and to develop a more capacious sense of care grounded in a recognition of our shared humanness and potential for suffering. This kind of pedagogy does not result in a "professionalism" that can be measured, quantified, and assessed, but rather in a way of being in the world—a posture of openness toward others, an ability to face uncertainty, and the capacity to extend care to patients even when "nothing else can be done."

In the epilogue, I conclude by synthesizing the broader themes of *Afflicted*, emphasizing the need to address the normalized and taken-for-granted epistemology of medicine and its preoccupation with calculative thinking and technical notions of care that (re)produce the perspective that only what can be empirically verified is true or real. I reiterate how the narrow focus of modern medicine serves to numb doctors to existential anxiety—their patients' and their own—in the face of suffering and to deafen them to the call to authentically face the suffering other, and how acknowledging its dehumanizing effect on the care they provide reveals the need to offer doctors in training new, more expansive narratives about medicine that account for the lived experience of illness and suffering.

Some Closing Preliminary Comments

Taking seriously Bakhtin's and Gadamer's conviction that truth is shared and that it emerges within a polyphony of voices offered by multiple interlocutors, *Afflicted* is enriched and supported by the voices and stories of medical trainees who generously shared with me their experiences within medical education and practice. With approval from the Institutional Review Board at the University of Texas Medical Branch (UTMB), I interviewed ten medical trainees—nine third- or fourth-year medical students and one first-year resident—about what they thought of their medical training, their experiences with patients and mentors, and what they believed it means to become a doctor.[38] The point of these interviews was not to gather and analyze "verifiable" or generalizable data (a project that would, no doubt, be guided by calculative thinking), but rather to inform my own perspective and guide my own (meditative) thinking, as well as elucidate for my readers the lived experience of medicine and medical education.

I spent years living and learning closely alongside my friends and loved ones while they endured medical school, and the opportunities I have had to teach and mentor premedical and medical students and residents have provided me invaluable insight into medical education. For this project in particular, I wanted to take the time to formally ask and document the questions that I have been exploring over the years. My hope is that the experiences of these medical trainees are reflected in the pages that follow and that this project itself can contribute to the important work being done toward creating educational environments that cultivate broader notions of care—for the sake of both future doctors and their patients. And it is my hope that such work can create an educational culture that begins to recognize and value the lived, embodied, phenomenological experience of illness, a culture that embraces what sociologist and medical educator Arthur Frank calls a "pedagogy of suffering"—the idea that "the ill offer others a truth," especially those practitioners who authentically encounter them.[39] I believe this is true not only for current and future physicians, but also for all who work or will work in other areas of healthcare, including nursing, occupational and physical therapy, and surgical, respiratory, and radiologic technology, to name a few. Witnessing and responding to the testimony of patients opens up the possibility for personal transformation; made aware of their own vulnerability and brokenness by entering into the suffering of others—either face-to-face or imaginatively through stories or art—those who offer care to patients may come to see that suffering is not merely a puzzle to be solved or controlled, but an undeniable part of the human condition.[40]

1 Exploring the Shortcomings of a "Scientific" Medical Education

The face [is] a source from which all meaning appears.
—Emmanuel Levinas, *Totality and Infinity*

Young physicians may focus so much on trying to acquire the science of medicine that they ignore the art—the human face—of medicine.
—George E. Dickinson and Robert E. Tournier, "A Decade Beyond"

For decades, scholars, practitioners, ethicists, and educators have attempted to make the internal morality of medicine and the ways students are educated to become "ethical" or "professional" more conspicuous. If recent statements and actions of professional medical organizations, journals, and accrediting bodies for medical schools and residency programs are any indication, then American medicine seems to have become more introspective about the moral weight of its practice and the effect training has on future clinicians.[1] There are those, however, who maintain that, by the time medical students reach professional or medical school, they are adults with fully formed ideals, perspectives, and political leanings, and any attempts to change them during their medical education are likely in vain.[2]

The argument that curricular changes should be made as early as possible in medical students' development is important and valid, yet it should not lead us to conclude that by the time they reach medical school, it is impossible to change or expand their moral bearings. Recent research has shown that students do, in fact, change during medical school, albeit usually for the worse: often idealistic and enthusiastic when they start medical school, most experience a decrease in empathy and some even "ethical erosion" as they progress through their medical education.[3] However disheartening or discouraging these findings may seem, they suggest that most students at least *start* medical school with open minds and hearts. As a fourth-year medical student told me, "I think very few, if any, medical students are 'bad' people with bad or selfish intentions. I think most go into medicine for good reasons, and they want to help people. But, I think medical school does a poor job of recognizing and developing that part of them" (MSIV-1).

What is it about medical school, then, that allows students' altruistic intentions to fade or even erode despite the profession's proclaimed ideal that doctors ought to be compassionate and virtuous? According to some scholars, the problem lies not so much with the education the schools provide, but with their admission policies, which disproportionately favor applicants' Medical College Admission Test (MCAT) scores, grade point averages, and success in narrow, science-based premedical courses.[4] The scholars argue that, despite most applicants' altruistic desire to help others, few have been exposed to a rich liberal arts education that might encourage them to think critically about social issues and power constructs or deeply and broadly about the human situation. These applicants are therefore not well prepared to contend with what they will encounter as medical students and doctors, especially since "medicine necessarily engages with almost every aspect of the human condition."[5]

If this is the case, then it certainly presents a problem since most students entering medical school are trained almost exclusively in the sciences. A 2007 study showed that, of the 17,759 students who matriculated in medical schools in the United States, nearly 70 percent majored in the biological and physical sciences, whereas only 4 percent majored in the humanities.[6] This is not to say that being trained in the sciences and learning to think critically or respond appropriately to human suffering are mutually exclusive. There are, of course, many applicants who majored in the sciences who understand the depths of human suffering and who are keen to point out some of the shortcomings of modern medicine or reductionistic scientific research. Nevertheless, most applicants are not admitted to medical schools based on their desire to change the social and economic forces that shape medicine or on their capacity to authentically empathize with others and engage in conversations about the existential struggles that severe illness can give rise to.

The problem with admission policies is more complex than it seems, however. If you ask those involved in medical education, including those who participate in the admission process, they will more than likely say that future physicians ought to be compassionate, personable, and deep-thinking people, not mere technicians.[7] And yet this espoused ideal is often belied by a selection process and a four-year curriculum that "implicitly reward a narrow intellectual range and a superficial focus on grades and test scores [that is] counterproductive in preparing them for the real world of the practice of medicine."[8] What is more, there is a perception that certain medical specialties are somehow "exempt" from needing doctors who know how to respond to the emotional suffering of patients and their families. Students interested in specialties such as surgery, radiology, anesthesiology, or pathology, so the argument goes, need not be concerned with the need to respond to emotional pain, to care for the dying, or to facilitate difficult conversations with patients and their families. It is therefore reasonable to accept applicants who exhibit narrow interests in the technical or scientific aspects of medicine, especially since they will likely score well on Board exams throughout medical school and residency: such applicants will fit well within more technical medical specialties, which involve little patient interaction. What this argument fails to consider, however, is that, regardless of specialty, an encounter with death and suffering is virtually inevitable in medical training and practice. However essential their technical skills may be, surgeons are called to be more than technicians: when a patient dies on the operating table, it is most often the surgeon who has to deliver this news to the family. What is more, even specialties that appear to be far removed from interactions with patients and their families are not that way inherently, as a pathologist recently made clear to a class of my medical students. He explained to them how hard it was to have to tell a mother that an autopsy was unable to uncover the cause of death of her young son, how he tried to comfort her, how he cried with her.

The problem of selecting appropriate applicants, then, is complicated by the fact that we are unclear about what we expect of doctors and, even if we were clear, whether we would call on all doctors to live up to those expectations. We might say that we want physicians who are empathic and altruistic, yet the students accepted to medical school simply need to prove that they can succeed in a program that largely ignores the development of such qualities and perpetuates ideas about those who won't *actually need* to respond to existential suffering. It is precisely this way of thinking that contributes to notions of medicine being little more than an "interesting" and lucrative career choice. When I ask medical students why they decided to pursue medicine as a career—something I often do—most of them reply that they have always enjoyed science, and medicine seemed like an "interesting" way to make a living. Though not a "bad" reason to go into medicine, I have found that, as students progress through their training, they rarely question or reflect upon this reason, and it continues to influence their decisions about residency. When I asked a fourth-year medical student what he thought was driving most medical students' decisions about their specialty choice, he responded: "Prestige, money, lifestyle, passion, no particular order. Depends on what the student values, and that's different for everyone" (MSIV-2). And for some students, prestige, money, and lifestyle clearly rank higher than passion in their order of values. A third-year medical student told me that his top contenders for specialties were dermatology and plastic surgery because he aspires to be a small business owner, and these specialties are particularly conducive to the development of a smart business model.

One could argue that there is nothing inherently wrong with this business-minded perspective, that there will always be those with such an outlook, and that there are places in medicine where doctors with this perspective will not only do well for themselves but will also make their patients happy. Although this may be true, it seems that, instead of simply accepting this perspective as inevitable and even fitting for business-minded students, we might encourage students to think more deeply about what it means to be a doctor and to reflect on the differences between a career and a calling.[9] Physicians Richard Gunderman and Steven Kanter maintain that "those who treat their career as a business proposition will be among the first to treat their knowledge and skill as their own personal property" and that "these habits undermine medicine as a profession, leading us to regard patients as customers and healthcare as a commodity."[10] With that in mind, instead of guiding students who tend to see medicine as a technical career or business endeavor into areas of medicine where such perspectives are widely accepted, we should instead ask those students to reflect on what will bring them not just a paycheck but also meaning and purpose in their life of medicine. This, however, is not the focus of most medical education programs.

It is precisely the incongruity between what most educators claim they want to see in medical students and physicians and what the system actually encourages and rewards that subjects students to what Johanna Shapiro and colleagues refer to as an "intellectual bait and switch."[11] Indeed, calls for vulnerability, empathy, and reflection in usually sporadic or "tacked on" medical humanities courses seem strange to students when most of them

> enter medical school having internalized the view that medicine is an objective, scientific pursuit based almost exclusively on factual knowledge and technical skills. This perspective is understandable because it reflects the prevalent image of medicine in American culture and is reinforced by the narrow prerequisites of premedical majors and entry requirements for medical school that prioritize quantitative and scientific performance.[12]

It is therefore too simple to say that the problems of medical education lie primarily with the "type" of students who are admitted to medical school. Most students simply aim to satisfy admission requirements and complete the kind of undergraduate education that appears to be valued most within the culture of medicine.[13] Even though medicine has become increasingly introspective and reflective about the moral weight of its practice, its goals and ideas about what doctors are called to do remain unclear, even to those who choose to pursue medicine as a career.[14] It is no surprise that medical students are resistant to cultivating their moral character and their capacity to address existential suffering when they have committed themselves to what appears to be a scientific and technical field in need of objective scientists and technicians.

A Closer Look at Medical Epistemology

It seems unfair, then, to place the onus entirely on medical students to become compassionate, empathetic, and socially conscious healers when the culture and system that shapes them does not, generally speaking, foster such qualities. As noted above, students usually enter their medical training with good intentions, regardless of a narrow undergraduate education; but nurturing these positive qualities is not a priority during medical school. According to sociologist Frederic Hafferty, medical education is more than training—it is a *socialization process*, one that has the power to influence and shape students' values and beliefs.[15] The underlying dimension of socialization is personal transformation, which is what differentiates "training" from socialization.[16] As spaces of personal transformation, medical schools and residency programs "are formidable—and formative—settings that structure and shape how future physicians will think, act, and identify themselves with core occupational values."[17] In other words, students don't simply adopt new attitudes and behaviors during this time, which are "added on" to an already formed self; instead, socialization or resocialization involves some aspects of students' selves being *"replaced* by new ways of thinking, acting, and valuing ... a dual process of moving into the new and moving away from the old."[18] Or, as Hafferty concludes, "It is a process—for better and/or for worse—to change hearts *and* minds."[19]

Nevertheless, medical students are rarely told explicitly that the education they are undertaking will have as much to do with their character as it will with their intellect.[20] And given the fact that medical education and practice are rarely viewed as sites of personal transformation, this transformative process is largely left unaddressed at the level of the formal curriculum and is instead "taught" via the "hidden curriculum"—through the messages students receive and the experiences they have with patients, peers, and mentors, which powerfully communicate what it means to be a doctor. This type of learning is particularly problematic, given that the hidden curriculum is largely shaped by the epistemology of medicine—what doctors know and how they come to know it.[21] Within medicine, what is "knowable" are the observable and measurable (usually empirical, scientific) facts, and how doctors come to know those facts is through their observations or measurements, lab tests, microscopy, imaging, and so forth. As Paul Komesaroff notes, traditional accounts of medicine are dominated by a discursive system grounded in an epistemology that views the body as an anatomical, physiological, and biochemical structure best known and understood through the methods of science and through the impartial observations of the physician.[22]

On its face, the assumption that medicine is a scientific endeavor may appear reasonable, considering that clinicians often rely on technology and scientific modalities (e.g., lab results, CAT scans) to "reveal" the workings of the biological body. But, as Kathryn Montgomery argues, this epistemology, which emphasizes objectivity and neutrality in practicing "good science," ignores the fact that clinical practice is inherently uncertain and reliant on experiential knowledge.[23] Moreover, an epistemology carries with it a certain kind of ethos, shaping ideas of the specific dispositions and values that allow us to properly secure knowledge.[24] The contemporary epistemological "virtues" of science, for example, include notions of objectivity, rigor, and detachment. The notion of objectivity specifically has its own set of values, rooted in a cultivation of a particular "scientific self" that attempts to suppress or negate aspects of one's subjective self—a kind of "willed willessness"—in the quest for "Truth."[25] In becoming or embodying this particular scientific self, knowing and knower are melded together, and the knower becomes one who must resist the temptations of imagination and subjectivity. In the pursuit of objectivity, people's values are concretized through repetitive engagement in certain ways of seeing the world around them. Thus, when medicine is conceived of as an applied science, and when one of the epistemological virtues of this science is objectivity, students and doctors may come to see the adoption of an objective stance toward a patient and the patient's illness as good, noble, or right—even though scientific objectivity can disregard the very human elements of illness and medicine, resulting in narrow and insufficient care of the suffering other.

In their recent ethnographic study that examined healthcare workers' perception and embodiment of professionalism and care in an urban hospital, Ester Carolina Apesoa-Varano and Charles Varano found that a technical, scientific orientation still dominates in the hospital, even though medicine is not *actually* practiced that way, which may be a result of the epistemological assumptions of medical training and practice.[26] One surgeon reflecting on his training, explained to them: "I think that one of the things that is not readily apparent to the nonmedical public is that medicine is by no means a clean, pure science.... I can give you a multiple-choice test and say, 'Wow, you really know a lot about this fancy pathology, etc.' But what is not so easy to test is your ability to apply that at the patient's bedside. It turns out that patients don't present with multiple-choice type questions."[27]

The misconception of medicine as an impartial science reinforces ideas about the need to remain "professionally detached" in the face of suffering and death. As a result, some doctors, especially those who see themselves as scientists, may avoid difficult questions that cannot be answered with the kind of certainty that science offers and many patients seek.[28] They find it easier to comport themselves as technical experts of the body and disease than to face the complexities of suffering. One fourth-year medical student who believed that a firm foundation in the basic sciences was essential for clinicians, especially for novices who lack clinical experience, and who also recognized the limits of such training, hinted at the benefit of viewing oneself as a "scientist" in the face of human suffering: "Some days I think [medicine] is an applied science[, but] I've been on pediatrics for the last month, and you see all these sad stories, and then you really want to pretend it's a science" (MSIV-3). This "pretending," it seems, is both useful and futile; no matter how much one would like to view medicine as an applied science, the reality of human suffering inevitably forces itself into the clinical space. And yet, pretending to be the detached scientist is safer and easier than acknowledging and responding to such suffering.

In a similar vein in *The Anticipatory Corpse*, Jeffrey Bishop finds that medicine, despite its scientific underpinnings, has a metaphysics, though it is largely unacknowledged.[29] He describes this metaphysics as one of material and efficient causation; following Aristotle's Four Causes (formal, material, efficient, and final), Bishop argues that modern Western medicine is primarily concerned with the efficient cause.[30] In other words, doctors almost exclusively see their purpose as intervening or "doing something" to the material of the biological body, rather than as concerning themselves with the final cause of human beings, which involves questions about meaning or purpose. Using the work of Michel Foucault, Bishop also argues that, in medicine, life is seen merely as matter in motion, and the body as merely an animated corpse. Medicine is thus concerned with ways of controlling and manipulating the material of bodies, and "the purpose of knowing—the end of knowing—is to bring about desired effects" in the material world.[31] Within this paradigm, existential questions become irrelevant, and making meaning of illness and suffering is not viewed as the proper end of medical knowledge. Moreover, this commitment to a metaphysics of efficient and material causation is rooted in practitioners' medical training, and it encourages them to respond to patients by "first seeing the loss of function and responding to that functional loss."[32] The problem, Bishop tells us, is that the training doctors receive actually prevents them from perceiving suffering beyond function since medical students and doctors are presented with the idea that attending to the physical body is the best and perhaps even the only response to suffering.[33]

Although the epistemological assumptions of medicine are normalized and, for the most part, rendered invisible, they manifest themselves in clearly recognizable ways within medical education and practice. As Eric Cassell famously articulated decades ago, modern medicine is still guided by an anachronistic mind-body dualism and a "division of the human condition into what is medical (having to do with the body) and what is nonmedical (the remainder)," which, he says, has caused medicine to narrow its perception of "its calling."[34] According to Cassell and many others who have written after him, medicine is eager to take the biological workings of the body under its purview, but it considers most forms of suffering other than bodily pain to be outside its domain. It follows that many of those working within medicine do not feel inclined to attend to "the remainder" of the patient in front of them.[35]

One consequence of distinguishing between medical and nonmedical forms of suffering, which is sustained and reinforced by modern medicine's science-based epistemology, is the frequent conflation of care and cure. As Edmund Pellegrino sees it, the biomedical model that chiefly drives American medicine defines itself "simply as applied biology," which perpetuates the idea that "the primary function of medicine is to cure, and this requires the physician to be primarily a scientist. This model ... focuses on *things* to do for a particular disease that are measurably effective."[36] The distinction between cure and care is an important one to make, especially in the context of chronic or incurable diseases. Because curing is often equated with "things to do," a physician's actions can be significantly limited when faced with intractable or terminal illnesses—that is, for patients for whom it is believed "nothing else can be done." When physicians conceive of themselves as purveyors of biological cure and attendants to the technical, mechanical, physiological workings of the body, the existential suffering of the terminal patient is left unacknowledged. What is more, physicians who feel that their only job is to cure may feel that caring for dying patients is not their responsibility and may simply hand off their patients to a hospice or palliative care team.[37] Or they may, instead, prioritize the eradication of disease over all else, even when further treatment is not in their patients' best interest.[38] Indeed, patients may receive aggressive treatment up until the day they die, with little focus on palliation, which can result in physical and emotional suffering, as well as missed opportunities for acknowledging and making sense of their impending death. Whether it is because of overtreating or undertreating, when doctors believe that medicine is concerned almost exclusively with curing the biological body, the suffering of patients that extends beyond the purview of technical experts becomes undeniably conspicuous, at least to outsiders and especially in the care of the dying.

In *The Wounded Storyteller*, Arthur Frank confronts this division between care and cure and the consequences that arise from it. In discussing the taken-for-granted assumptions of medicine, Frank employs the trope of "narrative plotlines" to describe the dominant discourse of contemporary Western medicine.[39] The "restitution narrative," he explains, highlights medicine's capacity to identify biological dysfunction, intervene appropriately, and ultimately restore health.[40] This oversimplified plotline communicates the modernist expectation that there exists a remedy for every ailment, and because this narrative requires a mechanistic understanding of the body, it is quite palatable to modern medicine. According to Frank, "restitution requires fixing, and fixing requires such a mechanistic view."[41] Perhaps the ultimate limitation of the restitution narrative and its "single-minded *telos* of cure" is that death and dying—because there is no hope for cure or physical restitution—cannot be a part of the plot.

The dominance of the restitution narrative in mainstream medicine and its failure to appropriately account for the reality of death are made clear in the story Frank tells of his own family. Neither his mother-in-law nor he and the rest of the family confronted the reality of her impending death until two days before she died, due in large part to everyone focusing on the "incremental remedies that medicine continued to offer" that allowed the issue of mortality to be evaded.[42] This experience made it clear to Frank that a narrative plot outside the restitution narrative was required to address death and mortality. Nevertheless, the restitution narrative continues to prevail in medicine, despite the existence of suffering to which it cannot speak. Thus one fourth-year medical student seemed to define the primary goals of medicine within the plotline of the restitution narrative. "I'm not sure if I would distinguish 'healing' from 'curing' . . . to me, healing seems like curing," the student told me. "I'm not sure what else I could do for a patient who no longer responded to treatment" (MSIV-3).

The Intersection of Epistemology and Pedagogy

Sherwin Nuland argued in 1995 that the "rescue credo of high tech medicine" and the largely curative ethos of the 1980s to which Cassell and Pellegrino brought attention still pervaded the culture of modern medicine. A former surgeon and medical educator who died in 2014, Nuland emphasized the very real pressure he felt from peers and colleagues to follow the "clear duty to save life."[43] In his best-selling book *How We Die*, Nuland described the guilt he felt after convincing an elderly patient to undergo invasive surgery, in part because he knew what his colleagues would say if he had instead advocated forgoing treatment. "Had I let Miss Welch have her way," Nuland explained, "I would have had to defend the result at the weekly surgical conference (where it would certainly be seen as *my* decision, not hers), before unbending colleagues to whom her death would seem a case of poor judgment, if not downright negligence of the clear duty to save life."[44]

Nuland argued that this perceived duty to cure and save lives, and the misperception of medical practice as an applied science were perpetuated within both hospital culture and the contemporary medical school curriculum—a curriculum that tended to enchant students with "the solution of 'The Riddle' of disease."[45] The emphasis of "The Riddle" in medical education—which might be described as a preoccupation with the identification and amelioration of biological disease states that tended to ignore the actual patient with the illness—had the potential to "transmute [a student] unawares into the embodiment of a biomedical problem-solver."[46] Nuland found this pedagogical approach exceedingly problematic, especially since he believed that a preoccupation with The Riddle was directly at odds with providing quality care, especially for those at the end of life.[47]

Some of those concerned about the perceived detachment of doctors point to the failure of medical schools to cultivate the capacity to confront suffering and manage reactions to it, and they suggest that clinical detachment starts early on in students' education. Many have suggested that the emphasis on test scores and the memorization and regurgitation of scientific and clinical information that is the major focus of the first two years of medical school communicates to students early in their training that their primary concern should be to understand the scientific workings of the human body, abstracted from the lived experiences of patients. In an online blog post that began circulating on social media websites in September of 2014, an anonymous female medical student writes about the disconnect between the first two years of medical school (which include only intermittent interactions with patients) and the reasons why most students choose to go into medicine, which usually include engaging with people in order to help them.[48] She describes her experiences during her first two years of medical school as being saturated with studying and standardized test taking and almost entirely devoid of patient interaction. "If my university believed in one thing," she says, "it was that there was no human enterprise on Earth that could not be held to a rubric. They had yet to fail in their quest to quantify, to measure all of the qualities of an ideal doctor."[49]

Along with the focus on test scores and rubrics, the most obvious example of the detachment that is implicitly encouraged early on in students' medical training is the common practice of requiring students to enter the anatomy lab and cut into a human cadaver on the first day of medical school, with little or no open discussion about death and dying, personhood, embodiment, or the ethics of willing one's body to science. Looking back in 2007 at her residency training decades before, physician Katharine Treadway wonders how she and her fellow residents had so easily detached themselves from the reality of suffering and death:

> Where did we learn this detachment? For most of us, the first lessons came very early in medical school, when we were confronted with the dissection of a human body—conveniently called a cadaver, as though that made it something different from a person who had died.... We learned to bury our fear of death in an avalanche of knowledge. We learned the trick of silencing the parts of our brain that really didn't want to be this close to death.[50]

Although Treadway notes that it is sometimes necessary to detach oneself, especially in emergency situations, she suggests that medical training does very little to help students develop discernment about when it is and is not appropriate to maintain emotional distance for the sake of patients and, instead, tacitly encourages detachment as a kind of default position. As ethicist William May points out, the early placement of anatomy in the medical curriculum "presents the young professional with a cadaver before he or she ever sees a living patient [and] suggests that one's science must not diverge from its appointed tasks into the complexities of the relationships to the living."[51] The passive and diseased body thus becomes the normative body in medical training and practice.

In her 2010 essay "A Piece of My Mind: The Good Doctor," medical student Shekinah Elmore wonders about some doctors' inability to imagine what their patients are feeling.[52] Shortly before starting medical school at the age of twenty-seven, Elmore was diagnosed with metastatic breast cancer. After receiving the diagnosis, she sat alone in the exam room crying. A few minutes later, after being comforted by the medical assistant, she overheard her oncologist approach the assistant outside the room and ask in a whisper, "Why is she crying?"[53]

This experience haunted Elmore, who wondered when it was during their training that doctors like her oncologist—who undoubtedly began medical school as "kind and concerned human beings"—came to be so detached from the lived experiences of patients.[54] As she progressed through medical school, her belief that medicine was "holistic and humanistic and . . . infused with genuine care," emphasized so strongly during her white coat ceremony at the beginning of the school year, began to falter.[55] Though this did not surprise her, she was struck by how quickly the focus of her training changed, and how the initial emphasis on empathetic care degraded "not slowly, as I expected, but rapidly, declining with a speed inversely proportional to the rise of basic and clinical sciences. In anatomy lab, in the name of efficiency, we move feverishly around and through the bodies of our donors, focusing on nerve, muscle, bone, attachment."[56] Alluding to how the hidden curriculum reinforced ideas about medicine being a rigorous science, rather than an encounter between human beings, she explains: "The same holds in lecture halls and tutorial rooms and at laboratory benches. We are overwhelmed with pathogens, seduced by physiological mechanisms, intrigued by drug names. We begin to speak more and more cryptically, learning the incantations to unlock the approval of attending physicians."[57]

Elmore suspects that this rapid change in focus is the reason why doctors, who start medical school intent on helping others in their times of vulnerability and crisis, become so intrigued with biological disease processes that they lose sight of how a difficult diagnosis or the realities of a serious illness can affect the life of a patient.[58] As physicians Susan Block and Andrew Billings suggest, "the hidden curriculum of contemporary medicine—especially [during] the hurried, disease-centered, impersonal, high-throughput clinical years—still tends to undermine the best intentions of students and faculty members and the best interests of patients and families."[59] Even though there are "subjective" aspects to the practice of medicine, such as clinical intuition, practical experience, and the ability to relate to and engage with other people, these are largely eclipsed by the need for objectivity and a narrow focus on biological disease. As a result, when students eventually find themselves on the wards with patients who suffer in ways beyond biological dysfunction, they feel ill prepared to confront the realities of illness. The pedagogical structure of medical education, which is shaped by and perpetuates an epistemology that deems human suffering secondary (if not extraneous) to fixing the body, serves the needs of neither patients nor the students and doctors who are called to care for them.

Why This Epistemology Persists

If the epistemology of contemporary Western medicine fails to account for the lived experience of illness and has such negative consequences for so many in the medical system, why does it persist? Despite the addition of ethics and humanities to medical curricula, the biomedical paradigm reigns supreme in medical education. One reason for this may be that "empathy training" and courses in the medical humanities are often tacked on to the curriculum in ways that do not challenge the prevailing objective, medico-scientific paradigm of medicine and medical training. Because of the tendency of medical education, in the words of doctor and philosopher Reidar Pedersen, to "not challenge or critically discuss the objectivity of biomedical understanding,"[60] and because of the near-universal acceptance of this biomedical paradigm, students receive mixed messages about what it means to care for patients. They may be told initially or sporadically that empathy and compassion are required for humane care, but this "requirement" is belied by a curriculum that emphasizes objectivity, rubrics, measurable or quantifiable data, and scientifically reductionistic understandings of illness and health. As Pedersen points out, "if objectivity is taken for granted, then there is little or no need for empathy, reflection, and dialogue."[61] The message that empathy and connection matter is overwhelmed by the perceived need for clinical objectivity.

Although it is important to recognize the limitations of mainstream medical epistemology and the effects this has on pedagogy and on learners, doctors, and patients, it is even more important that we work to understand *why* this epistemology is so seductive. In part, the dominant epistemology of medicine is so attractive because, to put it simply, it *works*. The scientific methods employed within medicine yield a certain kind of truth, one that is seen as definite and reliable. Test results and visual images of internal pathology offer verifiable explanations of illnesses, and scientific research can and does lead to very real and very useful advances in clinical care—it has helped to ease pain, to virtually eliminate some diseases, and to improve social welfare.[62] Although it would therefore be inappropriate to consider all scientific approaches to medicine as reductionistic or otherwise inimical to quality patient care, the assumption that scientific inquiry is the most reliable—and perhaps the only—way of approaching truth significantly limits students' and doctors' understandings of care. As Shapiro and colleagues point out, doctors and students tend not to ask "metaquestions" about what it means to be a doctor, about the subjective experiences of their patients, or what it means to care for patients as persons because, in general, they view medicine as atheoretical, as a "permanent 'Truth' with a capital T, a constant reality that simply *is*."[63] Despite the efforts of those who have theorized medicine from biopsychosocial, phenomenological, feminist, narrative, and postmodern perspectives, the notion of medicine being atheoretical is widely accepted.[64] This is hardly surprising, given the belief in science's supreme ability to glean objective and verifiable truth about the world, a belief bolstered by the fact that science offers practical—albeit narrow—answers to some of our most pressing questions. Indeed, as Linda Wiener and Ramsey Eric Ramsey argue, its practical answers and its claim to reveal or point to the "truth" grant science "considerable power and influence and helps deflect criticism from those without scientific credentials"—a problem no doubt for many proponents of the medical humanities.[65]

Heidegger and Epistemology

The philosophy of Martin Heidegger can help us think more carefully and deeply through this issue of medical epistemology and its relationship to "scientism"—a worldview defined by the desire to frame every question and answer within the scientific paradigm while disregarding alternative views as wrongheaded, culturally relative, or inaccurate.[66] Heidegger moves us beyond, or rather, *before*, epistemology and toward *ontology*. He distinguishes between three types of inquiry or modes of investigation: "ontic" inquiry, "ontology," and "fundamental ontology."[67] Ontic investigations are primarily concerned with describing the *characteristics* of human and nonhuman beings and entities—their functions, attributes, qualities, and so forth. This type of inquiry is particular to the ontic sciences (biology, physics, etc.). In contrast, ontology aims to uncover the *being* of these entities, their essence or essential makeup, rather than merely listing their characteristics. Although ontology gets closer to understanding being, Heidegger contends that its investigations still fail to consider what it means to *be* at all.[68] He is more concerned with what he calls "fundamental ontology," which asks about the *meaning of being* in general, and how and why beings make sense to us at all, rather than focusing primarily on *beings* (entities) in the world.[69] More specifically, in his highly influential text *Being and Time*, Heidegger asks us to consider the being who interprets the world (*Dasein*, or human being), not simply the nature and characteristics of the entities this being encounters.[70] With that in mind, Heidegger sets out to show that even though scientific-empirical investigations of the ontic sciences can and do tell us valuable things about the world, they often miss what is most fundamental. According to Heidegger, "subjecting the manifold to tabulation does not ensure any actual understanding of what lies there before us."[71]

Heidegger's philosophy breaks with the Western philosophical tradition in holding that the question of being is prior to any other philosophical issue, especially epistemology, which, according to Heidegger, begins its inquiry too late.[72] Heidegger asserts that there is a fundamental assumption or presupposition that undergirds all contemporary epistemologies, no matter how divergent they may otherwise be, an assumption that privileges *presence*.[73] Understanding being, according to these epistemological theories, requires only descriptions of objects; being is reduced to "being extant," something available for human perception, measurement, and manipulation. As Heidegger states in *Being and Time*, "the question of [our] Being has remained forgotten . . . this Being is rather conceived as something obvious or 'self-evident' in the sense of the *Being-present-at-hand* of other created things."[74] For Heidegger, this understanding of being as that which is present-at-hand or extant is an inadequate ontological starting point.[75] We cannot possibly uncover all there is to know about something simply by observing it "objectively" and listing its characteristics or physical properties. But what is more important, we cannot fully understand human experience through explanatory theories, quantitative measurements, or positivistic approaches alone. As Heidegger reminds us, "the person is not a thing, not a substance, not an object."[76] The human *being*, in other words, escapes quantification and exceeds precise articulation.

According to philosopher Charles Guignon, Heidegger seeks to dislodge Western philosophy from its preoccupation with an epistemology primarily shaped by and perpetuating what Guignon calls the "Cartesian model"—a model that interprets the world as "consisting of minds and matter, a picture of truth as correct representation, and a belief that intelligibility is to be rooted in rationality."[77] Guignon cites events that occurred around the lifetime of René Descartes (1596–1650), such as the appearance of Martin Luther's Ninety-Five Theses and the publication of Michel de Montaigne's *Essays*—which highlighted the everyday person's role in the interpretation of truth (interpreting Scripture, for example) and the relativistic nature of truth and morality—as representative examples of the cultural and social upheaval out of which Descartes's philosophy emerged. In response to it, the work of Descartes attempts to overcome relativism and reinstate the intelligibility of the world, as the previous framework that dominated during the Middle Ages and early Renaissance (e.g., the lived world as a reflection or microcosm of the immutable and perfect cosmos) began to give way.[78] According to Guignon, what Descartes needed to "overcome the ravages of relativism" was a method that would "lead us to certain and indubitable truths."[79]

Heidegger questions the taken-for-granted assumptions of the whole Cartesian inquiry that has grounded thinking for the past four centuries—an inquiry that is derived from the methods of physical science and views human beings as subjects wholly distinct or separate from the world of objects that they come to know.[80] In bringing us back to the question of being (and what it means to be) and to broader possibilities for interpreting ourselves and our experiences, Heidegger shows us that Cartesian thought is just one approach among many for understanding our world.[81] The Cartesian model, championed during the scientific revolution and the Enlightenment and reappropriated today in contemporary medicine, views objects—including the body—as matter that is wholly distinct from us. This model reduces and equates "truth" with correctness and logical correspondence and believes that such truth is ascertained through logically sound judgments and quantifiable measurements.[82] As philosopher Charles Taylor puts it, this epistemology sees knowledge "as correct representation of an independent reality."[83] But, for Heidegger, empirical investigation, quantification, and scientific calculation are secondary phenomena; they are but one form of world disclosure that is grounded within and derivative from our more primordial, everyday way of being in the world.[84] Interpretation of our world is not something that occurs once we bracket our subjective experience and objectively observe what appears before us; rather, we are always already interpreting and understanding our world.

In fact, according to Heidegger, "to be" means to interpret.[85] We always already dwell concernfully and understandingly in the world in which we have been thrown: "To exist as Dasein," says Heidegger, "means to hold open a domain through its capacity to receive-perceive the significance of things that are given to it."[86] It is our lived experiences, then, and not scientific facts that are the most concrete starting place for understanding ourselves and our world.[87] According to Wiener and Ramsey, contrary to popular belief, it is not "subjective" theory, philosophical pursuits, or inquiries about the human condition that are detached or "abstracted" from reality, but science itself: "Science is one of the most abstract social practices because it can and . . . is obligated to bracket the lived experience so as to have room to do its work."[88] Science and its methodologies appear to be directly linked to "Truth," yet their tendency to ignore the texture of the lifeworld means that scientific answers can only ever offer partial, and often decontextualized, explanations of phenomena.

Heidegger argues that this notion of bracketing our lived experiences in order to interpret phenomena accurately is not just an abstraction; it is an impossibility. We cannot simply bracket our situatedness—our unique cultural, historical, and experiential backgrounds—in order to interpret phenomena "accurately." As Taylor points out, Heidegger's philosophy reorients us toward hermeneutics, and the thesis of most post-Heideggerian hermeneutics is the idea of "self-understanding." This means that our understanding of ourselves and the world is informed by what Taylor calls a "background of distinctions of worth," by where we find ourselves (our respective languages and cultures, for instance), which, in turn, informs what we value, what we find irrelevant, what we incorporate into our self-perceptions, and what we ignore—though this background is not always visible to us.[89] Given the complexity of self-interpretation, which involves a dynamic interaction between a person and the person's social environment, and given the inevitable relativity and subjectivity involved in the constant creation of the self, our being or personhood can never be understood absolutely or treated scientifically in the same way we approach an understanding of material objects in the world.[90] Who we are and how we see ourselves are always shaped by our social, historical, and experiential backgrounds.

Making full use of the irremovable lens through which we interpret ourselves and our worlds, Heidegger offers a recapitulation of the traditional notion of truth. Instead of accepting truth as the total transparency of natural forms or the correspondence between thought and reality, he returns to the Greek word *aletheia* (uncovering, unhiddenness, or unconcealment) to describe truth.[91] For Heidegger, truth is not some verifiable fact to be ascertained, nor is it based on a conformity between an abstract, universal representation and what is represented (i.e., propositional truth); rather, truth

Exploring the Shortcomings of a "Scientific" Medical Education

is a *process* of uncovering, revealing, or "letting show" what is only ever partially transparent to us in our situatedness. Within this understanding, human beings become the primary locus of truth since it is we who do the uncovering.[92] We can only ever interpret our experiences in terms of the context of the situation at hand and in relation to things within our world.

Heidegger often describes craftspersons in their workshops to elucidate this point. Thus, according to Heidegger, painters understand a paintbrush, for instance, not merely as an object or in terms of its physical characteristics, but rather in terms of what it does for them in the context of their situations or, put simply, in terms of its "use." Because they already have a "fore-understanding" of what a paintbrush is and how it is used in the world, painters interpret it not as an arrangement of molecules or even as a slender piece of wood with bristles, but rather as something they use to apply paint or to create a piece of art, as that which will help them complete their projects.[93] Thus, while using the paintbrush in their projects, the brush "disappears" within the context of their work. The craftspersons comport themselves within their projects prereflectively or precognitively; they already "know" what the paintbrush is and how to use it and do not have to cognitively register what it is and then "tell" their hand to use it to apply brushstrokes. In this way, Heidegger draws our attention to the fact that all understanding is an interpretation, and all interpretation is informed by our everyday understanding of the world and the situation at hand. Because one of the fundamental constituents of being human is "being-in-the-world"—the idea that humans and human understanding are inseparable from the world itself—we always already dwell in the world understandingly.[94] As such, interpretation is akin to a circle or spiral: the meaning of a phenomenon is always interpreted in relation to our fore-understanding of the world, and we then reinterpret the phenomenon in light of our new understanding of the world (of which this phenomenon has now become a part).

Ultimately, Heidegger shows us that we are always already "caught up" in the world. We already know the world and come to know it more fully simply by *being* in it. The world discloses itself to us, first and foremost, through our everyday lived experiences. Our interpretations of "truth" are therefore inevitably embedded within the context of our lives, and approaching truth involves a constant uncovering of phenomena as they appear within the intricate collage of our experiences, assumptions, and biases, which inevitably influence our perceptions and cannot ever be bracketed.

Any interpretation or description that is offered is inextricably encumbered in the web of significance in the world as we see it; the things we encounter and the words we use are always already "world laden."[95] For Heidegger, it makes no sense to abstract the paintbrush from the lifeworld of the human being in order to show, for example, that the brush *really* is a collection of molecules. The brush ceases to exist as brush if there is no human being to use it.[96] In other words, meaning and interpretation—our everyday ways of being in the world—presuppose and undergird this kind of technical information. Nevertheless, we continue to perceive abstracted, scientific descriptions as more accurate and ultimately more "true" than anything else, rather than seeing technical or scientific thinking as simply *one form* of world disclosure that is abstracted from our prereflective understanding of the world.

Calculative and Meditative Thinking Heidegger's philosophy intends to show that truth is not factual correctness or logical correspondence, but rather letting something "show itself" as itself. Truth is not merely an assertion, nor is it a matter of either-or; it is more a matter of degree, an illumination of or a shedding of light on something.[97] Contemporary science and medicine, however—despite the influential philosophy of Heidegger and his contemporaries who wrote in the phenomenological tradition—rarely let things show themselves and instead seek to reduce nature and the body to the components that fit within their chosen paradigms. One of the reasons for this is that science and medicine are dominated by what Heidegger calls "calculative thinking,"[98] which has come to dominate nearly all thinking in the West and which calculates and "computes . . . even if it neither works with numbers nor uses an adding machine or computer."[99]

Though not a Luddite per se, Heidegger warns us of the dangers of technology understood in the traditional sense—as technical gadgets and equipment. Similar warnings are not uncommon among contemporary medical practitioners. Physician William Bynum, for example, argues that technology all too often distances doctors from their patients in clinical encounters and that "helping our learners to master these new technologies without sacrificing their ability to connect with their patients will undoubtedly be one of the great challenges of educating the next generation of physicians."[100] Though Heidegger would agree that a dependence on technological equipment has pernicious effects on our ability to engage authentically with others and that we run the risk of "fall[ing] into bondage" to "technical devices," his critique runs deeper than this.[101] It is not merely technology as technological equipment that presents a problem, but rather the dominance of technical or calculative thinking as a hegemonic form of world disclosure, the ubiquity of technical equipment being merely one of its manifestations. Heidegger is concerned about why and how it is possible for the doctor to become, in Bynum's phrase, "an automated medical kiosk" in the first place.

Because calculative thinking "works" and because, as Heidegger points out, "technical devices . . . challenge us to greater advances," it is tempting to see calculative thinking as the effective, right, and best way of seeking answers. As a result, whether it employs technological devices or not, calculative thinking sets forth the criteria needed to assess whether an answer is correct—or whether the question is even "thinkable"—before the investigation ever begins.[102] In Heidegger's words, technology and calculative modes of thought pervade and "enframe" all of our thinking.[103] That is to say, calculative thinking frames how we see the world and how the world is revealed to us, and holds that all things are amenable to and best understood through scientific investigation. Guignon alludes to this enframing when he describes the predominant Cartesian worldview that Heidegger critiques: "When a worldview becomes firmly entrenched, it tends to perpetuate a set of problems that are taken as natural and obvious. The possibilities of thought become calcified; the same questions and the same types of futile answers are repeated along the guidelines laid out by the grid that structures our thought."[104]

Within this framework, we see the world as something we can set our gaze upon in a predefined way in order to "discover" the certifiable answers we seek, and we take the reasons for such an approach to be self-evident.[105] In medicine, for instance, doctors often enframe the patient as a diseased body-object in need of medical intervention, thereby overlooking the myriad ways that an illness can affect a person and the person's everyday way of life. And, paradoxically, a patient might expect or even desire such an approach. The way our modern world is enframed by calculative thought is so pervasive and normalized that some patients accept medicine's objectifying gaze and consent to invasive technological intervention, believing this to be the best way to identify and subsequently remedy an illness.

One of the reasons why such approaches to medical care persist despite their obvious limitations is that, according to Heidegger, we have lost sight of the original meaning of technology, as revealed through the Greek word *technē*, which is closer to the kind of truth described by the term "aletheia" discussed above.[106] As opposed to the common way "technology" is used today, usually as a technical imposition onto the natural world (for the production of energy or the extraction of useful resources, for example), "technē" speaks to a means of unconcealing, revealing, or letting something show itself. "Technē" allows for a "bringing forth" of something ("poiesis"), and artists, craftspersons, or scientists assist in this bringing forth in ways that do not "challenge forth" nature in order to expose what they intend to find.[107] But modern science, having lost sight of the original conception of "technē," can be said to challenge forth the world because it sets its methods over and against the world in order to glean particular, verifiable data, even though some phenomena resist such objectification and cannot be fully explained through this mode of investigation.[108] As Heidegger tells us, reality cannot fully be captured by a description; phenomena always exceed the descriptions we give of them.[109] Seeing the objective, measurable, and tangible or corporeal characteristics of nature and of the body is only one way these phenomena disclose themselves to us. But because this form of world disclosure is accompanied by some measure of certainty and verifiability, it easily masquerades as the apogee of our investigative ability or the ultimate revealer of truth—and all other aspects of life that resist such objectification and calculation risk being dismissed as trivial or even nonexistent.[110] So, even as calculative approaches reveal some "true" aspects of phenomena, they also conceal or cover over truth in the larger sense.

Calculative Thinking and the Clinical Gaze Heidegger claims that this "technical" relationship between humans and the world appeared first in Europe during the seventeenth century, a product of the far-reaching ideals of the Enlightenment.[111] This calls to mind Foucault's historical analysis of the development of modern medicine in *The Birth of the Clinic*. Bishop explains that, focusing on eighteenth- and nineteenth-century French medicine as it was practiced in the Paris School, Foucault's analysis centers around the perceptual shifts occurring in medicine and medical education at the time, particularly the transition from diagnosing patients based on the personal description of their symptoms to diagnosing patients based on the doctor's ability to "verify" and articulate the presence of disease through knowledge about the pathophysiological interworkings of the body—a shift that Foucault believes occurred alongside the introduction of pathological anatomy.[112] Foucault suggests that, as a result of this shift, medical knowledge became increasingly rigid and structured, and disease categories began to be organized and arranged in tables to aid in the diagnostic process.[113] The physician or student-physician would simply compare the patient's symptoms with those listed in the tables in order to verify and label a particular disease state. Medical practice thus became a practice of mapping a disease onto the body's surface.[114] According to Foucault, this transition has resulted in the patient becoming quite literally "patient"—the passive object of what he calls the "clinical gaze": the mythical belief that physicians can, with their gaze, see through to the underlying reality, the hidden "truth" within the patient's body, a gaze that often results in the dehumanizing separation of the patient's body from the patient's person.[115] Or, as Foucault himself explains:

What was fundamentally invisible is suddenly offered to the brightness of the gaze, in a movement of appearance so simple, so immediate that it seems to be the natural consequence of a more highly developed experience. It is as if for the first time for thousands of years, doctors, free at last of theories and chimeras, agreed to approach the object of their experience with the purity of an unprejudiced gaze.[116]

Foucault goes on to say that the analytic technique of diagnosis is similar to that employed during autopsy; disease is revealed by the penetrating gaze much in the same way it is revealed by cutting open the cadaver.[117] It is in this way that the dead or unanimated body—abstracted from the lifeworld of the patient—"becomes the epistemologically normative body" in medicine, as Bishop puts it.[118] The "truth" of the illness is reduced to uncovering its pathological foundation within the human body. In a recent article exploring the professional training of medical students in the gross anatomy lab, Mark J. Kissler and colleagues—though they don't refer to Foucault's clinical gaze—note how several students described a transition to a new way of knowing defined by "a figurative new power of sight" or "X-ray vision."[119] "We gain the confidence we need," as one anatomy student in the study put it, "a sort of X-ray vision that allows us to see beneath the skin. Maybe it's this sixth sense that helps with our diagnosing, but also being sensitive to the problems that lurk below."[120]

Philosopher Christian Hick suggests that Foucault's analysis points to the development of the "closed" scientific way of seeing reality in contemporary medicine. This perceptual pattern falls within the frame of calculative thinking, for it prioritizes and relies on "absolute" knowledge and presents itself not as one possible description of reality but as *the* description of reality. Within this frame, both illness and the body are challenged forth to fit into predefined categories and labels, and illness—the lived experience of being sick—is reduced to biological disease. It should be noted that such categories are useful and necessary in medicine; indeed, it is difficult to offer the correct treatment without identifying the disease, and some patients' pain can be significantly alleviated once they discover the source of that pain.[121] Nevertheless, the problem lies in the fact that identifying pathology and its corresponding remedy have come to stand as medicine's raison d'être. The patient's body, rather than the experience of the person suffering illness or "dis-ease," becomes the primary focus of medical care.[122] For this reason, among others, we can see why some students so easily conflate healing with curing: intervening at the level of biology seems to be the definitive characteristic of medical care.

In many ways, seeing the world in technical, rational, measurable, and curable terms offers a false sense of security and control. As Nuland pointed out in 1995, the modern profession of medicine has become a place where the doctor attempts to create order from chaos and exert control over disease, nature, and "his personal universe."[123] Medical intervention, even when futile, becomes a means of controlling the chaos of embodiment and being human, not only for patients, but for doctors as well. Heidegger's critique, notes Guignon, is aimed at this very assumption of technical and calculative thinking—that is to say, the idea that "we can gain final control over Being by making it fully explicit and intelligible."[124] The problem with this assumption is that it is guided by the idea that being is materially present and therefore subject to manipulation, which covers over and conceals questions of *meaning*.[125] Therefore, even though science can in many ways explain *what* we are, it cannot explain *who* we are and *why* we are. And yet the ubiquity of calculative thinking and the perception that "science is a road to a happier human life" continue to endure.[126] Scientific and naturalistic understandings of the self are appealing because they make us believe that we can disengage and detach from our world by objectifying it,[127] which offers us a sense of freedom, agency, and power that seems unencumbered by outside forces. Thus, despite their espoused "neutrality," scientific and reductionistic understandings have a kind of "moral appeal," presenting themselves as the best, most sound, and most complete way of understanding the world and ourselves.[128]

Instances of such thinking abound in medical, academic, and lay communities alike. In a poignant and rather troubling example of this thinking, a 2014 *Business Insider* article announces: "IBM's Watson Supercomputer May Soon Be the Best Doctor in the World." Watson offers treatment options for patients based on its ability to "mine patient data" and then combine it with other sources of information, such as evidence-based treatment guidelines, peer-reviewed research, and clinical studies. The supercomputer is described as being "already capable of storing far more medical information than doctors, and unlike humans, its decisions are all evidence-based and free of cognitive biases and overconfidence."[129] The article goes on to quote researcher Andrew McAffee, who lauds Watson for its accuracy, affordability, and consistency: "Given the same inputs, Dr. Watson will always output the same diagnosis. Inconsistency is a surprisingly large and common flaw among human medical professionals, even experienced ones. And Dr. Watson is always available and never annoyed, sick, nervous, hungover, upset, in the middle of a divorce, sleep-deprived, and so on."[130]

Both of these statements assume that doctors might be able to free themselves of their biases, an assumption that Heidegger suggests is misguided and biased in and of itself, a mere vestige of Cartesian and Enlightenment thought. But perhaps more disturbing is the assumption that patients would or should *prefer* a disaffected, objective supercomputer like Watson over a flesh-and-blood doctor. Not only does this assumption fail to consider that an algorithm can never stand in for the clinical intuition, personal experience, and ineffable perceptions that so often go into a physician's ability to diagnose and treat patients, but it also overlooks the fact that patients suffer in ways that extend beyond biological dysfunction—a supercomputer cannot interpret and attend to the *meaning* of the illness within the context of the patient's life. This technology represents a total disconnect from technē as a revealing of truth. Instead, truth—in this case, a diagnosis—is delimited and determined by an algorithmic calculation. Watson can only "reveal" what it is designed and predetermined to produce, which is likely a narrow and purely biologic description of the patient's illness.

The creation of Watson and the discourse surrounding its potential contribution to clinical care may seem like an absurdly hyperbolic manifestation of medical reductionism, but, within the calculative paradigm that enframes the way so many see the world—including illness and health—Watson appears as the natural next step in the journey of medical and scientific "progress."[131] After all, a supercomputer like Watson can challenge forth the body and fit it into predetermined schema more perfectly and more exactly than any human. It is precisely this thinking that creates the conditions for a physician to become the "automated medical kiosk" mentioned above—conditions that are bigger, less conspicuous, and more complex than the simple introduction of technological equipment and the electronic medical record into the clinical space.

Heidegger's ideas about calculative thinking reveal how it shapes our perception of the "real" and "true," even outside medicine. They show us that the problems with medicine cannot be remedied simply by replacing its misguided epistemology with a "better" one, especially considering that nearly the whole of the West's philosophical and epistemological inquiry of the past 400 years has been dominated by calculative thinking. In this way, Heidegger helps us see that a fundamental problem of medicine, and contemporary Western society more generally, is an ontological one: human beings have lost sight of the fact that we are primordially not calculative but *meditative* beings,[132] to whom the world always already presents itself as meaningful. We recognize beauty when we see it, we know when we feel pain and experience betrayal, and we do not need technical explanations of these things in order to understand them or believe they exist. It is meditative thinking, which deals with questions that do not have exact answers and which remains open to wonder and complexity, that brings us closer to understanding the lived experience of things like joy, suffering, loss, and love.[133] But in a world enframed by calculative thinking, we engage in a flight from meditative thinking and, as Heidegger says, we "forget to ponder . . . we forget to ask: What is the ground that enabled modern technology to discover and set free new energies in nature?"[134]

This way of framing the world, which manifests itself so obviously within medicine, covers over the lived experience of illness and suffering and can render these experiences extraneous or superfluous. The notion of truth as aletheia or uncovering, which allows existential suffering to be perceived as just as true or "real" as anything that can be measured or quantified, is lost in favor of tangible, measurable reality—even though the lived experience of the body is the primordial grounding that makes abstract definitions of disease categories possible in the first place. The benefits of biomedical perspectives of illness and techno-scientific approaches to care are undeniable—indeed, we often *need* them in order to bring physical healing to patients—but scientific and biomedical understandings of the body and illness have become totalizing. Indeed, it is the ubiquitous and unquestioned acceptance of scientific authority that have set the stage for physicians to "artificially circumscribe [their] task in caring for the sick," as Cassell described it.[135] The word "artificial" is important here, for it suggests that doctors do not *have* to comport themselves as technicians, even in an environment so caught up in technical thinking. Though the narrow biomedical paradigm too often becomes the default approach to care, this approach is not the only approach—physicians can, in fact, choose to expand their understandings of what it means to care for the other. The question that remains, then, is why do they fall into such narrow conceptions of care when their patients suffer in ways that clearly extend beyond their physical bodies?

All told, the ubiquity of calculative thinking helps explain why this is so. And its power and pervasiveness help explain the disconnect between the expressed, desired qualities of the ideal clinician or medical student and the qualities that are actually reinforced during the medical school selection process and subsequent training. Scientific acumen and technical skills override intuition, humility, and openness to the unexplainable or indefinite, which are perceived as "soft" qualities secondary or subsidiary to the "real" skills needed for doctoring.

There is, however, more to the story. Why we tend to force the world to present itself to us in particular ways and why we value certainty, clarity, and control require further examination. Drawing on the insights of Kierkegaard, Nietzsche, Heidegger, and Merleau-Ponty, chapter 2 will explore what it is about being human that draws us toward certainty and away from vulnerability—namely, our desire to disburden ourselves from the reality of our frailty and mortality. And it will examine the consequences of this disburdening for both patients and physicians and how it tends to leave the phenomenological experience of illness largely unaddressed.

2 The "Remainder" in Modern Medicine: The Lived Experience of Illness and Existential Anxiety

When the body breaks down, so does the life.
—Arthur W. Frank, *At the Will of the Body*

Proximally and for the most part, Dasein covers up its ownmost Being-towards-death, fleeing *in the face* of it.
—Martin Heidegger, *Being and Time*

Heidegger's contention that we have forgotten that we always already dwell meaningfully in the world in a way that precedes any scientific examination of that world, though revolutionary in many ways, was by no means new. Heidegger's early philosophy, especially the ideas presented in *Being and Time*, was inspired by the writings of Danish philosopher and theologian Søren Kierkegaard (1813–1855).[1] Like the writings of Heidegger that would appear nearly a century later, those of Kierkegaard expressed disillusionment with much of the philosophical and theological inquiry of his time, which he believed was preoccupied with an intellectual abstraction that lost sight of the perspectives and commitments of flesh-and-blood human beings.[2] He was suspicious of the speculative thinkers, especially those in the physical sciences, who set themselves "outside" the world in order to contemplate existence from a privileged, objective vantage point. Though Kierkegaard believed that this kind of detached inquiry was suitable for some investigations, he was concerned when it exceeded its proper limits and was used to explain or ignore unanswerable, usually metaphysical, questions concerning faith, suffering, or the human condition.[3]

Arguing that the desire to engage in "pure thinking" represents a "dubious beginning" that makes a person's existence "trivial," Kierkegaard emphasizes that abstract questions are inextricably connected to the existential.[4]

Nevertheless, abstract, technical inquiries reigned supreme in his time, and Kierkegaard saw this trend as evidence of the tendency of human beings to turn away from— to "forget"—the realities of existing in the everyday and instead to turn toward abstract explanations of the world that, according to Kierkegaard, "remove the difficulty by omitting [the existential] and then boast of having explained everything."[5] The misguided belief that such inquiries could, in fact, explain everything was precisely the problem for Kierkegaard, who believed this unbridled faith in scientific knowledge divested individuals of their ability to choose for themselves the meaning of existence: "To think abstractly is easier than to exist . . . truly to exist, that is, to permeate one's existence with consciousness . . . that is truly difficult."[6] Ultimately for Kierkegaard, "people have entirely forgotten what it means to *exist*, and what inwardness is."[7] That is to say, abstract inquiry has indeed overstepped its appropriate bounds, presenting itself as the only means of revealing the "truth" of existence.

Friedrich Nietzsche (1844–1900) expresses a similar critique in *On the Genealogy of Morals* (1887). Although Nietzsche's philosophy is viewed as essentially irreligious, whereas Kierkegaard's is seen as perhaps primarily religious, their philosophies converge in their suspicion of far-reaching abstract, scientific thinking and of the unyielding faith in science's ability to produce truth.[8] In *On the Genealogy of Morals*, Nietzsche implores us to reexamine our valuation of truth and to question our assumptions about the infallibility of scientifically derived facts, going so far as to claim that our faith in science is parallel to a faith in religion: "It is still a *metaphysical faith* that underlies our faith in science."[9] In other words, science is predicated on an unquestioned faith in its ability to uncover objective truths about the world, which ultimately requires a faith in science's power to do so. What is more, this unquestioned faith is grounded in an uncontested understanding of just what one means by "truth" in the first place.[10] Nietzsche argues that the value of truth itself needs to be called into question, for this unbending faith in absolute truth is nothing more than another iteration of the ascetic priest's unremitting faith in an absolute God: "That general renunciation of all interpretation (of forcing, adjusting, abbreviating, omitting, padding, inventing, falsifying, and whatever else is of the essence of interpreting)—all this expresses, broadly speaking, as much ascetic virtue as any denial of sensuality."[11] In other words, the ideal upon which the value of scientific truth rests is one that can never be empirically verified or proved.[12] Because of this, Nietzsche advocates a dynamic "perspectivism," in which we acknowledge that all accounts of truth or phenomena are unique perspectives that we cannot escape or rid ourselves of. Perspectivism points to the limits of our situated knowledge and to the fact that we cannot view reality from a singular, privileged vantage point. This position is a far cry from the usual stance we take toward the facts uncovered by scientific methodologies, facts that we most often hold to be inherently and irrevocably true. As Nietzsche laments, "There is *only* perspective seeing, *only* a perspective 'knowing;' and the *more* affects we allow to speak about one thing, the more complete will our 'concept' of the thing, our 'objectivity,' be. But to eliminate altogether, to suspend each and every affect, supposing we were capable of this—what would that mean but to *castrate* the intellect?"[13]

It is this kind of narrow, scientific thinking that has come to dominate medical culture for the past three centuries, carrying with it vestiges of Cartesian dualism that sustain the view that the suffering of the biological body (usually conflated with bodily pain) falls within the purview of science and medicine, whereas the care of the subjective, unquantifiable, and "less real" aspects of the mind (or nonbodily suffering) falls within the purview of nonmedical entities, such as the church, social services, family unit, and the like.[14] As a result of this compartmentalized and dualistic thinking, the doctor's calling is narrowed to technical treatment of biological dysfunction, whereas tending to the intangible suffering of the patient is conceived as (naturally) belonging to those outside the practice of medicine properly understood.

One consequence of this implicit assumption about what rightly falls within the purview of medicine is that issues such as existential suffering and death, though almost always present, are seldom discussed in medical practice and education. When the body is conceptualized as a biological entity, then there appears nothing else to which the doctor is called to attend besides biological dysfunction. But, as philosopher Theodor Adorno observes, "Objects do not go into their concepts without leaving a remainder."[15] In medicine, after the body is subjected to the clinical gaze and conceptualized in terms of its biology or pathology, the remainder left over can be significant and strangely conspicuous, especially to the patient and the patient's loved ones. Most often, this remainder is the lived experience of illness, the changes in the way one goes about the everyday, as well as potential fear, uncertainty, emotional suffering, and feelings of meaninglessness that can ensue. A preoccupation with tending to the biological body obscures what it means to *live* in that body, what it *feels* like to be ill or injured, what it is like to experience the world differently as one's embodiment shifts and changes. As Kierkegaard warned us, the proliferation of scientific and technical inquiries can lead to an intellectualization of feelings and emotions—human qualities that become obscured or rendered insignificant by scientific explanations.[16]

Embodiment and the Lived Experience of Illness

As stated in chapter 1, the primary focus of medicine is physical, functional restoration. Although restoring function to the body is often desired and often even achieved, in the instances where this is impossible or simply not sufficient, patients' suffering can be overlooked, or even worse, intensified. As Jeffrey Bishop points out: "Human life cannot be reduced to functionality, to material and efficient causation, without doing violence to the other features of being-in-the-world."[17] The other features of being-in-the-world to which Bishop is referring most notably include the phenomenological experience of illness and suffering—the often overlooked lived reality of being ill. Thinkers in the existential and phenomenological traditions, inspired by the philosophies of both Kierkegaard and Nietzsche, have been keen to point out that, in order to understand who and how we are, we need to start with our lived experiences, the precognitive understanding of our lives.[18] Perhaps nowhere is this more important than in our attempts to understand what it means to be ill. According to philosopher S. Kay Toombs, who not only writes about illness but also lives with multiple sclerosis, looking at illness phenomenologically can "effectively mitigate some of the dehumanizing aspects of medical care" because it draws attention to the lived experience of illness and does not "abstract the body from the person whose body it is."[19] Likewise, Swedish philosopher Fredrik Svenaeus points out that thinking about illness and the body phenomenologically—that is to say, starting one's "investigation" in everyday life—can reveal the *meaning* of the illness experience.[20] This does not mean that determining how patients interpret their illnesses is the most important component of clinical encounters, nor does it deny that it is sometimes necessary and even preferred to abstract a patient's body from the patient's illness experience.

But, considering that the anatomical-physiological body is only one facet of the unity of a person's life, it is nearly impossible to uncover how patients suffer and what illness means to them without an understanding of the lived experience of illness.

What Is Phenomenology?

Much like the medical humanists and bioethicists who would appear on the scene several decades later, early philosophers in the phenomenological tradition sought to reclaim what they perceived had been lost through the overreliance on empirical or scientific investigations within the realm of human life.[21] Phenomenology is both a method and a philosophical movement, and phenomenological thinkers and applications of phenomenological methods are extremely diverse.[22] That said, phenomenology might be defined—generally speaking—as a philosophy of experience that describes the world as we live it.[23] More specifically, phenomenology is concerned with uncovering and describing phenomena that present themselves to us in our everyday, concrete lived experience. For the phenomenologist, the fundamental source of all meaning lies in the structures of lived experience or the "lifeworld" (*Lebenswelt*) of people themselves.[24] Edmund Husserl (1859–1938), who is often cited as the father of phenomenology, attempted to bring philosophy back from abstract metaphysical speculation and toward "the things themselves." Husserl maintained that the focus of phenomenology was on the world as experienced or *lived* by a person, rather than the world as an object or as something separate from or "outside" the person.[25] He claimed that the study of lived phenomena—things that often are experienced prereflectively or pretheoretically—would allow us to reexamine taken-for-granted assumptions and to uncover new meaning. And directing our focus toward things and fully grasping phenomena as they appear to our consciousness—while bracketing or suspending any assumptions that distort such phenomena (Husserl would call this "suspending the natural attitude")—would allow us to describe particular realities.[26]

According to Husserl, all consciousness is intentional, and to experience something is to be conscious of it, to be "directed towards it in an act" (looking, touching, smelling, thinking, reading, etc.).[27] "Bracketing" or suspending our presuppositions about a phenomenon—that is, laying aside any philosophical, scientific, cultural, or religious theorizing about an entity—frees us to perceive the entity as it appears to us and how "it obtains meaning" for us.[28] Once we have bracketed all preceding scientific and philosophical theories about a phenomenon, we can then focus simply on a "purified" experience of it.

Heidegger, who studied under Husserl, extended and critiqued Husserl's phenomenology, and, with the publication of Heidegger's *Being and Time* in 1927, phenomenology came to be understood in terms of both thinkers' contributions.[29] Recognizing that not all lived experiences are conscious or intentional (habitual patterns of behavior, desires, and anxieties, for example, are not), Heidegger did not limit his phenomenology to conscious experience, and refrained from using the terms "consciousness" and "intentionality" altogether.[30] Though both philosophers set out to describe the way in which the world appears to and through human beings, Heidegger's phenomenology takes a distinctly ontological turn: it focuses not on the intentional structures of consciousness, but on the meaning of being in general and what it means to be human specifically.[31]

Heidegger's phenomenology also differs from Husserl's in its emphasis on hermeneutics. Phenomenology becomes hermeneutic when its method is understood as interpretive rather than merely descriptive.[32] Although hermeneutics began as a branch of theology concerned with the interpretation and exegesis of scriptural texts, over the course of the eighteenth and nineteenth centuries, it expanded to become a theory of understanding in general,[33] largely focusing on the problem of "distance" between person and object or person and person that renders meaning or understanding opaque. Within the hermeneutic tradition, existential phenomenologists like Martin Heidegger and Hans-Georg Gadamer seek to uncover human experience as it is lived, yet they argue that completely "bracketing" presuppositions and judgments is impossible: we cannot stand outside our understanding of, or situatedness within, the world. Rather, we interpret our experiences in terms of the context of the situation or our relation to things within the world around us.[34] All understanding is always already "in" the world, alongside beings and entities that we already understand in some capacity. Thus hermeneutics might be seen as the attempt to make the structure of situatedness more conspicuous, even if it is presupposed in the very attempt to explicate it.[35] So, whereas Husserl contends that our main connection to the world is through cognition, Heidegger sees humans as always already wrapped up in the world, feeling and understanding the world first and foremost precognitively. And because we are already caught up in the world, all understanding (both cognitive and precognitive) carries with it our particular interpretive perspectives that both reveal and conceal the phenomena we encounter. In other words, our understanding of the world and what we encounter in it is interpretive from the start.[36]

This focus on explicating or "laying bare" our situatedness and its inevitable effect on our basic understanding is where hermeneutics becomes one with phenomenology.[37] Hermeneutic phenomenology's emphasis on our situatedness (historical, cultural, social, familial, and so forth) and how it influences the way we interpret the world as we see it and our experiences in that world has resonated with those interested in the experience of medicine and illness. Especially for those who see "objective" biomedical accounts of illness as narrow explanations that conceal more than they reveal, approaching health, illness, and the body phenomenologically offers a richer and more penetrating look at such phenomena.

Phenomenology and the Body

In her phenomenological analysis of illness, Toombs argues that illness is "first and foremost a subjective experience" that cannot be reduced to the presence or absence of biological disease.[38] Thus, to understand the nature of illness and the experiences of their patients, physicians must bring their attention to the lived experience of "embodiment." Toombs's work is heavily influenced by the early phenomenologists, especially the French philosopher Maurice Merleau-Ponty (1908–1961) and his conception of embodiment. Rejecting the longstanding Cartesian mind-body separation, Merleau-Ponty developed a phenomenology that underscored the role of the body in human experience.[39] He aimed to show that, far from being simply a physical entity "operated" by the mind, a person's lived body *is* the person in "engaged action" with the things and the people that person perceives.[40] For each of us, the body already has a tacit know-how of making its way in the world; our everyday existence and ability to move about or comport ourselves this way or that is already understood prereflectively by the "habit body."[41] Moreover, this prereflective understanding of the world comes (necessarily) "before" any scientific understanding of our bodies and the world, for we are always already embodied in the world before we ever come to investigate such things scientifically.

As set forth in his Zollikon seminars, delivered to a group of doctors and medical students in Switzerland between 1959 and 1969, Heidegger's rich phenomenological description of the body is not unlike Merleau-Ponty's.[42] In a 1965 seminar, Heidegger claims that "perhaps one comes closer to the phenomenon of the body by distinguishing between the limits of a corporeal thing [*Körper*] and those of the lived body [*Leib*]."[43] This understanding of the body as a kind of dual phenomenon is critical for Heidegger, who believes that a singular conception of the corporeal body (*Körper*)—an entity that "stops with the skin"—cannot fully capture the phenomenon of the lived body. Though the body is a corporeal thing, its thingness does not wholly constitute it; the body is also a *lived* body (*Leib*), an ecstatic phenomenon that extends beyond the skin and engages in a "bodying forth" into our projects, our travels, our engagement with others in the world.[44] It is the lived body, which cannot be measured or studied like the corporeal body, that is always already spatially attuned to and engaged in the unobtrusive everydayness of life—that climbs stairs, walks away, makes room, and cozies up.[45] It is this lived body that allows us to "get on" in the world and lets us project ourselves into our projects.

This distinction helps us to see that a narrow focus on the dysfunctions of the corporeal body alone might obscure the lived body, thereby abstracting pain or disease from the lived experiences of such phenomena. This is especially true in medicine where the physical body so often takes precedence over the lived experiences of illness. As Heidegger remarks in that same 1965 seminar:

Because you are educated in anatomy and physiology as doctors, that is with a focus on the examination of bodies, you probably look at the states of the body in a different way than the "layman" does. Yet a layman's experience is probably closer to the phenomenon of pain as it involves our body lines, even if it can hardly be described with the aid of our usual intuition of space.[46]

Though our layperson's description of our pain may not fully represent the physiological workings of the corporeal body, it speaks to the truth of our lived body and our lived experience. When we refer to the "shooting pain down my leg every time I stand up," this can reveal more about our particular illness or injury and what it means to us in our particular lifeworld—what it prevents us from doing and the disruption it creates in our routine—than the CT scan that reveals a compressed sciatic nerve. And even though a precise understanding of the biomechanics of the corporeal body is critical when choosing appropriate medical interventions during the breakdown of that body, by allowing this perspective to obscure the realities of the lived body, physicians may exacerbate rather than relieve the suffering of their patients.

The Lived Body and Illness

In good health when all feels as it should, the corporeal body usually "disappears" or becomes inconspicuous. Gadamer refers to this as the tacit or "natural equilibrium" of the body.[47] But when we become seriously ill or injured, the lived body and the corporeal body intrude on each other, and the body presents itself as object, even as we remain in our lived embodiment in the world. In other words, the taken-for-granted interrelation or synergy of body and world begins to break down, and a "disturbance" is created in something that previously escaped our attention almost entirely.[48] Suddenly, the corporeal body—which usually fades into the background of everyday life—forces itself into awareness. As Gadamer says: "The sick person is no longer simply identical with the person he or she was before. For the sick individual 'falls out' of things, has already fallen out of their normal place in life."[49]

As the natural equilibrium of the lived body is disrupted by the corporeal body's dysfunction, the body-as-object is brought into conscious awareness. And it is precisely the change in the average everydayness of their lives wrought by illness or injury that matters most to patients. People with multiple sclerosis, for example, know their illness not only as an autoimmune disease affecting the central nervous system, but also as something that interrupts their everyday ways of being in the world. Their bodies become noticeable and draw attention to their taken-for-granted functioning, and habitual tasks that were once given little thought force themselves into view: stairs become unclimbable, holding their child becomes unbearable, or commuting to work impossible.

In her illness narrative *Cancer in Two Voices*, coauthored with her life partner, Sandra Butler, Barbara Rosenblum eloquently describes the experience of living in "an unstable body" after receiving a cancer diagnosis—a body that holds her "hostage to [its] capriciousness" and "sabotages [her] sense of a continuous and taken-for-granted reality."[50] Explaining what it is like to live in and through her ever-changing body, Rosenblum points to the sudden intrusion of the corporeal body into the everyday experience of her lived body:

What is it like to live in a body that keeps on changing? It's frightening, terrifying, and confusing. It generates a slavish attention to the body. . . . One becomes a prisoner to any perceptible change in the body, any cough, any difference in sensation. One loses one's sense of stability and predictability, as well as one's sense of control over the body. . . . Predictability ends. One grieves over its loss, and that further complicates the process of adjustment to an unstable body. Time becomes shortened and is marked by the space between symptoms.[51]

The imposition of the corporeal body onto Rosenblum's taken-for-granted way of being in the world is clear: her knowledge of her biological disease changes her interpretation of bodily sensations and functions. In this way, her body and its functioning have not only become noticeable; they have also become a problem. Her corporeal body—or perhaps her diligent attention to it—has come to control her and mediate her interpretation of the world around her. Rosenblum's changing corporeal body alters her lived, bodily experiences; she has fallen out of the world she once knew and has entered what Susan Sontag famously called "the kingdom of the sick."[52] She knows herself, her world, her body, and her relationships in a new way. Any accustomed sense of predictability eludes her, and her experience of time and her ability to project herself seamlessly into the future is disrupted.

Rosenblum's description of the lived experience of illness reveals that the body does not simply become a conspicuous problem when we are seriously ill or injured, but that its doing so causes our entire way of being to change, including the way we make (or can no longer make) sense of the world around us. Serious illness can dissolve any semblance of a coherent life trajectory, intensifying experiences of the present and alienating the sick person from that person's future.[53] Indeed, the future Rosenblum alludes to becomes uncertain and is no longer guaranteed. Approaching illness phenomenologically, then, reveals that a patient cannot be understood as a self-contained corporeal body separate from the context in which the patient dwells.[54] In other words, it exposes the primary reason why a doctor could never be replaced by an IBM supercomputer, for such a "doctor" could neither discern nor address the breakdown in a patient's lifeworld.

Svenaeus uses Heidegger's philosophy to explicate the life breakdowns that can occur during illness, describing them as experiences of "unhomelike being-in-the-world."[55] According to Heidegger, we always already understand the world into which we are thrown.[56] Most of the time, our ability to dwell in the world understandingly is seamless and unbroken, and the world seems homelike, relatively stable, and comfortable. Health, for Svenaeus, represents a homelike being-in-the-world, where the lived body comports itself with ease, unaffected by corporeal dysfunction or bodily breakdown.[57] The connection between body and world is harmonious, and we feel at home in the world around us.

Serious illness or injury, however, "breaks in on us," and such serious intrusions resist meaning and can threaten our homelike being-in-the-world.[58] Because illness disturbs our meaning-making processes, it is not only our body that becomes alien or uncanny, but also our entire way of being. What is more, this disruption of meaning—as well as the plans, expectations, and relationships that change or fall away—can occasion feelings of fear, isolation, and anxiety. In his moving and insightful illness narrative about experiencing a heart attack at age thirty-nine and receiving a serious cancer diagnosis the following year, Arthur Frank speaks to the way illness can alter aspects of one's entire life, leading to the experience of unhomelikeness. Though he points out that different illnesses "set in place different possibilities" for everyone and that how we each interpret our illness will vary, Frank maintains that there appears to be a "common core of what critical illness does to a life."[59] As he describes it: "Critical illness leaves no aspect of life untouched. . . . Your relationships, your work, your sense of who you are and who you might become, your sense of what life is and ought not to be—these all change, and the change is terrifying."[60]

The analysis of illness as unhomelike being-in-the-world, so clearly presented by Frank, draws attention to the fact that when medicine preoccupies itself primarily with the corporeal body and overlooks the ways in which the lived body suffers, it also overlooks the dynamic illness experience that extends beyond even the lived body. When illness strikes the lived body—which is inextricably connected to the world and how we make our way in it—our whole being is affected. As Frank puts it: "What happens when my body breaks down happens not just to that body but also to my life, which is lived in that body."[61] This suggests a need for healthcare professionals to attune themselves to the phenomenological experience of their patients and the ways in which illness creates an unhomelike quality for them, shifting their world in unfamiliar ways.[62] And part of attuning themselves requires the ability to distinguish "disease"—which Svenaeus describes as a disturbance of the biological functions of the body that is usually identified and described from the third-person perspective of the doctor—from "illness" (or what Toombs calls "dis-ease"), which affects patients' everyday ways of being and speaks to the human experience of being ill.[63]

Although "illness," as opposed to "disease," speaks to the changes patients experience in their everyday lives, it is often the case that what Frank calls "disease talk" drowns out the voice of "illness talk" during the clinical encounter. As Frank describes it:

> Because the disease terms refer to measurements, they are "objective." Thus, in disease talk *my* body, my ongoing experience of being alive, becomes *the* body, an object to be measured and thus objectified. "Objective" talk about disease is always medical talk. Patients quickly learn to express themselves in these terms, but in using medical expressions ill persons lose themselves: the body I experience cannot be reduced to the body someone else measures.[64]

The way in which things are discussed or left undiscussed in the discourse of medicine creates and informs both physicians' and patients' reality and how they interpret their experiences. Such domains of discourse, which determine what counts as experience and who count as actors, are what Michel Foucault describes as "discursive regimes," for they frame the ways in which we come to know our world and how we interpret and understand our experiences.[65] Although things such as sensations, ineffable feelings of the body, and spirituality exist "outside" discourse proper, we make meaning out of life events and experiences (even the intangible) discursively, through narrative.[66]

Over the years, scholars have pointed out how healthcare providers almost exclusively "talk in stories," whether presenting cases in formal settings such as grand rounds or discussing patients anecdotally.[67] But clinicians often fail to see the "storied" nature of medical practice; they resort to and privilege impoverished technical narratives—those in patients' charts, for instance—wherein illnesses are abstracted, medicalized, and "dehistoricized."[68] Thus, within the discourse of medical institutions—namely, the language, images, metaphors, and narratives through which medical institutions produce and circulate knowledge—people learn to understand themselves or "experience" themselves as diseased or insufficient bodies in need of medical or surgical intervention.[69] And the complexities of the illness experience are reduced to the presence or absence of disease.

For Frank, this dominant discourse of medicine significantly limits the responses of both patients and doctors when they are confronted with the

The "Remainder" in Modern Medicine

kind of suffering or embodied breakdown that cannot be distilled into the language of disease. Frank writes:

> Medical treatment, whether in an office or hospital or on the phone, is designed to make everyone believe that only the disease—what is measurable and mechanical—can be discussed.... I know I am supposed to ask only about the disease, but what I feel is the illness. The questions I want to ask about my life are not allowed, not speakable, not even thinkable. The gap between what I feel and what I feel allowed to say widens and deepens and swallows my voice.[70]

What Frank and phenomenologists concerned about illness and health are attempting to do is bring attention to the fact that illness is not a uniform, unambiguous phenomenon that can be described from a biological or scientific standpoint. Much like Nietzsche's perspectivism, phenomenological accounts of illness and embodiment underscore that there is no one "real" understanding of illness and suffering, that the lived experiences of illness are just as "real or "true" as scientific explanations of disease.[71] Nevertheless, we live in a time when reductionistic explanations of biological dysfunction continue to dominate and delimit medical diagnoses and treatment, foreclosing broader conceptions of illness and suffering. As Bishop puts it: "The coldness of medicine is because in not restoring function, or even in restoring it, medicine has not understood that something other than function is being lost or returned. This something is embodied ontologically and is deeper than functionality."[72] The loss that runs deeper than functionality is the loss of our previous ways of being in the world, the (sometimes dramatic) changes in our lives, including our roles, relationships, or feelings of comfort, security, and predictability. As Frank says:

> My body is the means and medium of my life.... No one should be asked to detach his mind from his body and then talk about this body as a thing, out there. No one should have to stay cool and professional while being told his or her body is breaking down, though medical patients always have to do just that. The demand being made of me was to treat the breakdown as if fear and frustration were not part of it, to act as if my life, the whole life, had not changed.[73]

It is undeniable that serious illness involves much more than bodily breakdown, and yet many physicians overlook this reality in practice. One could argue that recognizing the lived experience of illness and existential suffering is not a requirement for all physicians, only for those who practice in certain areas of medicine—such as oncology, geriatrics, or palliative care, for instance. That there is much more at stake when existential suffering is overlooked among patients being treated in these fields does not mean, however, that the ability to recognize how patients' lives are affected by illness should be limited to only those physicians who choose such fields. We may want to believe that there is no need for future pathologists or anesthesiologists or radiologists to recognize the phenomenological experience of illness, but the reality is that all of these specialists work with people who suffer. There is something to be said about the pathologist who wonders about the grieving widow who was married for sixty years to the man whose body now lies on the autopsy table, or the radiologist who, looking at the inoperable tumor on the scan of a twenty-year-old woman's brain, wishes it weren't so. These are very human responses to the kinds of tragedies that occur in medicine. Yet such responses are implicitly (and sometimes explicitly) discouraged in a medical culture dominated by narrow, technical descriptions of disease and dysfunction. As a result, those who are asked to extend care to others during times of vulnerability turn away from the realities of illness, choosing to conduct themselves simply as professional experts or purveyors of cure.

If it is the case that illness and suffering involve so much more than fixing and curing, then why is it that some practitioners choose to acknowledge only the corporeal body, or perhaps worse, why do they pathologize existential suffering as biological dysfunction itself? Why do so many of us, including patients and nonclinicians, avoid living in the messiness and uncertainty of the everyday—as Kierkegaard says we do—by relying on abstract explanations of illness and suffering?

Why We Turn away from Suffering

The complex and profound suffering that is basic to the human condition—whether physical, mental, emotional, spiritual, or otherwise—is something few of us are willing to confront.[74] Most of us would prefer not to dwell on the unpredictability of illness and death or the vulnerability of the human mind and body, and with good reason: levity and lightness are hard to come by in a world filled with such realities. And yet those in medicine encounter pain and suffering rather frequently, though they likely feel no less inclined than the rest of us to turn away from them.

Because serious illness or injury can affect so much more than the body, some clinicians may find such suffering overwhelming. As Frank suggests, the voices of patients can be hard to hear, for they "bespeak conditions of embodiment that most of us would rather forget our own vulnerability to."[75] Indeed, suffering can have a powerful effect on those who witness it and may even threaten them with personal "dis-integration." The suffering of patients may force physicians to confront their own mortality and potential for suffering, something many if not most of us would rather turn away from. As a defensive posture, a doctor may choose to ignore the existential reality of embodiment, pain, and mortality, and, acknowledging only the biological reality of illness, may instead engage in a "medical 'doing something' to deny the hovering presence of death."[76]

Indeed, Johanna Shapiro—who argues that medicine is predicated on the modernist assumption of restoration of health—claims that medicine works to reassure both patients and doctors that they will not *really* become ill—and if they do, there is still little to fear, for they undoubtedly will be cured and restored.[77] Because of this, diseases that do not conform to this ideal, especially chronic or terminal illnesses, are "frustrating and frightening," and patients with such illnesses are likely to encounter physicians who distance themselves or who even withdraw entirely from them.[78] Frank's own illness experience speaks to this. Looking back on his time as a patient, he writes: "Continuing suffering threatens [the medical staff], so they deny it exists. What they cannot treat, the patient is not allowed to experience."[79] Although developing a "thick skin" and occasionally turning a deaf ear to suffering are understandable forms of self-protection, they do not, as Annette Baier points out, count as "functional virtues" in medical practice.[80]

There are certainly exceptions to these generalizations. Many practitioners—especially those who work in palliative and hospice care—remain critical of the dominant curative ethos of mainstream medicine.[81] Perhaps this is because when dying patients become "untreatable," medicine's implicit assumptions about cure and restoration become rather obvious. When restoration is impossible and physicians who see themselves as "curers" retreat, the existential suffering of terminal patients is left largely unaccounted for. In his most recent book, *Being Mortal: Medicine and What Matters in the End*, physician Atul Gawande recounts some of his final encounters with a dying patient that speak to this point. "We had no difficulty explaining the specific dangers of various treatment options," he says, "but we never really touched on the reality of his disease. . . . We could never bring ourselves to discuss the larger truth about his condition or the ultimate limits of our capabilities, let alone what might matter most to him as he neared the end of his life."[82]

When treating patients' biological disease is no longer an option, medicine's narrow focus comes into view, and we begin to see the rather limited ways medicine addresses the various and complex ways people experience illness. But if Frank is right that it is hard to recognize the ways patients suffer because such suffering is threatening to caregivers and reminds them of their own embodiment, it is easy to understand why it might be difficult to face those who are dying since this is the ultimate reminder of human vulnerability. In fact, Bishop argues that a claim could be made that the whole of Western medicine is founded on the dream of deferring death indefinitely, "for death and the disease that is its harbinger are the most brutal reminders of the radical finitude of human existence. Death is the end of all meaning in and of (this) life. And because of this, humanity dreams the dream of eternal life, health, and youth."[83] For Bishop, medicine clearly is complicit in perpetuating this dream.

Medicine and the Denial of Death

Humanity's dream (at least in the West) of deferring death indefinitely or even defeating it altogether is not new. Although a thorough examination of the complex philosophical, social, psychological, cultural, and historical influences that contribute to our apparent fear and denial of death is beyond the scope of the present work, it is important to look at some of the scholarship in this area, particularly as it relates to modern medicine.

The "denial of death thesis" was first advanced in the social, psychological, and medical literature between 1955 and 1985.[84] One of the most influential "death denial" scholars during the late 1960s and early 1970s was Ernest Becker. In his 1973 book *The Denial of Death*, Becker suggests, contra Sigmund Freud, that our most basic drive is rooted not in sexuality or aggression, but rather in the terror of self-aware beings who know that they will die.[85] In other words, the conscious and unconscious motivation for virtually all human behavior is the need to control or deny our basic anxiety: the terror of death and our undeniable mortality. In his foreword to Becker's text, Sam Keen writes that "Becker taught us that awe, fear, and ontological anxiety were natural accompaniments to our contemplation of the fact of death."[86] For Becker, this leads us to a futile search for ways to transcend death by engaging in something meaningful and of lasting worth in order to palliate our anxiety, be it practicing a religion, building a family, constructing a monument, or instigating a political revolution.[87]

This particular conception of the denial of death has led other scholars to make similar claims about the death-fearing culture of the West and its relationship with modern medicine. Medicine and medical technology can serve as talismans in the face of inevitable death, with doctors and patients as "accomplices in staging a kind of drama in which we pretend that doctors have the power to keep us well," especially in a world that has grown increasingly irreligious.[88] In 1970, Paul Ramsey argued that medicine's ethical quandary over the prolongation of life at all costs is, at least in part, a manifestation of an increasingly secular worldview: "It may be that it is quite natural that in an atheistic and secular age the best morality men can think of is to make an absolute of saving life for yet a bit more spatiotemporal existence."[89] According to some historians, medicine's ability to offer the "hope of secular healing" in a modern world grown increasingly rationalist and irreligious has helped to legitimize both the role of the physician and the ever-expanding position of the hospital in society, especially in relation to care for the dying.[90]

There are others, however, who argue that the medicalization and institutionalization of death are not indicative of society's denial of death, but rather manifestations of how society has decided to *deal with* death's reality. For these thinkers, death has been medicalized, institutionalized, bureaucratized, and technologized not because we are a society in denial, but because we are a society that has so thoroughly privileged scientific values—and, in particular, calculative thinking. That is to say, society in general and the medical profession specifically have decided to deal with the *scientific reality* of death by accepting death as a biological phenomenon and attempting to control it through scientific interventions.[91]

This does not mean, however, that there is not a denial of the *existential reality* of death within the practice of medicine—a denial that manifests itself psychologically and relationally between doctors and patients and, Howard Stein claims, one caused in part by an inter- and intrapsychic response to the threat of personal disintegration and the confrontation with their own mortality evoked in physicians by the suffering of their patients.[92] Much like Shapiro, Stein argues that, for many involved in the practice of medicine, the purpose of patient care is to comfort the *medical staff* by reassuring them in their pursuit of the eradication of disease.[93] Other scholars argue that not only psychological qualms and anxieties about death but also personalities defined by the fear of failure and the desire for control and certainty can lead physicians to undertake medical interventions that conceal the inevitability of death, rather than help patients confront the reality of their situations.[94]

A broader look at the research surrounding physicians' psychological responses to suffering and death suggests physicians are more fearful of death than are either patients or persons in good health.[95] Some studies indicate that this greater death anxiety among doctors might prevent them from breaking bad news to patients—although most patients say they want to know the truth about their prognoses—or that it might even lead doctors to avoid suffering patients altogether.[96] Sandra Kocijan Lovko, Rudolf Gregurek, and Dalibor Karlovic found that medical staff in oncology departments more often distanced themselves psychologically from very sick and dying patients than did staff working on general medicine floors.[97] Furthermore, following Robert Plutchik's theory of emotion—which suggests that basic human emotions evoke particular ego defenses (e.g., denial, displacement, intellectualization, repression)—Lovko, Gregurek, and Karlovic assert that some hospital workers, especially those who deal with dying or severely suffering patients, may resort to "neurotic" defense mechanisms.[98] One such mechanism they mention is intellectualization, which can take the form of focusing on the biological reality of death or the physical processes of pain and suffering in an attempt to control emotional responses to them. Indeed, as psychiatrist Peter Maguire notes, some of those providing medical care to terminal patients readily acknowledge that their emphasis on pain control and biological symptom relief could "be the most effective distancing tactic of all."[99]

In the late 1960s, Herman Feifel, Susan Hanson, and Robert Jones, after finding increased death anxiety among the surgeons, internists, and psychiatrists they interviewed, suggested that an elevated fear of death might be a relevant variable for choosing medicine in the first place.[100] Perhaps those with greater death anxiety, they argued, might be drawn to a career that is oriented toward controlling death and dying. Taken together, such research indicates that increased death anxiety among some clinicians can manifest itself in the desire to control illness and death, or even in futile attempts to postpone death indefinitely. It would appear, then, that mainstream medicine has a clearly paradoxical orientation toward death—one that accepts death as a biological reality, on the one hand, but that denies death as an existential reality, on the other. Such a culture is created by—and also creates—physicians who approach and manage dying and death as biological happenings, while at the same time distancing themselves from death as an ever-present possibility not only for their patients, but also for themselves.

Heidegger and Death Anxiety

Heidegger's phenomenological description of death and anxiety in *Being and Time* is critical for a deeper understanding of medicine's paradoxical approach to suffering and death. Although the studies mentioned above indicate that physicians may have increased death anxiety, Heidegger's work reveals that anxiety about death, or our potential for "no-longer-being-able-to-be-there," is a fundamental and inescapable constituent of being human.[101] In other words, this anxiety, which manifests itself psychologically, emanates from a deeper, existential, and ontological condition that is a part of all of us, not just those who choose medicine as a career. "Only because Dasein is anxious in the very depths of its Being," Heidegger explains, "does it become possible for anxiety to be elicited physiologically."[102]

Heidegger's explication of death anxiety clarifies exactly what it is that makes us anxious. He distinguishes "existential death"—the possibility "of the utter impossibility of existence" as we know it—from the similar concepts of "perishing" (*Verenden*) and "demise" (*Ableben*).[103] What most of us would normally call "death" (the cessation of our biological functions), Heidegger refers to as "perishing," the death of living things.[104] He further distinguishes "perishing" from "demise," an affective experience particular to human beings that involves the "collapse of our intelligible world" that can happen as we perish.[105] If we are aware that we are perishing, for example, we would also know that we are "demising," and that the world as we know it is coming to an end. However, it is possible that we could, in fact, perish without demising if we were to perish quickly or suddenly without knowledge of its happening.[106] Dying suddenly or dying without knowledge of its approach (in an automobile accident, for instance) precludes the possibility of awareness or recognition of the collapse of our existence in the world.

For Heidegger, however, death—or more specifically, *dying*—is not only physical perishing and existential demise, but also an authentic recognition of "the impossibility of every way of comporting oneself towards anything."[107] In this sense, our dying is equated to world collapse—the experience of the world as we see it ceasing to make sense, thus making it impossible for us to project ourselves forward into such meaninglessness.[108] When we can no longer project ourselves into our futures, we come face-to-face with ourselves—with the recognition that, at bottom, our connection to the world is tenuous and our existence is finite.[109] What we are afraid of is not the biological perishing of our bodies—though this is very frightening to many—but the possibility of no longer being able *to be* at all. Death is not a biological, or even a biographical, event that is "not yet" and will occur sometime in the future. Rather, death is a phenomenon that is always already with us, the potential for no-longer-being-here that can occur at any moment.

Our anxiety, then, is not about the fact that we will one day die. Rather, it is a lucid recognition of our human frailty, which both emanates from and *reveals* the precariousness of our existence. Heidegger's explication of anxiety as that which results from (and points to) the precariousness of being-in-the-world is largely influenced by Kierkegaard's explication of "dread."[110] For Kierkegaard, "dread" is a shared condition of being human that is directed at nothing and no one in particular.[111] This dread or despair, which Kierkegaard says virtually everyone experiences, feels "inexplicable"; it is an "anxious dread of an unknown something" that alienates us from our projects in the world.[112]

Because this anxiety or dread is "of nothing," it should not be confused with an emotion like fear, for fear takes an entity in the world as its object. Emotions like fear usually are directed at things in the world (one is afraid of the man in the dark alley, for instance, or the wolf howling in the night), whereas anxiety or dread is what Heidegger calls a "ground mood" (*Grundstimmung*) or "attunement"—a "state-of-mind" that is not directed toward any "thing" specifically.[113] Although anxiety emanates from and reveals our tenuous connection to the world, this tenuous connection is not a "thing," but rather an ontological structure of our being-in-the-world. And because anxiety reveals our ever-present potential for suffering and world collapse, it "feels" uncanny or unhomelike, as if we no longer fit in the world the way we did before. This makes sense since anxiety is an ontological attunement that arises out of our being-in-the-world itself, entirely coloring how we see the world around us.[114] As Heidegger says: "Dying is not an event; it is a phenomenon to be understood existentially."[115] Death anxiety, then, is not anxious in the face of some thing or some happening; rather, it is anxious in the face of the pervasive possibility of our lives collapsing into something foreign and senseless.

Death as Collapse of Identity Philosopher Iain Thomson further distinguishes between Heidegger's ideas of death as demise—collapse of the world as one knows it—and death as an ontological phenomenon revealed in world collapse.[116] For Thomson, Heidegger's notion of death as the impossibility of existing cannot refer to a biographical point in one's life when one dies because such an event can never be realized.[117] Once we die, we cannot experience our impossibility of existing because we are no longer "here" to experience anything at all. What we are really anxious about, according to Thomson, is not the *terminal* collapse of our world, but *being here to experience such a loss*. Thus Heidegger must not be referring to a terminal end of one's life when he speaks about "death." In Thomson's view, what Heidegger means by "death" is not perishing or terminal demise, but rather a death or collapse of one's identity that *one lives through*. It is this kind of death of self—events that cause the "death" of our identity as a teacher, parent, spouse, caregiver—that leaves us in a shattered world that forecloses future possibilities. Because this kind of death threatens our identity and our understanding of ourselves and our world, it is something from which we would rather turn away.

Thomson's reading of Heidegger on death has interesting implications for those in the health professions. Because healing is so often conflated with curing, when physicians are unable to cure, this can cause what most of the literature in this area describes as feelings of personal "failure."[118] If, however, Thomson's reading of Heidegger is correct, then patients whose illness is incurable present an even bigger problem for physicians defining themselves primarily as persons who intervene to eliminate disease. Not only would encounters with such patients represent potential personal "failures" for them, but numerous such "failures" could threaten their identities as physicians. And if it is the case that such threats to their sense of self could potentially result in world collapse, where they are no longer able to project themselves into their possibilities as physicians, then it becomes understandable why they would try to distance themselves from patients suffering from incurable illnesses. These patients not only remind the physicians of their own embodiment and fragility, but their presence also threatens to dismantle the identities the physicians have assumed.

Whether death for Heidegger means a recognition of the end of our existence altogether or the end of our particular identities, the common thread in both interpretations of death is the idea that death anxiety reveals or, more precisely, *is* the unhomelike nature of being. That is to say, it discloses the precariousness of our existence as we know it right now. Whether it is a particular life project that is coming to an end (being a father or mother, a doctor, a friend) or the entire project of our lives that faces terminal collapse, we can no longer project ourselves into our possibilities the way we did before, and the world as we once knew it is different and incoherent.[119] As I see it, however, terminal death—understood as the ever-present possibility of the *final end* of our total existence—is the most palpable, obvious, and frightening example of the fragility of our being and the foreclosure of our possibilities. This kind of death reveals our undeniable frailty and vulnerability and the unnerving reality that a fundamental constituent of our being is our potential for no-longer-being-able-to-be-there at all. It is the final collapse of our being-in-the-world. Thus the constant presence of death in the practice of medicine and the complex ways that the lived body suffers (which are often harbingers of eventual demise) are likely to stir significant anxiety within physicians. Even suffering patients who are not at the end of their physical lives but who have trouble making sense of the world as they see it—something that occurs often in the illness experience—may be hard for physicians to engage with, for the suffering of these patients points to the ever-present potential for the world as the physicians know it to become suddenly and intolerably unhomelike.

It is for this reason that the suffering or death of the other can, at least in my view, evoke one's own world collapse. Although Heidegger contends that death "reveals itself as that *possibility which is one's ownmost*," this does not mean that *another's* death cannot cause one's own ontological-existential anxiety.[120] Indeed, Heidegger himself says that the death of the other is "impressive" and makes death "objectively accessible" to us; it offers us "an experience of death, all the more so because Dasein is essentially Being with Others."[121] Because a fundamental constituent of being human is being-with-others—we only know and understand ourselves in relation to others in the world—the suffering of the other reveals something about us, pointing toward aspects of our being that we all share, despite our irreducible differences: fragility, impermanence, pain, fear, loneliness, and so forth. Because of this, the suffering or death of the other can reveal our own potential for such experiences.

It is not often, however, that we allow the reality of these shared possibilities to penetrate our consciousness. The potential for anxiety in the face of mortality and vulnerability may be universal, yet true anxiety—the kind that awakens us to a more authentic existence—is, according to Heidegger, "rare" and often remains hidden to us.[122] In fact, some of us expend much energy relieving or "disburdening" ourselves of such anxiety in a "manner of evasive turning-away," which is particularly easy to do in our modern, technology-saturated Western culture.[123] The *potential* for experiencing anxiety about our finite existence—though shared by every human being—is thus seldom actualized since we usually turn away from anxiety, and feelings of uncanniness get "dimmed down."[124]

Anxiety and Disburdening

Though it is possible to respond to anxiety *authentically* by recognizing the precariousness of our being and releasing attempts to control this precariousness, the most common response to such anxiety is an *inauthentic* turning away from this anxiety and turning toward what Heidegger calls the "they"—in other words, turning toward an understanding of things (like death) after they have been "leveled down" through public interpretation.[125] Often, our response to anxiety involves, as Kevin Aho puts it, "a 'flight' back into the illusory stability of our daily routines as a 'they-self.'"[126] Heidegger's understanding of inauthenticity and the "they" or the "they-self" is largely influenced by Kierkegaard, who argues that those who appeal to socially accepted codes of conduct without determining for themselves how or who they would like to be run the risk of "falling victim" to inauthenticity and employing diversions to conceal from themselves the despair that haunts them.[127] These diversions might be obvious—escaping reality by self-medicating or engaging in self-destructive behavior, for example. Yet such inauthenticity is not always noticeable or perceived as pernicious. Indeed, Kierkegaard tells us that some who are in despair and distract themselves in "worldliness" can live "perfectly well in the temporal" and may even be publicly "honored and esteemed" for it.[128] Such distractions might take the form of keeping busy or engaging successfully and productively in society without considering that the definitions of "success" and "productivity" have been determined by someone or something other than oneself.

Inauthenticity, escapism, and the "leveling down" of ideas through public interpretations of what is "right" or "good" are for Kierkegaard, first and foremost, ethical issues.[129] Yet Heidegger claims that his own explication of inauthenticity and "falling" has no "negative evaluation."[130] For him, being inauthentic is simply our everyday way of being; we cannot help but be inauthentic since our world is public and shared, and we come to know such a world in relation to those around us. An indispensable part of being human is being-with-others-in-the-world, and, accordingly, our lives, identities, and understandings are shaped by those with whom we share our world.[131] As Heidegger points out, to exist means to be "thrown" into a world that already has meaning, and, as a result, we are already "fallen to"—or absorbed in—the way the "they" interprets the world.[132] Without the "they," it would be difficult for us to interpret phenomena, make decisions, or understand things at all.[133] If we did not have shared language and interpretations, for example, it would be quite difficult to get on in the world. For Heidegger, then, we most often dwell as a "they-self," and being authentic is a rare and fleeting modification or a derivative mode of our more common, inauthentic, everyday selves.[134]

So how is it that the very familiar "they" serves to "tranquilize" us and disburden us of our anxiety? The "they-self" may be indispensable and inescapable, but it can have a strong—though often invisible—hold on how we engage with the world. This is because we are not any persons or group in particular, but we are everyone and also no one. I might believe that *this* is good or *that* is distasteful based on what the "they" deems pleasing or ill mannered. Thus the "they" is others, but also myself (hence, *they-self*), insofar as I do and think as "they" do and think, and feel as "they" feel.[135] In adopting the perspectives of the "they," we inevitably engage in ambiguous "idle talk," simply repeating passed-along phrases on what the "they" deems as right, good, fashionable, appropriate, and so forth.[136] The "they" strips us of our responsibility, for we simply are doing and saying what the "they" prescribes as reasonable and appropriate, which is particularly problematic when so much of today's discourse is dominated by technoscientific explanations of the world around us.

What is most dangerous about such idle talk or "chatter" is that it deceives us into thinking that matters are settled and that there is no need to look further.[137] We need not dwell on what it means to be "successful" in society or how to respond to someone in grief, for example, because such things already have been socially and culturally determined. And we certainly need not worry about suffering, death, or world collapse since "they" say these are remote possibilities that might happen to us in the distant future and are of little concern to us now.

The "They" and Inauthentic Understandings of Death Perhaps the most dangerous chatter of the "they" surrounds the issue of existential death and anxiety. Because, as Heidegger says, we desire to "cover up" our "ownmost Being-towards-death [by] fleeing *in the face of it*," we can easily run toward the tranquilizing interpretations of death that the "they" offers.[138] So, even when anxiety reveals to me that my existence is tenuous and not guaranteed, the "they" covers over the reality of my *own* death.[139] Although the "they" might agree that everyone dies, it treats death as a remote possibility, something that happens to other people in the world but not to me.[140] Heidegger says it best:

The "they" has already stowed away an interpretation for [death] . . . as if to say, "One of these days one will die too, in the end; but right now it has nothing to do with us.". . . In such a way of talking, death is understood as an indefinite something which, above all, must duly arrive from somewhere or other, but which is proximally *not yet present-at-hand* for oneself, and is therefore no threat. . . . The "they" gives its approval, and aggravates the *temptation* to cover up from oneself one's ownmost Being-towards-death.[141]

In talking about death as an "event" or "thing" that is always yet to happen, the "they" covers over our ever-present possibility for death or for the kind of suffering that collapses our meaningful world. In so doing, the "they" transmutes ontological anxiety "into fear in the face of an oncoming event."[142] This tendency to see death as that which happens to others and not to ourselves is perfectly captured in Leo Tolstoy's masterful 1886 novella *The Death of Ivan Ilych*. Peter Ivanovich, one of Ivan's closest "friends," who, like nearly everyone else, is indifferent toward Ivan's death, is suddenly struck by the reality of his own mortality after hearing of Ivan's acute and prolonged suffering in the days before he died: "'Three days of frightful suffering and the death! Why, that might suddenly, at any time, happen to me,' he thought, and for a moment felt terrified."[143] Peter's epiphany, however, is short lived:

> The customary reflection at once occurred to him that this had happened to Ivan Ilych and not to him, and that it should not and could not happen to him, and that to think that it could would be yielding to depression which he ought not to do. . . . After which reflection Peter Ivanovich felt reassured, and began to ask with interest about the details of Ivan Ilych's death, as though death was an accident natural to Ivan Ilych but certainly not to himself.[144]

Distilling anxiety into "fear of something" and death into a thing or event that is "not yet" makes these world-shattering phenomena appear as though they might be controlled. And because the "they" is entrenched in a distinctively modern epistemological framework that views "beings" as various subjects and objects that are most fully known through calculative thinking, such a view of death as a self-contained event—as an observable, measurable, and perhaps controllable "thing" that occurs to us later on in life—seems natural and perhaps even progressive and enlightened. Indeed, stripping death and suffering of their spiritual, religious, or metaphysical moorings by characterizing them as biological occurrences might appear to some as the most reasonable and justified way to attend to such phenomena. As Heidegger points out, our "plunge" into the "they" remains hidden to us "by the way things have been publicly interpreted, so much so, indeed, that it gets interpreted as a way of 'ascending' and 'living concretely.'"[145] Verifiable, scientific understandings of death and suffering, though they cover up so much of the lived experience of such phenomena, present themselves as the best way to think through and "manage" such issues. What remains hidden, however, is why such narrow approaches are so appealing—we fail to see that we adopt these approaches because existential suffering and demise are safer and easier to confront when sanitized by "they-self" notions about the ability to control such "things." Nevertheless, such narrow approaches are something that science and medicine have become exceptionally good at employing and perpetuating.

Disburdening of Anxiety and Reductionistic Medicine

As discussed in chapter 1, the epistemology of medicine is predicated (however tacitly) on the need for scientific acumen and clinical objectivity. And though scholars who consider "scientific medicine" to be more like a *practice* than a science have been quick to criticize it for overlooking important aspects of caring for patients who suffer in any number of ways, few have attempted to unearth *why* medicine remains so firmly rooted in its current epistemology.[146] It may be true that medicine holds to the indispensability of calculative approaches simply because they *work*—they yield verifiable data shown to have "incalculable benefit" in promoting healing.[147] Yet it is precisely because such calculative approaches work and are publicly interpreted by the "they" as best suited to reveal "the truth" that the deeper motivation behind them remains hidden. It is my view that the reason practitioners cling so strongly to the epistemological assumptions shaping patient care is that these assumptions serve *to disburden them of their ontological anxiety in the face of death.* Being ill is a stark reminder of our shared potential for experiencing a world collapse, and reductionistic understandings of illness as biological disease allow practitioners to disburden themselves of their own vulnerability by reducing illness and suffering to discrete pathophysiological ailments that medical science might remedy. Rather than face the uncertainty and unpredictability of existence, practitioners interpret or reinterpret illness and suffering as something that might be treated and controlled, allowing many if not most to turn away from their ownmost experience of unhomelikeness in the world. As Kierkegaard suggests, by remaining in the realm of dogmatic certainty, whether that of science or religion, one escapes the need to engage authentically in a contingent and uncertain world. Nietzsche holds a similar view, though he makes an even bolder claim than Kierkegaard about our need to privilege the work of science and objectivity:

Science today is a hiding place for every kind of discontent, disbelief, gnawing worm, *despectio sui*, bad conscience—it is the unrest of the lack of ideals, the suffering from the lack of any great love, the discontent in the face of involuntary contentment.

Oh, what does science not conceal today! how much, at any rate, is it meant to conceal! The proficiency of our finest scholars, their heedless industry, their heads smoking day and night, their very craftsmanship—how often the real meaning of all this lies in the desire to keep something hidden from oneself! Science as a means of self-narcosis: *do you have experience of that?*[148]

For Nietzsche, science—or in this case, the whole of "detached" scholarship and higher learning—serves as form of "self-narcosis," a means of disburdening those who believe in or practice it of the difficulty of the everyday world. Much like intellectualizing emotional responses to suffering patients, choosing to conduct themselves as scientists or technicians in the clinical space may serve as "a hiding place" that protects physicians from their patients' suffering and their own potential for suffering.

Embracing calculative understandings of illness and suffering is pervasive not only among seasoned physicians, but also among medical students, who pick up on the "need" for distance, abstraction, and intellectualization early on. Looking back on her experience as a medical resident, Katharine Treadway writes:

> Early in our training, bending over our cadavers, we learned to silence a part of ourselves. We learned the power of humor as a means of avoiding hard conversations about more complicated feelings. Often we kept those feelings to ourselves, rarely giving voice to them as we proceeded through far more challenging situations during our clerkships—a newly diagnosed lung cancer, a 2-year-old with an inoperable and therefore fatal brain tumor, a young man with quadriplegia from diving into shallow water. We discussed the medical management and the complications in detail and with intense care, but we could not give voice to the feelings these events evoked, often reducing them, in the formal case presentation, to the single word "unfortunate."[149]

It is easier to confront the "unfortunate" reality of human frailty through "medical management" than it is to face and give voice to it, and it is this particular posture toward suffering and death that is so often taught and modeled to medical students. Thus Gawande explains in *Being Mortal* that, despite a weekly "Patient-Doctor" seminar during medical school, his time as a student was focused almost exclusively on learning "the inner process of the body, the intricate mechanisms of its pathology. . . . We didn't imagine we needed to think about much else."[150] It was not until, in the course of his surgical training and practice, Gawande encountered patients who were facing the realities of suffering and mortality that he realized "how unready I was to help them."[151]

Some of the students I interviewed reported similar experiences in their training. They felt unprepared for their encounters with suffering and death, and once they began seeing patients, they received little guidance from their clinical mentors. Asked if there was any discussion with her medical team following her first experience with a patient death on the wards, a fourth-year medical student gave a quiet laugh. "No," she replied. "There was no discussion. I think the next day the attending [said,] like, 'Well, the patient died overnight. Okay.' I think there was seriously maybe one or two lines and then, like, 'On to the next patient'" (MSIV-3). Similarly, a third-year student alluded to how hard it was for some clinicians to stop treating those patients who opted to discontinue curative care. When discussing one of his first encounters with a patient at the end of life, he explained:

> The patient chose to go home with palliative care, though most members of the team advised her to stay in the hospital for treatment. Although staying in the hospital would have extended her life, she didn't want to die in the hospital and wanted to die in the comfort of her own home. The medical team tried to persuade her to stay and even considered getting a psych eval to assess if she had the capacity to make such a decision (MSIII-5).

Not only did the medical team in this instance resist stopping curative treatment, but their considering a psychiatric evaluation to assess whether the patient had the capacity to make such a decision suggests a discomfort with patients who were willing to confront their own impending death. Indeed, however problematic, the perception that a patient who is emotionally ready to die must have a psychiatric or neurological problem (requiring medical intervention in itself) is not uncommon. As former surgeon Pauline Chen explains in her 2007 book *Final Exam*, wavering between the "dramatic heroics" of curing and the "well-worn pattern of denial" is something medical students start to do early in their training as they learn to "suppress" their "anxieties" while dissecting cadavers.[152] Over time, medical students and doctors "come to believe so deeply" that curing illness and avoiding death "make us better doctors that some of us will skip around the very word ["death"] during our conversations with terminal patients. We will work almost maniacally to forestall the inevitable but then stubbornly, when death becomes inescapable, refuse to face it for fear of losing our focus in the goal of cure."[153]

This "goal of cure" serves an important function for clinicians who have a need to escape their anxiety: focusing on the pathophysiology of ailments that might be cured or treated is much easier than confronting a patient's existential suffering or impending demise.[154] Or, as researcher Craig Earle and his colleagues suggest, proposing or initiating new lines of treatment—even after multiple therapeutic failures—may, at least in some cases, be a physician's way of avoiding difficult conversations about a patient's prognosis.[155] Indeed, physicians who see themselves as scientists or technicians may be tempted to avoid existential questions that cannot be answered easily or with certainty.[156] It is in this way that "illness talk," as Frank points out, becomes "disease talk," and "*my* body" becomes "*the* body," to be analyzed and intervened upon.[157] A dysfunctional body that requires medical intervention is much less anxiety producing than a person whose existence has become conspicuously precarious.

Most attempts by doctors at disburdening themselves of the reality of suffering and demise, however, are not consciously planned. Doctors seldom suggest more treatment options simply to avoid difficult conversations. Instead, narrow approaches to care that are focused on controlling and manipulating bodily disease are embedded within the epistemology of medicine itself. In other words, dominant medical epistemology—which is grounded in notions of scientific objectivity and impartiality—is guided by and perpetuates a flight from the ontological reality of suffering and death. Yet so pervasive and normative is this epistemology that its relationship to ontological anxiety and disburdening is all but invisible. What most doctors and medical students fail to recognize, then, is that most approaches to care have already been "decided upon"—they cannot see the way that the "they" has determined things for them and relieved them of "the burden of explicitly *choosing* these possibilities."[158] Thus, in caring for others as the "they" deems professionally or medically appropriate, "Dasein makes no choices, gets carried along by the nobody, and thus ensnares itself in inauthenticity."[159] The idea of being "carried along" becomes apparent when doctors, students, and patients alike complain of "getting caught up in the wheels of medicine" or "falling victim to the system." The anonymous medical student who posted an online article about her disillusionment with medical education in 2014 writes poignantly there about the painful dissonance between her expectations of medicine and her actual experience:

I never understood the trend of loss of empathy during medical training. Until now. See, when you're in so much pain that if you thought of your life past this moment, this singular point in time, you would implode, pain seems as natural as breathing. Pain is part of life. Pain is nothing. You can't stop to nurse your own wounds, you can't talk about how much you hurt. So how could you possibly have enough room in your broken heart to take on someone else's pain? So you don't. You cover your bases and survive. You become that machine that you swore you'd never become. Because it hurts too much to feel, and it's so much easier to float than swim.[160]

The medical system and its underlying epistemology leave little room for clinicians to attend to their own pain and anxiety—feelings that can arise from participating in a system that discourages them from approaching the suffering and anxiety of others. As a result, personal survival becomes paramount, "they-self" notions about distance and detachment become increasingly more appealing, and floating does indeed become much easier than swimming.

Patients' Own Disburdening
It is not only the case that clinicians disburden themselves of their anxiety through curative or technical approaches. Patients wanting to turn away from their own vulnerability may also see in these approaches ways to disburden themselves of their own anxiety. Some patients very near the end of their lives, for example, may choose to continue curative interventions even when these are of little or no benefit or may actually intensify their suffering.[161] Even after a terminal diagnosis, if a patient's doctor merely mentions the possibility for a "cure," the patient and family may hear this as an option that must be explored.[162] This is not surprising since, as Gadamer describes it, "there is a deep connection between the knowledge of death, the knowledge of one's own finitude, that is, the certainty that one day one must die, and, on the other hand, the almost imperious demand of not wanting to know, of not wanting to possess this sort of certain knowledge."[163] Accepting that we all must die one day is, of course, different from accepting our ownmost death as an ontological reality that can present itself at any moment.

Although part of our ontological structure is the desire to flee in the face of our anxiety—an anxiety that can be most palpable during an illness crisis—it is simplistic and dismissive to assume that most patients who continue to seek treatment are simply "in denial." Speaking from his own experience, Frank works to sharpen our understanding of patients' perceived denial, stating that it is not always the case that patients are unwilling to face their vulnerability. Rather, they are simply embodying the role that the medical world prescribes for them. It is "too convenient," Frank says, to assume that denial comes solely from the patient, for it allows clinicians to ignore that "they are cueing the patient."[164] When a patient's response is labeled as "denial," it appears as if the denial is "the need of the patient" and not the "patient's *response* to his situation"—a situation that has been defined by objectivity, avoidance, and disease talk.[165] This is similar to Maguire's perspective that the preference among clinicians for dealing with the body and its physical problems can lead patients to believe they should not even mention any psychological or emotional issues they may be experiencing.[166]

In a context where biological intervention is prioritized and healing is conflated with curing, nearly any treatment option proposed by the physician has the potential to extend medical interventions, eclipsing opportunities for meaningful discussions about the existential, psychological, and spiritual needs of the patient. So, although some patients—as one medical student told me—"want a complete fix . . . a quick fix" (MSIV-3), it is misguided to deem such a desire irrational or unreasonable when it occurs in a medical environment that privileges intervening and fixing. It might be true that pressures for efficiency and productivity, coupled with limited time and medical resources, create a system where deciding whether to treat patients becomes the primary focus of medical care, and discharging them becomes the hospital's top priority. As the same student said later, "I think [the desire to fix] might be the nature of the hospital; the goal is to get patients discharged." If their experience in the hospital is suffused with talk from others about medically intervening (or not) and then sending them on their way, then it is shortsighted to view patients' desire for a cure or fix as a manifestation of their own "need." Although the time and resource constraints of a medical system that is becoming increasingly corporatized undoubtedly exacerbate the problems clinicians face in providing care, claiming that their inability to engage authentically with patients who are suffering is *solely* the result of the pressures these constraints create can obscure the larger and deeper issue at hand—namely, that our medical culture has become exceptionally adept at evading the ontological reality of death and suffering and at making this evasion ever easier.[167]

Estrangement from Ourselves

I have made the argument that, during serious illness, patients suffer in ways that go beyond the dysfunction of their corporeal bodies; for some, the illness experience can arouse ontological-existential anxiety and evoke a profound realization of their vulnerability, ultimately shattering their understanding of themselves and the world as they see it. Moreover, because an elemental part of our being is being-with-others, witnessing the intense suffering of another who is experiencing such a world collapse can result in our own desire to turn away from this suffering person in order to disburden ourselves of our own anxiety. This perspective helps explain what physician and writer Danielle Ofri describes as the "awkward relief" she feels on coming home after a hospital shift, leaving behind the graphic reminders of what could "befall [her] own body."[168] Somewhere deep down, she says, is the need to convince herself that doctors are invulnerable to such suffering and are "a different species from our patients," though she knows her attempt to do so is futile.[169] For some medical practitioners, fleeing from suffering and death can take the form of focusing on only the physical aspects of illness, reducing suffering and death to "things" or events that can be objectified, measured, and perhaps even controlled—and such disburdening both reifies and is perpetuated by modern medical epistemology.

Taking a calculative approach to illness, suffering, and death might feel safer and might even be lauded by the "they" as the best way to manage them; yet, such an approach covers over the *meaning* behind these phenomena. The "indifferent tranquillity" that the "they" offers physicians in the "decree" that death or world collapse is merely an event that happens to others and is always "not yet" for themselves prevents them from authentically facing both the suffering other and their ownmost potential for suffering. Such an approach to care covers over the human experience of living and dying and creates a chasm between those who need care and those called to offer that care.[170] As Gadamer puts it: "Modern science and its ideal of objectification demands of all of us a violent estrangement from ourselves, irrespective of whether we are doctors, patients, or simply responsible and concerned citizens."[171] Objectification obscures the potential for meaningful connection, thereby distancing us from ourselves since we are beings whose being is inextricably bound up with others.

Kierkegaard argued long ago that approaching things abstractly and from a distance was much easier than consciously existing in a messy and unpredictable world. Today our current medical epistemology offers an easy means to avoid the messiness of human suffering by allowing us to cling to ideas about certainty and control. Heidegger's philosophy helps us see that the problem of scientific detachment and calculative thinking that dominates medicine is not *primarily* an epistemological problem, but an ontological one. Although the challenges we face in medicine are therefore difficult to address—since they relate to what fundamentally constitutes *who we are*—recognizing that they present an ontological problem reveals that it is also a problem all of us share. And recognizing that those in the healing professions who are so often confronted with suffering are human beings like the rest of us—structurally inauthentic and anxious in the face of death—can help us extend them grace and understanding.

The question that remains, however, is how we might begin to end this estrangement from ourselves and from one another. The answer lies in authentically facing others in their suffering while releasing any desire to view such suffering as a thing present-at-hand that can be contained and controlled. In witnessing the vulnerability of others, physicians might become acutely aware of their own vulnerability, their own limits, and their own suffering. It is precisely when we begin to understand that the clinical encounter is a meeting of two *persons* who both suffer and who both participate in the quest to find meaning that we begin to see that such an encounter can offer both persons insight into themselves and into the human condition. This shared suffering need not create a sense of hopelessness, however. Witnessing others struggle to find meaning and purpose in their suffering might evoke compassion and create a sense of solidarity in our shared quest to make meaning in a life that is often fraught with existential pain.[172] In authentically responding to the call of suffering, physicians approach not only their patients but also themselves—their subjectivity is deepened and expanded with the recognition of their own potential-for-suffering that is always already at hand. Chapter 3 will take a closer look at what it means to engage in such authentic encounters with suffering and what we might reasonably expect from physicians who are confronted with the call to address it.

3 Turning toward Suffering Together

I want my doctor to tell me the medical meanings of my symptoms, to be sure, but I also want some help in grasping the personal significance of my malady. I want both to have my "otherness" acknowledged and to be recognized as still belonging to the tribe of the living.
—Ronald A. Carson, "The Hyphenated Space"

The being that expresses itself imposes itself, but does so precisely by appealing to me with its destitution and nudity—its hunger—without my being able to be deaf to that appeal. Thus, in expression, the being that imposes itself does not limit but promotes my freedom, by arousing my goodness.
—Emmanuel Levinas, *Totality and Infinity*

As unrelenting reminders of the inherent vulnerability and fragility of our being, intense suffering and death are realities we tend to avoid, and understandably so. Those in medicine, however, have a more difficult time avoiding such realities, not only because medicine is replete with sickness, suffering, and death, but also because there is an expectation or assumption that they are *called* to deal with these realities in ways that most of us are not.[1] And though it is true that doctors and other healthcare professionals attend to the sick, the injured, and the dying more regularly and more fearlessly than most of us, they are moved to do so more often by a perceived need to employ their technical expertise than by a call to face and alleviate their patients' suffering. This is not because of some personal or moral failing on their part, however, but because the notion of "calling" is largely eclipsed by calculative thinking within the medical culture itself, even though there are those who, at least initially, do feel personally called to enter medicine. Over time, the epistemological assumptions about the need for scientific rigor, certainty, and clinical distance come to define medical training, and ideas about a personal calling to provide care for the sick and vulnerable tend to get covered over. For, as William May points out, in the medical world, "those features of technical performance that lend themselves to measurement . . . tend to determine destiny."[2]

So, although we might want to answer the question, Why should physicians respond to patients' existential suffering? by saying that, as healers, they are *called* to do so, such an answer would carry little weight with professionals who might see themselves as *not* called to do so at all. Indeed, some might believe such a calling to be reserved for patients' loved ones or for social workers and chaplains. It is this lack of clarity about what exactly it is that doctors are called to do that Arthur Frank alludes to when he says, "Perhaps physicians and nurses should simply do what they already do well—treat the [biological] breakdowns—and not claim to do more."[3] Although Frank's extensive body of work about the patient-practitioner relationship makes it clear that he believes nurses and doctors should, in fact, do more than what they already do well, he is right to suggest that the call for healthcare professionals to do more than treat biological breakdowns is often drowned out within our contemporary medical culture, where technical expertise is so highly valued.

Making the argument that healthcare practitioners are called to respond to patients' existential suffering is difficult, but this chapter aims to do just that and to do it by making what I believe is the stronger argument, that facing suffering—both our own and that of the other—is what makes us more fully human, what allows us to exist with authenticity and intentionality. Choosing to face the vulnerability that is part of our shared ontological structure as humans creates the capacity for deep and abiding compassion and personal flourishing. It is my hope that an appeal to the fundamental constituents of being human that we all share—whether we are in the medical field or not—offers a more compelling reason for why doctors are called to respond to existential suffering.

Heidegger and Authenticity

As outlined in chapter 2, our existential anxiety comes from and reveals the fact that our existence as we know it is tenuous. We desire to flee from our anxiety—to turn away from the reality that our being inescapably projects itself toward death. It is understandable that we would like to disburden ourselves of this rather dark and hopeless-sounding reality. But, as Martin Heidegger sees it, our recognition of our being-toward-death—facing our existential anxiety—can, in fact, free us for "authenticity" by snatching us out of the clutches of the "they."[4] Heidegger's view that an honest confrontation of our potential for death or world collapse can bring us authenticity (however temporary) was inspired by Søren Kierkegaard's view that confronting despair liberates us from the grip of the world and frees us up to make a "leap of faith" or authentic religious conversion.[5] In Heidegger's secularized conversion narrative, confronting our anxiety—rather than disburdening ourselves of it—frees us from the grip of death anxiety and allows us to see and choose among our finite and everyday possibilities *for ourselves*. In authentically confronting our death, we no longer desperately need the "they" in order to distract or disburden ourselves from our anxiety, and we are free to be true to ourselves and decide for ourselves how we want to live. In this way, for both Heidegger and Kierkegaard, the anxiety that comes with the recognition of our ever-present potential for suffering and world collapse can be both limiting and liberating. Although such anxiety can be frightening and can cause us to lead diminished lives in our futile attempts to flee from it, it can also call us toward authenticity—if we are willing to respond to its call.[6]

The Call to Authenticity

This "call" that Heidegger refers to comes from no place and no one in particular, but rather from Dasein (our being) itself. The caller is our being in its uncanniness—the call comes from our own experience of unhomelikeness that results from being-in-the-world.[7] Our anxiety calls out to us, reminding us of the vulnerability of our existence, and we can choose to face it or turn away. It is because we are never wholly and irretrievably lost in the "they"—since the structure of our being is such that we always have the possibility for both authenticity and inauthenticity—that we have the capacity to choose authenticity.[8] It is the "residual awareness of [our] authentic self" that allows us both to call to ourselves and to respond to that call on occasion.[9]

The call to authenticity shows us that our death or world collapse is something we face alone. A recognition of this "non-relational character of death" lays a claim on us and pulls us out of the anonymous mode of the "they-self."[10] One begins to see that the attempts of the "they" to avoid or control suffering, death, and world collapse are unavailing, and one is therefore made "*free for* the freedom of choosing oneself and taking hold of oneself."[11] Perhaps this notion is best expressed by an example. It might be said that Frank, who experiences the total breakdown of his world during his illness, responds to the call to authenticity. As I see it, Frank's narrative expresses a willingness to confront both the existential anxiety brought upon by his being ill and his potential for a total world collapse, and this confrontation changes him: "The ultimate value of illness," Frank says, "is that it teaches us the value of being alive."[12] Death no longer appears to him as something to flee from, and Frank is free to develop his own interpretation of death: "Death is no enemy of life; it restores our sense of the value of living. . . . To learn about value and proportion we need to honor illness, and ultimately to honor death."[13] Though being seriously ill was frightening and exhausting for Frank, by not disburdening himself of the anxiety that pointed to the precariousness of his life, he instead was transformed by it. As a result of this transformation, his reentry into the "healthy" mainstream after his recovery was rather difficult, for he "now knew that the way [he] and others lived was a choice, and often not the best one."[14]

Though Frank and others who authentically confront their being-toward-death are freed from the "they-self" and distorted interpretations about their finitude or mortality, such moments of clarity are usually short lived. Heidegger describes the moment of insight that occurs when we respond to the call of authenticity with the German word *Augenblick*, which means "the glance of the eye" or "moment of vision."[15] He uses this word to express that the "being free" to see, know, and choose for ourselves is fleeting; even after responding to the call to authenticity, we are always at risk of once again falling victim to the "they."[16] This is because our usual and most comfortable everyday way of being-in-the-world is inauthentic—our daily lives are typically defined and circumscribed by the "they." We can see this in Frank's writing when he explains how, several years after his recovery, he often loses sight of what he learned from his being ill and begins to engage with the world in the ways he did before he got sick, before his anxiety illuminated a more authentic way of being:

I take my senses for granted, and I miss the joy I felt from suddenly hearing music or taking a walk or being in my own home or sleeping through the night. When I was ill I valued just being with others. Too often now I think of people as intruding on my work. I forget to ask myself if what I'm doing is so terribly important that I should allow it to crowd out all else.[17]

Although Frank has been changed by his confrontation with world collapse, he is surprised by how easily he "forgets" what he has learned and finds that he has to consciously remind himself of what it was like to have his world shatter, wishing he could live "a bit more like I did then, without having to have cancer."[18] Living authentically, however, is difficult for anyone to do once the acute anxiety experienced in the face of a potential world collapse begins to recede. "It is therefore essential," Heidegger explains, "that Dasein should explicitly appropriate what has already been uncovered, defend it *against* semblance and disguise, and assure itself of its uncoveredness again and again."[19] Since our default mode of being is inauthenticity, even those of us who have confronted our existential anxiety in the past must repeatedly return to the moment of authenticity, uncovering our own truth time and again.[20] As Richard P. McQuellon and Michael A. Cowan point out, none of us returns unchanged from an authentic confrontation with death, yet we cannot sustain a "full encounter" with immanent death over a long period of time since mundane, everyday tasks "invariably interrupt brooding obsession with mortality."[21]

But, Heidegger argues, it is not obsessing or "brooding over death" as "something that is coming" in the future that reminds us of our potential for being authentic.[22] Rather, the insight we gained in our previous authentic response to anxiety opens us to the possibility of *anticipation for death* (rather than brooding about death), which ultimately leads to authentic existence.[23] Our being is temporal and, because it is, we can project ourselves toward the future into the possibility of no-longer-being-able-to-be-there. That is to say, our "being-towards-death" colors our present, reminding us that we always already face a potential world collapse at any moment. We then anticipate or "run ahead" into our death, facing our possibility of no longer having any possibilities at all.[24] But this authentic awareness of our inevitable finitude is not a macabre obsession with death and mortality. Rather, it is a genuine acknowledgment of the finite nature of our identity or existence that "pervades and shapes [our] whole life," freeing us *for* death, and thus freeing us for authentic living.[25] In recognizing (and then anticipating and reminding ourselves) that our world as we know it has the potential to shatter at any moment, we might begin to appreciate and deepen our present being-in-the-world. Philosopher Jerome Miller puts it this way:

> The authentic anticipation of this "not," i.e., the traumatizing possibility of death, is not an existential dead-end. On the contrary. It throws us open to the possibility of authentically appreciating [being], instead of taking it for granted, as we do when we operate in a "world" that represses the "not." The traumatizing "not" does not "outstrip" our capacity to exist authentically; it actually opens us to, and opens to us, the possibility of authentic existence. Our capacity to exist authentically enables us to assimilate the traumatizing possibility of nothingness into a way of living that is care-full toward [being].[26]

When we remain in authentic anticipation of our possibility for "nothingness" or total world collapse, we can begin to live in a way that is more intentional, "care-full," and "resolute." For Heidegger, to be resolute means to hear the call to authenticity that comes from ourselves and then respond to this call by living in anticipation-for-death and opening ourselves up to new truths that are illuminated by this anticipation.[27] In being resolute—which comes with facing one's vulnerability and then anticipating the possibility of world collapse—"one becomes free *for* one's own death, one is liberated from one's lostness in those possibilities which may accidentally thrust themselves upon one."[28] When we are authentically resolute, we wrench ourselves loose from the tenacious grip of the "they" since we no longer need to disburden ourselves of the anxiety that we have now faced, and we open ourselves up for new ways of being.[29] Such resoluteness, however, is still an "anxious" resoluteness, for anticipating our ownmost possibility for death is not, as we might imagine, the most tranquil of experiences. Yet, despite the anxious and fleeting nature of being resolute, the authentic anticipation that allows for resoluteness, is "an impassioned freedom towards death—*a freedom which has been released from the Illusions of the 'they,' and which is factical, certain of itself, and anxious.*"[30] Authenticity and anticipation, then, leave us with the sober realization of life's frailty and sheer contingency, but this realization is liberating. We are free to decide for ourselves what is most significant, pressing, or worthy of our energy and care. It is this kind of freedom that allows physicians or medical students, for instance, to open themselves up to the possibility of entering into a patient's suffering and sharing this world, rather than disburdening themselves of anxiety by relying on calculative thinking and offering care as technical experts who are concerned only with the physical aspects of being ill.

Such an approach to patient care is made possible because the authentic resoluteness that opens us up for new ways of seeing and interpreting the world involves a letting go or "releasement" (*Gelassenheit*) of any attempt to control or exert our will over being.[31] In being resolute, we relinquish calculative attempts to disburden ourselves of death anxiety by engaging in the world in the belief that we might control the uncontrollable. Hans-Georg Gadamer reminds us that "the need for security is intimately bound up with this knowledge which promises mastery and control," even though such a promise is an empty one.[32] The suffering and angst that can come with recognizing that our being is groundless and precarious can, for both patients and doctors, shatter our ideas about our ability to control and order our lives in the way our modern technical age would like us to think we can.[33] Thus, when we are authentically resolute, we can see that attempts to contain our anxiety by reducing patients' suffering to no more than physical breakdowns, for example, are simply attempts to evade an authentic confrontation with our own inescapable fragility and mortality.

When we are authentically resolute, then, we engage with the world meditatively; we are able to "let" beings reveal themselves as they are, rather than attempting to master them by forcing them into ready-made conceptual categories. In other words, we do not "cling one-sidedly to a single idea, nor . . . run down a one-track course of ideas," but, rather, we remain open to other ways of being.[34] In remaining open, we can see the utility of calculative thinking and employ calculative approaches when they are appropriate, but we can also freely let go of them when they are no longer called for or when they are poorly suited for the project at hand. For doctors, this might mean redefining their ideas about care, recognizing that they can embody the qualities of proficient technicians when it is called for and also let go of their relationship to technology and technical care when that relationship is no longer useful. Heidegger refers to this ability to "say 'yes' and at the same time 'no'" to technology and technical thinking as "releasement toward things": "Releasement toward things and openness to the mystery belong together. They grant us the possibility of dwelling in the world in a totally different way. They promise us a new ground and foundation upon which we can stand and endure in the world of technology without being imperiled by it."[35]

For medicine, this "new ground and foundation" of releasement and openness would mean acknowledging the benefits of technical approaches to care, while at the same time allowing for a more expansive perspective that recognizes that illness and suffering cannot always be controlled. As Frank says: "One lesson I have learned from illness is that giving up the idea of control, by either myself or my doctors, made me content. What I recommend to both medical staff and ill persons, is to recognize the wonder of the body rather than try to control it . . . wonder and treatment can be complementary."[36] Heidegger's use of "mystery" (*Geheimnis*) and Frank's use of "wonder" are critical here. Whereas "curiosity" is typically seen as a positive attribute of a competent and scientifically rigorous clinician, "mystery" and "wonder" sound rather strange in the context of medical care.[37] And yet openness to mystery and wonder allow for a relative comfort with uncertainty, something few of us, especially doctors, have. Western medicine's emphasis on test results, checklists, and statistical evidence perpetuates the notion that medicine is an exact science, despite what Kathryn Montgomery calls the "radical uncertainty" in clinical practice when it comes to determining what is best for an individual patient.[38] Not only do diseases manifest differently, but patients make sense of their experiences in different ways and have different expectations and goals. But because the "clinical gaze" is unable to discern the mysteries of the lived body, Montgomery defines medicine as a "learned, rational, *science-using* practice that describes itself as a science even though physicians have the good sense not to practice that way."[39] So, even though most doctors recognize that there exists a degree of uncertainty in the care of every patient, the epistemological framework of medicine rarely acknowledges this uncertainty, let alone embraces wonder at the body or the mysteries of suffering.

On the other hand, physicians and other healthcare providers who are willing to face the uncertainty and precariousness of being and release their attempts to control the mysterious nature of life and death might begin to embody a kind of humility in the face of illness and suffering. Rather than turning away from suffering and uncertainty because these serve as reminders of their own existential contingency, physicians who are able to open themselves up to the awe-filled force of the mystery of their being-in-the-world might unearth a capacity to authentically enter into the lived experiences of their patients. As Kevin Aho puts it, the call to let go of our attempts to master or control being speaks to an "attitude that embodies gratitude, awe, and humility in the face of mystery, and this humility is itself freeing because it releases us from our own prideful and egotistic concerns."[40] In slowing down to wonder at the workings of the human body, the lived experiences of illness and suffering, or the uncertainty of life and unpredictabilty of death, doctors are reminded of how much they share with the patients before them.[41]

This is not to say that pride and ego are the only, or even the major, concern with physicians. The problem, rather, is that a preoccupation with definite, unambiguous answers and specific medical treatments limits the kind of care a doctor might offer. As Frank points out, "A physician who does not have [a] sense of wonder seeks only to cure diseases. Sometimes he succeeds, but if cure is the only objective, not achieving it means he has failed."[42] Because doctors who primarily identify as those who cure or restore the body might be threatened by intractable disease or impending death, they must begin to acknowledge, and even be humbled by, the wonder of the human body and the unpredictability of the human condition—especially since medical trainees who are educated in a system that focuses primarily on control and restoration and who do not have access to a discourse that pushes against this system are more likely to manage distress by distancing and detaching themselves from patients.[43] Ideas about control, containment, and certainty might serve to disburden physicians and medical students from the painful realities of human frailty and suffering, yet these strategies can lead to feelings of personal failure and prevent authentic engagement with those who are most in need. Linda Wiener and Ramsey Eric Ramsey poignantly speak to the broader issue of our need for control and certainty:

We are again driven to ask, along with Nietzsche: why should we downgrade our experience and the contingency and uncertainty of the world just so we can feel safe and confident with the part of the world we are able to represent to ourselves through science? Why trade, in Nietzsche's words, "even a handful of 'certainty' for a whole carload of beautiful possibilities?"[44]

Being-with-Others

Although anxiety has the potential to open us up to new, and even beautiful, possibilities of being, both Kierkegaard and Heidegger have been criticized for focusing too narrowly on what appears to be the "stoic" individual. Some scholars have argued that Kierkegaard's emphasis on personal salvation overlooks the communal and compassionate aspects of authentic living.[45] And with all the talk about authenticity, individuation, anticipation, and resoluteness in *Being and Time*, it is no wonder Heidegger's work has received similar criticism. But, as Patrick Gardiner points out, these critiques often fail to take into account that Kierkegaard's later writings stress that, without the love of and for others, life is not worth living.[46] Similarly, a careful reading of *Being and Time* reveals that being authentic is nothing if not an authentic recognition of our *being-with-others*. As Heidegger says:

> Resoluteness, as *authentic Being-one's-Self*, does not detach Dasein from its world, nor does it isolate it so that it becomes a free-floating "I." And how should it, when resoluteness as authentic disclosedness, is *authentically* nothing else than *Being-in-the-world*? Resoluteness brings the Self right back into its concernful Being-alongside what is ready-to-hand, and pushes it into solicitous Being with Others.[47]

So, even though an encounter with existential anxiety individuates us, this does not mean that, at bottom, we are utterly alone; rather, such an encounter brings us face-to-face with our being-in-the-world and thus with the fact that we are *always already with others* in the world.[48] Indeed, a structural feature of Dasein is its being-with-others—even in being alone, we are "with" others since we only know ourselves and what it means to be alone in relation to others in the world.[49] Thus we are—inescapably—with others in a world that we all share together; we cannot engage with or understand our world as isolated individuals, for all interpretation is, in some sense, a public interpretation. In fact, we are so much "with" others that we rarely distinguish ourselves from the "they" in our everyday inauthentic mode of being,[50] where we are more often than not indifferent to one another—abiding with others as if they were simply other objects in the world, just "passing one another by."[51]

Being resolute and ready for anxiety, on the other hand, can push us into a more authentic and concerned being-with-others in the world.[52] Because the trappings of the "they-self" and its tendency to promote calculative thinking can "conceal from ourselves the need for human beings," facing our anxiety can release us from the "they," open us to new ways of seeing the world, and allow for new ways of being with one another.[53] Even the anxiety that comes with serious illness—however excruciatingly lonely being ill may feel—can remind us of our connectedness to others. "To be ill," Frank tells us, "to share in the suffering of being human is to know your place in that whole, to know your connection with others."[54] Recognizing our vulnerability and mortality can draw us closer to others since we all share the same potential for total world collapse. This realization can bring immediacy to our relationships and cultivate humility in the face of our shared, finite existence.

When we are resolute, we recognize the precariousness of our being, and this recognition pushes us to a deeper and more intentional engagement with the world and with others in the world. Such resoluteness, moreover, not only reveals our potential for authentic being-with-others, but it also allows us to share this potential with others.[55] This means that we can "co-disclose" the call to authenticity and "let the Others who are with [us] 'be' in their ownmost potentiality-for-Being."[56] If Heidegger is right, this has very interesting implications for both patients and doctors. A patient's confrontation with world collapse might personally affect the doctor caring for the patient, for example, and might even reveal to the doctor his or her own potential for world collapse and thus also for authenticity. As McQuellon and Cowen see it, even though when a patient faces the end of life, only one person is actually dying (or perishing), the doctor who enters into the patient's experience is facing death as well,[57] "vicariously" experiencing his or her own potential for world collapse through the patient.[58]

Our authentic engagement with another—which, according to Heidegger, occurs when one or both of us have confronted our anxiety—can be transformative for those who bear witness to it.[59] This means that physicians and medical students who enter into the suffering of their patients and remain open to the uncertainty of being ill might be reminded of their own potential for suffering and thus also their own potential for authentic being. And it is this shared recognition that can lead to more authentic care for the other. Indeed, as Johanna Shapiro reminds us, "without acknowledging their shared mortality, frailty, and vulnerability, students will not be able to make much sense of truly caring for others."[60] Entering into the experience of a patient and being-with the patient's suffering in a way that does not attempt to control it can reveal the shared mortality and vulnerability to which Shapiro alludes. In other words, a person's experience of world collapse *through another* can be transformative, provided the person remains open to it.

Philosopher Eleonore Stump highlights the unique knowledge that is gleaned from what some philosophers are now referring to as "second-person experience."[61] Unlike a first-person experience where one is only directly and immediately aware of oneself, or a third-person experience where one has knowledge about the states of other people but does not directly interact with those others, in a second-person experience one interacts directly, consciously, and immediately with another person who is also aware of one. This direct interaction of the second-person experience is key for Stump, for she believes it offers "knowledge of" another person. Stump differentiates between "knowledge that," which refers to descriptive, analytical, or propositional knowledge, such as knowing *that* a flame is hot or *that* one's mother is a lawyer, and "knowledge of," which is nonpropositional and acquired through personal, and sometimes ineffable, experiences.[62] In this sense, one could know *that* one's father loves one, but one might not know *of* his love until one has experienced it in a second-person sense.

In terms of pain and suffering in the context of illness, there is a difference between knowing that persons experience pain and suffering and knowing of this suffering. Although it is important for physicians and medical students to acquire scientifically sound knowledge of pain and suffering in order to alleviate symptoms, they should also have an understanding of suffering in a different, deeper sense—what suffering or dying *means* to patients—in order to provide the best care possible. Acquiring this kind of understanding of suffering can be made possible through a direct, second-person experience of another's suffering. This deeper understanding not only leads to better care for patients, but it also can be personally transformative for doctors and medical students. As physician and professor Rita Charon notes, "Medical practice requires the engagement of one person with another and realizes that authentic engagement is transformative for all participants.... Through authentic engagement with their patients, physicians can cultivate affirmation of human strength, acceptance of human weakness, familiarity with suffering, and a capacity to forgive and be forgiven."[63] Charon goes on to suggest that, in caring for sick and dying patients, reflective physicians can "make sense of their own life journeys."[64] It is through this kind of engagement that personal familiarity with suffering and confrontation of anxiety lead to authenticity for both of those involved. And if this is so, then medical professionals are uniquely positioned for such second-person transformation: in caring for others who might be experiencing a world-shattering illness, they are reminded constantly of their own potential for death and world collapse, and they can be brought back to authenticity and can "assure" themselves of their "uncoveredness again and again."[65]

Turning toward the Other: Levinas's Phenomenology of the Face

Though Heidegger's philosophy emphasizes our inherent "being-with" and our mutual dependency on one another, it still offers no direction on what we "do" in our resoluteness or how we might specifically choose to live in our authenticity.[66] Facing our existential anxiety might free us to be-with others more authentically, but we might wonder what "authenticity" actually means. Despite the ethical baggage that words like "authenticity" and "resoluteness" carry, Heidegger resists the idea that he is offering any kind of ethics—if we understand "ethics" to mean a set of normative principles or prescriptions for "right" conduct—and he does not give us advice on how to live our lives, even after we break free from inauthenticity.[67] In fact, he does not even make it clear whether resoluteness is morally "better" than irresoluteness and only suggests that in resoluteness, our choices become our own rather than those of the "they."[68] According to Heidegger, the call to authenticity "asserts nothing, gives no information about world-events."[69] For this reason, Heidegger's position on resolute authenticity has been criticized not only for its stoicism, as mentioned above, but also for its lack of explicit ethical content, which some scholars have interpreted as a kind of quietism.[70] So, although Heidegger's philosophy shows us that doctors might be called to authenticity through their engagement with patients' suffering, in terms of answering the question of whether, why, or how doctors *ought* to respond to the existential suffering of the other, Heidegger's analysis does not take us far enough.

Emmanuel Levinas (1906–1995) encountered Heidegger at Freiburg University and was greatly influenced by his philosophy. That said, he responded to the conspicuous absence of any indication of what constitutes "authenticity" in Heidegger's writings by arguing that what is most primordial about being human is our *ethical encounter* with the other.[71] In this way, Levinas's philosophy—though in many ways made possible by Heidegger's groundbreaking fundamental ontology—takes us further than Heidegger's, for it holds that responding to the other in his or her suffering is what constitutes our being. For Levinas, the call to authentic living and resoluteness comes not from ourselves in our being-in-the-world, but rather from the face of the *other* whom we encounter. The other, according to Levinas, is what calls the self into question.[72]

Levinas's Phenomenology
A French philosopher of Lithuanian ancestry and a survivor of the Holocaust, Levinas gained popularity in the mid-twentieth century with his work in Jewish studies, existentialism, ethics, and ontology. Though his philosophy draws heavily on Talmudic doctrine, he does not consider himself primarily a religious thinker, nor does he ground his philosophy in Scripture. As Levinas tells us in *Is It Righteous to Be?*: "I illustrate with verse, yes, but I do not prove by means of the verse."[73] To be sure, Levinas's philosophy is not ethics but rather a phenomenological and hermeneutical description of the human encounter with the other—that is, an exploration of the *conditions of possibility* for any concern we might have about "doing good" or living well at all. In other words, it is a description of the precognitive, affective, and intersubjective experience of encountering another in the world, of being called by and responding to the other—an encounter that precedes any kind of codifiable ethics.[74]

This distinction between ethics and philosophy is rather arbitrary, however. For Levinas, our encounter with the other—which his phenomenology attempts to illuminate—is undeniably and imminently ethical. As social beings, our relationships have an ethical quality that determines our existence with others in the world. Ethics, therefore, is not a theory, system, or cognitive schema—it is simply what "goes on" between human beings in the world.[75] According to Levinas, ethics is "a comportment in which the other, who is strange and indifferent to you, who belongs neither to the order of your interest nor to your affections, at the same time matters to you."[76] The fact that our encounter with the other, before anything else, demands of us some kind of response—even if it is to let the other simply "be" and to make room for that other in the world—reveals to Levinas that "ethics is first philosophy," as he often puts it. This means that at the bottom of any account of human existence lie matters of good and bad, right and wrong—that is to say, human existence is ethical "all the way down."[77]

Levinas attempts to draw attention to a primary and primordial experience of our everyday existence that appears to have been forgotten, taken for granted, and covered over.[78] His core dictum is that all persons are responsible for one another, and this responsibility precedes all else; one is responsible before one is a thinker, an explainer, or a helper. This view is significantly different from saying we "ought" to respond to one another. For Levinas, this is not something we should do, but something *we cannot help but do*—we respond to one another every day, even if our response is diminished, corrupted, indifferent, or hurtful.[79] On the other hand, according to Levinas, attending to this usually unnoticed responsibility fundamental to our existence will allow us to become more fully human.[80]

Levinas employs the trope of the "face" to explain this responsibility. Though the human face encountered in the flesh is the most concrete expression of human suffering, for Levinas, the face means something more: it represents the "nakedness of the other"—the other's "misery" in his or her need.[81] According to Levinas: "If you conceive of the face as the object of the photographer, of course you are dealing with an object like any other object. But if you *encounter* the face, responsibility arises in the strangeness of the other and in his *misery*. The face offers itself to your compassion and to your obligation."[82]

The notion of "misery" is significant here, for Levinas claims that the encounter of the face of the other commands someone with its defenselessness and its need. This misery, or what I refer to as "vulnerability," is something that is crucial to the patient-doctor encounter, a point clinical ethicist and philosopher Richard Zaner draws attention to in his own work: "Vulnerability evokes—seems even to awaken concern, a wanting to care. . . . [It] awakens an otherwise dormant moral sense."[83] It is the vulnerability of the other that calls out to and draws the practitioner near: "I've found myself subtly taken over by that sense that, now, being here and not elsewhere, I've come into a special kind of responsibility, one that cannot be gainsaid."[84] In much the same way, the face for Levinas is "the commandment to take the other upon oneself, not to let him alone," and it is ceding one's place to the other and withdrawing one's own interestedness in being-for-oneself and answering the call to be for-the-other in the other's vulnerability that Levinas sees as ultimately ethical.[85] But the encounter with the face is not merely an idea or ideal; it is a concrete, affective happening, an event.[86] We encounter the other affectively, and though we often fail to see it as such, this face-to-face meeting calls out to us emotionally, demanding us to respond. The face, then, is not only vulnerable—it is, at the same time, powerful and demanding.[87]

Levinas refers to the act of responding to this call as "hospitality": "No face can be approached with empty hands and a closed home."[88] Such language is intriguing, not only for the intimacy it evokes, but also because of its intersection with Heidegger's ideas about the experience of anxiety, or unhomelikeness, that comes from our precarious being-in-the-world. If illness does, in fact, create an unhomelike state of being-in-the-world, then perhaps what the physician is called to do when called by the face of the patient is to be hospitable, to bring the patient back to a homelike state. As May contends, "The fully rounded work of healing reconnects the patient with the world," and it attempts to achieve a making whole and a making well, even when cure is impossible.[89] And sometimes, reconnecting the patient to the world does not take much. For Frank, bringing the other back to a homelike state simply requires an acknowledgment of the other, *recognizing* the other in his or her suffering. Although "recognizing" the other seems rather simple, it is something Frank says rarely happens in medicine: "I always assumed that if I became seriously ill, physicians, no matter how overworked, would somehow recognize what I was living through. . . . What I experienced was the opposite. The more critical my diagnosis became, the more reluctant physicians were to talk to me. I had trouble getting them to make eye contact; most came only to see my disease."[90]

Nevertheless, in a way that sounds undeniably Levinasian, Frank sustains a commitment to this idea of recognition: "When we know that someone recognizes our pain, we can let go of it. The power of recognition to reduce suffering cannot be explained, but it seems fundamental to our humanity."[91] Here Frank seems to allude to that taken-for-granted, though elemental, aspect of our being that Levinas's work draws attention to—namely, that recognizing and responding to the call of the other is precisely what makes us human.

Not unlike Heidegger's conception of the call to authenticity, the call that comes from the face of the other, though meaningful and understandable, precedes all speech, communication, or spoken exchanges.[92] Although unspoken, it nevertheless draws us in, beckoning us to respond. As Levinas sees it, this unspoken call is the "interpellation" of "the I" by the face of the other: "The epiphany of the absolutely other is a face, in which the Other calls on me and signifies an order on me through his nudity, his denuding. His presence is a summons to answer."[93] Ultimately, "to be I signifies not being able to escape responsibility," and the other puts the self into question.[94] This calling forth from the other is incessant; it holds us "hostage" to the other, and we are never done with our responsibility to the other's call.[95] Levinas therefore claims that *to be* means *to be for-the-other*, a "taking upon oneself the fate of the other."[96] This "taking upon" should not be interpreted, however, as a kind of slavery to the call that can be reduced to a Kantian deontological rule of disinterested love. Though it is easy to reduce the call to such a rule, doing so would run directly counter to the transcendent, ineffable *love* that compels one to turn toward the sufferer.

But the face of the other can also be distressing, for it reminds us of our own vulnerability. As I read Levinas, it is the face of the other, which he sees as constituting our being, that calls us into authentic living. It is the face of the other that reminds us of the other's and, by extension, *our own*, precarious existence. It is the face of the other that causes us existential anxiety, and it is the face of the other that we attempt to flee. And, most important, it is in responding to the face of the other that we become more authentically and resolutely human.

When considered in the context of medicine, this reading of Levinas helps unearth the nature of the clinical encounter that is so often covered over—namely, that the doctor who responds to the call of the other receives something in return. As Michele Carter contends, healthcare practitioners "possess a special moral privilege as they witness the efforts of patients who struggle to give their lives a sense of meaning and purpose in the face of disease or death."[97] The privilege, it seems, is that in bearing witness to the suffering and vulnerability of another, we become acutely aware of our own vulnerability, our own limits, and our own potential for suffering. When the facticity of our mortality forces itself into view, our own contingency becomes conspicuous. In responding to the call of suffering, then, physicians approach not only the patient but *themselves*—their subjectivity is deepened and expanded with the recognition of their potential for suffering that is always already at hand.

Carter suggests something similar in the context of what she calls our "shared existential loneliness." She points out that doctors and patients both suffer from a "genuine sickness" of loneliness, despair, and meaninglessness (though we are not always aware of such sickness), and she also makes the intriguing and seemingly paradoxical claim that within our loneliness—which is "intrinsic to what it means to be human"—the "treatment" lies in our ability to authentically acknowledge one another in our shared loneliness.[98] That is to say, in being interpellated by the face of our shared loneliness, suffering, or vulnerability, we receive something in return. In authentically recognizing the face of the other, we recognize ourselves, and somehow, we are less alone. As a result, both patient and physician might find themselves grateful for the encounter because, as many existentialist philosophers argue, both "depend on others to become more fully human."[99] Zaner suggests as much when he says, "It is with [the patient] that I am brought to myself. . . . Thus, it is understandable that otherwise odd sense of gratitude one feels in being able to help someone."[100]

The Other and Alterity Levinas's philosophy helps to illustrate what it is about the clinical encounter that calls the practitioner to do more for the other than attend to bodily dysfunction. In encountering the other, especially the other who is suffering, the face calls out and draws one near. The vulnerability of the face pleads for help, and when the face is that of the patient, the physician is responsible for answering. Levinas makes it clear, however, that, even though the face calls out in its vulnerability, and we are responsible to answer, we must always recognize the other's "alterity," that the other person is fundamentally different from us. Levinas uses the neologism "alterity" (from the Latin *alter*, meaning "other") rather than "difference" to describe a difference that is *prior* to differences—an otherness that precedes any physical, cultural, or economic attributes.[101] For Levinas, alterity is a fundamental aspect of being; it is that something that reminds us always that "you are other than I."[102] According to Frank, Levinas makes respect for alterity one of his core moral imperatives. "Seeing the face," Frank explains, "requires respect for alterity: I must recognize that there are aspects of your suffering that I can never imagine and that I can never touch."[103] One can only ever approach the suffering of the other; one cannot experience the same suffering in the same way.

So, although some might see Levinas's philosophy of the human condition as totalizing, Levinas works to show that it is anything but.[104] For him, human existence is a social existence, and the other whom we encounter in this shared existence is irreducibly other.[105] Having a different perspective, a different past, and a different subjectivity, the other person is irreducibly separate from the one who encounters him or her. So, although the call that comes from the other is essential in that it underlies any encounter with another person, it is also particular and particularizing. Our response might be guided by the fundamental call of the other to respond, but what we can and ought to do for the particular other is not a one-size-fits-all deontological command. It is, rather, contingent on the situation at hand.

This is one of the many reasons why I see Levinas's thinking as essential to medical ethics, especially contemporary medical ethics, which has been shaped so significantly by feminist theory. Much like Levinas's, a feminist approach to ethics, such as that proposed by Margaret Urban Walker, emphasizes the relational dynamics endemic to decision making, the "practices of responsibility" that define the range and limits of our accountability, and the need to attend to the specifics of the situation at hand.[106] In her seminal work *Moral Understandings*, Walker argues that moral theory has, for far too long, been dominated by a kind of master template that she calls the "theoretical-judicial model," which is preoccupied with autonomy, uniformity, and impartiality, and which is restricted to validating knowledge, uncovering codifiable or generalizable theories and principles, and developing moral theory that is functionally similar to a "scientific" ones.[107] She advocates instead for an "expressive-collaborative model" of moral theory that sees morality as relationally and socially embedded and takes seriously the ways in which people define their identities and responsibilities in their everyday lives, including intimate, familial, domestic, or "private" contexts. And because the care that takes place in such contexts is usually highly gendered (and raced and classed), traditional moral theory, which often overlooks the relational or collaborative context of morality, tends to perpetuate masculine and elitist conceptions of morality based on narrow understandings of individualism, autonomy, and personal agency.

Much like the feminist thinkers who would come after him, Levinas helps us to see that authentically recognizing suffering demands a response, one that is appropriate to the specific context at hand and the complex relational dynamics of those involved. This leaves some important questions unanswered, however. If the way we respond to the other is guided by the particular situation, how do we discern an appropriate response? And if the other is "irreducibly other," when that other is the patient, how can the doctor presume to know what the other needs at the outset? How can the doctor possibly come to know what exactly it is the other needs when the other calls out to him or her for help?

Responding to the Call of the Other:
Hermeneutics and Dialogue

According to Levinas, our obligations to the other are too often obscured by laws, regulations, and procedures, concealing the fact that our goal is not to enact a general rule or duty but to respond to another person in a specific way.[108] Even in the instances when we are called to perform an action guided by a rule or principle, the action is always interpersonal and is always shaped by the particular person and situation at hand.[109] Thus a doctor who responds to the face of the other and is guided by the ethical principle of beneficence, for example, would still need to ask: What form of goodness or care is needed here? What would benefit, what would harm, and how do I help this particular patient in front of me? And no abstract, general conception of beneficence will help the doctor answer these practical questions.

Fredrik Svenaeus's "medical hermeneutics" and Hans-Georg Gadamer's dialogue-based hermeneutics in which it is grounded can be helpful here, for both highlight the interpretive structure of medical encounters.[110] Gadamer's hermeneutics is particularly illuminating in the context of the patient-physician relationship because his approach to hermeneutics underscores that all interpretation is mediated by language and emphasizes "the dialogic meeting between persons who strive toward mutual understanding."[111]

A student of Heidegger, Hans-Georg Gadamer (1900–2002) draws attention to the inescapability of our historicity and situatedness and addresses our assumptions about "prejudice."[112] Gadamer believes that the idea that we might rid ourselves of prejudice and bias (a relic of the Enlightenment) is a prejudice in and of itself, for our view of the world is inevitably colored by the unique context of our particular lifeworlds.[113] But the impossibility of ridding ourselves of our unique perspectives on all phenomena, including other beings whom we encounter, does not mean that we will never approach a mutual or shared understanding. It is through what Gadamer calls a "fusion" of horizons of meaning, which can occur through dialogue, that we can begin to approach a shared perspective that incorporates both our own and the other's horizons of meaning.

Using Gadamer's notion of approaching the horizon of the other by remaining open to and attempting to understand the lifeworld of the other through dialogue, Svenaeus suggests that the clinician's goal is to try to understand the patient's interpretation of his or her illness and to resist the temptation to simply bring the patient within the horizon of the biomedical world. Physicians must remain open to their patients, allowing them to reveal their lived experiences and then incorporating these experiences within their own interpretations of patients' illnesses.[114] The clinical encounter is thus an "interpretive coming together of the two different lifeworld horizons of doctor and patient . . . [who] must through the gradual fusion of horizons ultimately reach to some extent a shared understanding."[115] This "shared understanding" and "gradual fusion" imply that both patient and physician work together to determine what is best for the patient. Rather than impose their "correct" clinical interpretations on their patients, physicians must instead recognize that their own interpretations are always partial and incomplete without the other's. They therefore learn from their patients by letting them share their interpretations—what the illness means to *them*—through open dialogue.

As an interpretive endeavor, the clinical encounter remains open ended and never asserts absolute meaning or what Gadamer would call "a definitive interpretation" but is always striving toward the best interpretation possible.[116] The physician and patient work together through dialogue, not to ascertain verifiable or definite truths, not to abstract the disease from the patient in order to "cure it," but to achieve the best interpretation possible to determine how best to bring healing (both physical and existential) to the patient within his or her particular lifeworld. Like Heidegger's conception of truth as "aletheia" or "uncovering," the dialogically guided clinical encounter does not presuppose that there is one "correct" interpretation to be discovered or one "right" decision to be made. Rather, the physician strives for a "good" or "authentic" understanding and recognizes that deciding what to do within this understanding is always particularized and dependent on the actual meeting of two different horizons.[117] That is to say, through interpretation, the physician must take into account the specifics of each patient's predicament—not only biological symptoms, but also the cultural, social, economic, and relational factors that are often "the root causes of personal [and medical] troubles"—in order to determine what is best for each particular patient within each particular situation.[118]

But the language of "merging" or "fusing" horizons must be used with caution, for it suggests that someone might come to know or "fully understand" the perspective of the other simply by listening closely and with openness. To some, such a notion smacks of hegemonic assumptions about identity and culture, assumptions that, in medicine as practiced in the United States, might ultimately lead to "colonizing" patients, especially patients who are unfamiliar with medical culture or American culture more generally. Because there are many who live on the margins, in the borderlands between worlds, or "on the hyphen," assuming that all patients are comfortable in the clinical space or that they interpret their illness or even what it means to be ill or healthy in the first place in the same way overlooks the struggle some patients face in trying to reconcile different and contradictory beliefs, norms, and cultural practices.[119] Although Heidegger helps us see that even if patients always already have an understanding of the world—they usually know, for example, why people seek the help of doctors and how patients might comport themselves in the clinical space, this does not mean that they are familiar with all of the practices of a culture that might be foreign to them, a culture that makes new demands on their interpretive existence. As Mariana Ortega explains:

If you are a white U.S.-born citizen and I am a Latin American born in Nicaragua, we will probably have different takes on what we experience in this room and we will have different takes on our experiences depending on the dominant norms and practices of the particular situation and how we relate to these practices given the contexts which dominate our particular interpretations.[120]

Given our irreducible differences, it is more helpful to see others not as unified, monolithic, fully knowable selves, but rather as complex, heterogeneous, multifarious (though still potentially unified) selves—what Ortega calls "'world' travelers"[121] The "world" traveler attempts to balance or align norms and practices between worlds, though this alignment is rarely neat, given that "world" travelers often are positioned on the borderlands of society or culture. Since they will inevitably encounter these "world" travelers in their practice (indeed, we all might identify as "world" travelers at different times), doctors must remain aware of any attempts to co-opt their patients' worldviews by submerging patients' interpretive horizons within their own. Levinas's notion of alterity is critical here; we can only ever approach the horizon of the other (and this approach must be carried out mindfully and diligently), and any attempt to subsume the other's interpretive horizon within our own fails to extend care to the other in the way he or she may need.

Hermeneutics and Phronesis

Given the interpretive nature of the clinical encounter, Svenaeus suggests Aristotle's conception of phronesis is indispensable to medical hermeneutics, a point that other scholars also have discussed in the medical literature. F. Daniel Davis, for example, argues that clinical reasoning involves choosing a course of therapeutic action in a concrete, particular situation that is pervaded by differences and uncertainty, which is a challenge very much like choosing right or good moral action in concrete situations.[122] Accordingly, it is phronesis, often translated as "practical wisdom" or "reflective discernment" and described as the intellectual virtue cultivated over time, that allows us to discern what choice is conducive to achieve the aim of the activity in which we are engaged—a wisdom or discernment that is critical for medical decision making.[123] If the telos of medicine is the good of patients—to help them and to extend *care* to them—it is phronesis that allows doctors to decide what the good of particular patients is in particular situations.[124]

Phronesis draws on the practical and experiential knowledge we have of other human beings, a knowledge that grows not from formal education or theorizing, but from our personal experiences and our encounters with others in the world.[125] As we have seen, medicine is not an applied science but rather an engaged praxis, an amalgamation of theoretical, technical, and practical knowledge. So, although physicians' knowledge about the patients before them will be informed by biomedical science, what ails these patients is always timely and particular; universal biomedical theory goes only so far since patients' clinical particulars usually "outrun" the scope of scientific theories and laws.[126] It is therefore physicians' clinical and practical discernment, a discernment developed over time and with experience, that allows them to see what the specific situation calls for and to make "good" judgments. In the practice of medicine, phronesis is essential for interpreting the situation at hand and determining how to respond to the face of the other; the physician—as a *phronimos*, or wise person—knows "the right and good thing to do in *this* specific situation."[127]

It is important to note that phronesis is cultivated through habitual practice and acquired over time; thus good mentorship is critical for the development of phronesis, a point emphasized and expanded upon in chapter 4. For now, suffice it to say that it is through dialogue and attention to the interpretive nature of the clinical encounter, refined by phronesis, that doctors come to know how to respond to the particular patients in front of them. But there is much more to dialogue and conversation than the exchange of words and ideas. As McQuellon and Cowen point out, engaging in genuine conversation is a turning toward something together,[128] a "bridge" that allows clinicians, students, and other caregivers to come to know and even share, in some way, the experience of the patient. For Ronald A. Carson, this bridge is represented by the hyphenated space in the doctor-patient relationship, a space that can be traversed together in conversation, even for those "world" travelers who might reside on the hyphen.[129] Though this space can separate the doctor and patient, it can also serve as a common ground where the patient's experience can be explored together. Such conversation can provide at least a *sense* of what it might be like to be in the situation of the patient.[130] Elsewhere, Carson writes:

> In expressing myself, I have also successfully placed what was heretofore on my mind and in my heart into the open, so that it is not just a matter for me to try to make sense of and contend with; it is a matter for *us*. . . . Having spoken, I am no longer alone; I am participating in a conversation with others aimed at making sense of what ails me. My experience is no longer mine alone but is now *our* experience. Language creates a shared vantage point from which we can view matters together.[131]

And, paradoxically, such connection may not even require anyone to speak. "Conversation," McQuellon and Cowan tell us, "is more than exchanging words; sometimes all it requires is silent, attentive presence"—a genuine recognition of the other's suffering that leads to mutual understanding.[132]

Determining what is required in a particular situation, whether it is silent presence or active treatment, requires clinical wisdom and genuine engagement with the other. Hermeneutic dialogue asks us to "remain open to the meaning of the other person" and that person's story and requires us to acknowledge our own situatedness and biases, recognizing that our interpretations of others and their stories are fluid and incomplete.[133] But such fluidity is not something to lament since it allows for the merging of horizons, and it is precisely the malleability and permeability of horizons that allow us to understand the other, despite his or her irreducible alterity.[134] Indeed, Gadamer argues that the idea of a closed horizon is an abstraction in the same way that "the individual is never simply an individual, because he is always in understanding with others."[135]

This idea about the individual as existing not in isolation but in some way constituted by the other—which appears in the writings of most of the philosophers mentioned above—runs counter to the modernist notion of the disengaged, monological, singular self.[136] Charles Taylor sees such modernist understandings of the self as a "stripped-down view of the subject," understandings that fail to account for the richness and variety of human culture.[137] For Taylor, human beings are inextricably connected to and absorbed in the world and with others in the world—we are always already engaged with one another *dialogically*. Our identity, in Taylor's account, is not defined by our individual properties but rather by how we engage in a social space.[138] But this does not mean that the self is a total social construct, formed solely by cultural and social norms or by the univocal and unilateral perspective of the other. Rather, the self is cocreated within dialogical action and conversation; our identity, which is always in flux, is shaped by our polyvocal encounters with others. Truly recognizing this, I would argue, can broaden our understanding of "medical hermeneutics": viewing the clinical encounter as a hermeneutic endeavor not only reveals the doctor's need for the patient in terms of helping him or her understand "what is the matter," but also exposes the doctor's *elemental need* for the patient: without someone to care for, the doctor (as healer) would cease to be a doctor at all.

Called into Becoming: Mikhail Bahktin's Dialogism The idea that we are fundamentally dialogical beings, which is suggested by Heidegger's "being-with-the-other," implied by Levinas's "being-for-the-other," and alluded to in Gadamer's conception of horizons, is explicitly addressed in the writings of Mikhail Bakhtin (1895–1975)—a thinker who spent his life developing his idea that human relationships are grounded in and made manifest through dialogue.[139] Bakhtin saw life as a never-ending, "unfinalizable" dialogue that takes place at every moment of lived existence.[140] This conception of dialogue, however, does not refer to the verbal interactions among two or more monads, which the term "dialogue" is often reduced to.[141] Much like Levinas's understanding of language, dialogue for Bakhtin is perceived as primordial phenomenon that is deeper than and precedes designative expressions.

Whereas, for Levinas, "to be" means to-be-for-the-other, for Bakhtin, "to be" means to communicate dialogically.[142] This communication is not merely an exchange of messages through the medium of language, however. According to Bakhtin: "To be means to communicate. To be means to be for another, and through the other, for oneself. A person has no sovereign internal territory, he is wholly and always on the boundary; looking inside himself, he looks into the eyes of another or with the eyes of another."[143] In this sense, what one "communicates" to the other actually *constitutes* the other's being. Because we cannot help but see ourselves with the eyes of another, Bakhtin says that we only become conscious of ourselves—in fact only become ourselves—while revealing ourselves "for another, through another, and with the help of another."[144] Dialogism, then, calls us to imagine what we look like to those around us and to grant those perceptions equal validity with our own.[145]

Ultimately, Bakhtin points to our *absolute* need for the other: "A human being experiencing life in the category of his own *I* is incapable of gathering himself by himself into an outward whole that would be even relatively finished."[146] It is in this way that Bakhtin's dialogism brings meaning to Frank's claim that the doctor, in escaping from honest dialogue with a patient, "escape[s] from himself."[147] Because physicians can only know themselves in a way that is "even relatively finished" through the dialogical encounter with the other, they are also only *called into becoming* by their patients.[148] Physicians are only physicians by virtue of caring for the patients before them; indeed, they could not "be" without their patients. It is for this reason that Jeffrey Bishop can claim that altruism "is simply not possible" when responding to suffering.[149] It is impossible because the responder receives something from the patient, a call to be there, a call that "constitutes [the responder's] purpose for being."[150] This is made clearer by Zaner's description of his encounter with a very sick patient, whose "presence there, in that bed . . . pull[ed] me out of myself and into concern for him, his sphere of life. . . . I had the sense then, and still have it now, that his being sick is what does this, and contributes to what I, this self, am."[151]

Calls for altruism are shared by virtually every code of medical professionalism and are variously defined as actions and decisions aimed at improving others' welfare and avoiding one's own self-interest and primarily emphasizing the abnegation of personal gain.[152] Although it is important to stress that healthcare professionals should never be driven solely by economic motives or the desire to obtain extrinsic rewards, the idea that physicians ought not to gain anything material from doctor-patient encounters obscures the fact that they are *constituted* by their encounters with patients.

A dialogical understanding of being, with its emphasis on the cocreation of the self, helps us to see how both interlocutors receive something from the patient-practitioner encounter. That patients are almost always perceived to be more vulnerable than physicians—whether due to physical illness or to the nature of the fiduciary relationship—does not mean that patients don't have something significant to offer those who care for them.

Bringing It Together: An "Authentic" Response to Suffering

Levinas, Svenaeus, Taylor, and Bakhtin show us that there exists within the phenomenological encounter of two human beings a call from one to the other, emanating from and communicating one's vulnerability. In responding to this call from the other within the patient-physician relationship, doctors *need* patients, not only for helping them determine what is the matter with their patients and how doctors can help them, but they also need patients in a more primordial way—in order to heal, in order to *be a healer*. As Heidegger would say, doctors need patients and their call outward toward them in order to become what they already are.[153]

It seems, then, that understanding what is required of the physician lies in our understanding of the clinical encounter as a meeting between two people who share in suffering and who work together in order to bring healing. Yet, as I have shown, healing requires more than attention to biology or pathology since the suffering that is the result of illness extends beyond the bounds of the physical. The doctor is therefore called to acknowledge the patient's existential suffering and attempt to alleviate it to the extent that this is possible. To this end, the doctor as healer must recognize and validate the other and authentically engage with him or her, something made possible through dialogue and genuine listening. Listening requires an understanding that we are not ourselves without the other, that "in listening for the other, we listen for ourselves," as Frank says.[154] And though listening and responding to suffering can be difficult and even frightening, it is, at least to Frank, "a fundamental moral act."[155]

Even when dialogue and listening are all that can be offered by way of treatment—for patients at the end of life, for example—the physician can still extend healing through witnessing the other. Witnessing allows patients to articulate and order their experience, which may, in and of itself, have some therapeutic value.[156] On the other hand, there are times when dialogue and verbal engagement are impossible or even undesirable. Yet, because dialogue—as Bakhtin reminds us—is extralinguistic or prelinguistic, authentic being-with is still possible without spoken language. It is this kind of extralinguistic engagement that Carter finds essential to caring for the dying: "In many situations involving terminal illness, the dialogue may be unspoken, captured more in expressions of tenderness, listening, and being with the other."[157] To put it simply, what the physician owes to the patient is a turning-toward the other—a "nonindifference" to the other's suffering, as Levinas might say.[158] What is required of the healer is to be-there-for-the-other in both the other's physical and existential brokenness.

Is This Asking too Much of our Doctors?
The ontological—and thus also ethical—constitution of the clinical encounter is such that the physician as healer is called to turn toward patients and respond to their suffering. But when it comes to engaging in a real way with patients, the sentiment heard in hospital hallways usually is to "let the social worker take care of that."[159] As part of the interprofessional care team, social workers—as well as nurses, case managers, and chaplains—do, indeed, fulfill critical and indispensable roles, engaging with patients and their families and connecting them to important resources that allow for holistic care—and often do these things better than physicians. Yet, to me, the idea that addressing the social and existential suffering of patients should be left to these team members is evidence of the pervasive and often noxious power dynamics that play out between doctors and patients, doctors and other healthcare professionals, and doctors and other doctors that can serve to relieve doctors of their responsibility. Often seated at the apex of medicine's power hierarchy, physicians have the distinctive privilege of choosing not to engage in the traditionally feminine, intimate, and emotional labor required for addressing existential suffering. This labor—which is decidedly *not* objective, rational, or scientific—can easily be dismissed as not the proper work of physicians and subsequently left to those in more subordinate positions. In this way, our perception of whether doctors are responsible for addressing the call of suffering, is inextricably linked to power—which is, again, linked to the epistemological norms and assumptions guiding medical practice.

This is not to say that all, or even most, doctors exploit their power in order to avoid their patients' suffering. There are many physicians, especially in primary care, who put forth much emotional labor attending to the complex needs of their patients. But we can't ignore the ways in which medicine's epistemology perpetuates the very power relations that sustain misguided assumptions about who is "really" called to attend to suffering. That said, I—like William May, who makes "no apologies" for emphasizing that the physician "wields immense power and creates the central problem in the healing enterprise"[160]—would argue that attending to existential suffering is, perhaps ultimately, the role of the physician. In my experiences both professionally and personally, I have found the doctor's words to be particularly weighty and significant, especially when it comes to diagnoses and prognoses. As Frank recounts his own experience: "The patient hangs on what brief words are said [by the doctor].... When the physician has gone, the patient recounts to visitors everything he did and said, and together they repeatedly consider and interpret his visit. The patient wonders what the physician meant by this joke or that frown."[161]

Given doctors' expertise and most patients' expectations concerning the role of their doctors, engaging honestly and authentically with another's suffering is not something that can easily be dismissed as falling outside a doctor's purview. Although each member of the patient's care team is integral to healing, the physician—whether or not he or she acknowledges it—represents something unique: the harbinger of hope, the bearer of unbearable news, a quiet comfort—or a conspicuously detached and imposing presence. The doctor is the expert; if there is anyone who can fix the problem, the doctor is that person. If there is anyone who can determine whether a patient is dying and there is nothing else to be done, the doctor is the one. At the very least, as McQuellon and Cowen argue, because of their training and experience, doctors are "rightfully expected to assume greater responsibility" for initiating and sustaining difficult conversations, especially if they are about the prospect of death.[162]

Realism or Idealism?

The philosophers discussed above appear to hold us all, and especially doctors, to impossible standards. Indeed, philosopher Hilary Putnam describes Levinas as a "moral perfectionist": "Such a philosopher is a 'perfectionist' because s/he always describes the commitment we ought to behave in ways that seem impossibly demanding; but such a philosopher is also a realist because s/he realizes that it is only by keeping an 'impossible' demand in view that one can strive for one's 'unattained but attainable self.'"[163] But Levinas and Bakhtin and those philosophers inspired by their work are not promoting naive idealism. They are realists in that they recognize the seemingly impossible demand of such ethical imperatives; and yet they stress the importance of striving toward these ideals nonetheless.[164] It is this reaching toward unreachable ideals that constitutes moral action. The imperative to do so is radical, yes, and Levinas acknowledges that to be radically for-the-other rarely occurs. But he reminds us that, as human beings, we are the only possible site for such far-reaching concern for the other, and, as human beings, we are responsible for striving to extend that concern to others:

The human in being is that possibility [of holiness or sacrifice]. The possibility of hearkening to the original language of the face of the other in his misery and his ethical command, this way of surmounting on one's own being one's effort to be interests me. . . . Evil is the refusal of that responsibility, the fact of letting this prior attention turn itself away from the face of the other man.[165]

Although Levinas is committed to the idea that being human is precisely what equips us for being radically for the other, he states that this unbounded ethical call is, nevertheless, limited by the particular. In our everyday lives, we are always other things in addition to being responsible.[166] Moreover, there are people in our lives to whom we respond in different ways and to different degrees, especially since our resources are limited.[167] And, finally, Levinas suggests that our responsibility is limited by the fact that we have our own needs and desires: if we did not stay attuned to our own embodied existence, we would have little or nothing to offer others.[168] Feminist thinkers, too, have pointed out the limitations of an ethics of care. While acknowledging that the kind of care women and other traditionally "feminine" groups offer is morally valuable, they are also committed to identifying and undermining the forces that perpetuate oppression. As such, most feminists believe that those who put forth the emotional labor required for caring should also remain attuned to social and political relations that such caring implicitly supports. Part of caring well for oneself involves distinguishing between circumstances in which it is appropriate to offer care and those in which care is better withheld.[169]

This attention to boundaries and to the care of the self is critical for all of us, perhaps especially for clinicians who are exposed to a concentration of human suffering. But, to see our responsibility to respond to others as "too much" or as an impossible sacrifice that diminishes our being is misguided. As Levinas sees it, the emptying of oneself for the other is liberating and leads to deep contentment. It is not a burden, but rather, as Michael Morgan puts it, "makes it possible for the self to fulfill itself by responding to, accepting and serving, the other person."[170] This giving of the self ultimately gives back to the self.

Such a response to the other does not call for physicians to lose sight of themselves entirely at the behest of their patients, but reorients their focus toward what they actually receive from caring for others. With this in mind, healers might begin to see encounters with patients as life giving, as that which brings deeper meaning and purpose to their careers—a perspective that might lessen the likelihood for burnout, not lead to it (a point that will be discussed further in chapter 4). Even caring for the dying, something that can be emotionally exhausting for physicians and fraught with existential anxiety about their own death, can offer them something in return. It can illuminate meaning and purpose for both patients and physicians, and being present with the dying can, as Pauline Chen argues, give "weight" to patients' experiences and allow physicians to become the doctors they "have always wanted to be."[171]

A Return Back to Ourselves

As humans, we are ontologically called toward the other, though we can choose to evade the call. We will never achieve being radically for-the-other, and yet in striving to do so, we become ourselves. The philosophical thinking presented above is not the stuff of medical ethics. It is, rather, an ethic of being human. As such, the physician *as person* is called toward this ethical comportment, especially considering that the call of vulnerability is so discernible in the clinical encounter. Healing, in its fullest sense, includes recognizing shared suffering, acknowledging personal limitations, and extending care for the other because of this shared suffering and despite these limitations. Indeed, the word "compassion" quite literally means "suffering together."[172] To answer the cry of vulnerability, loneliness, suffering, and pain implicit in the face of the other—whether one chooses to see it or not—is essential to the therapeutic relationship, a truth that has its foundation in what it means to be human and to share a world together. As Martha Nussbaum argues, compassion requires a sense of one' own vulnerability and a willingness to confront the idea that "this suffering person might be me."[173] Compassion requires a vulnerable openness to the other, a willingness to be present with suffering. In turning away from the world and the inauthentic ways care has been interpreted in it, deciding *for* ourselves what it means to care, and then turning back toward the world once again, we might begin to understand Heidegger's seemingly paradoxical call to "become what you are."[174] Recognizing that the core of caring and healing is responding to the other—really *seeing* the other's being—brings one back to oneself (a being who *is* being-with-others); it propels us toward what we can become, and thus informs who we are now. In choosing to be for-the-other, healers become who they always already were called to be.

Some might say that all of this is too emotionally demanding, impossibly utopian, and distressingly unrealistic. And because we are fallible humans who are structurally anxious and inauthentic, those who see it as such might be right. However, might we instead consider what has been laid out here as a heuristic of sorts, an ideal that gets us closer to a deeper and broader understanding of care for the other? We may never see a medical culture that acknowledges and embraces such a demanding call for the care of the sick, but perhaps we will see a culture that does not completely turn away from such a calling by unreflectively perpetuating an epistemology that reduces illness, suffering, and care to matters of pathophysiological breakdown and biological intervention. Perhaps we can start cultivating future doctors who recognize that patients who are ill might be facing a total breakdown of their lifeworld and that their sense of self hinges on the words of their doctors. As the great American writer Anatole Broyard once said after receiving his cancer diagnosis, "To most physicians my illness is a routine incident in their rounds, while for me it's the crisis of my life. I would feel better if I had a doctor who, at least, perceived this incongruity."[175]

What I am advocating is not so much a demand that doctors carry the weight of every patient's existential suffering, dwelling in the darkness of human frailty, heroically witnessing each individual's demise, but rather that doctors and medical students begin—at the very least—to recognize the incongruity between their daily routine and what is happening to their patients. All patients come to doctors for help because they experience some kind of disruption in their everyday way of being, and, for some, this disruption is the crisis of their lives. These patients are more than "interesting" cases or items on some medical to-do list; they are people in need of help, people who want their suffering to be acknowledged.

Truth be told, the failure of medical professionals to genuinely acknowledge individual suffering is not a new problem. It was well over a century ago that Leo Tolstoy wrote of the dejected and dying Ivan Ilych whose personal suffering was "for the doctor, and perhaps for everybody else . . . a matter of indifference," an indifference that "struck him painfully."[176] Like Broyard, Tolstoy speaks to the heart of the matter, drawing attention to the incongruity of the patient-doctor encounter that can be so destructive when we pretend it does not exist. The call for doctors to address existential suffering is not a nostalgic yearning to return to some idyllic medical professionalism of days gone by, when scientism was less pervasive. Yearning for such a time would ultimately fail us, not only because—as Tolstoy shows us—it very likely never existed, but also because the problem of contemporary medicine, as I have argued earlier, is not just an epistemological problem, but an ontological one. As human beings, regardless of our time and place, remaining impervious and indifferent to suffering is easier than confronting our shared vulnerability and mortality.

Fortunately for all of us, cultivating "nonindifference" is not impossible. In fact, according to Levinas, what makes us beings who care about others at all and what brings meaning to our shared existence is always already "there" for us, even if it is buried and forgotten.[177] The question to consider, then, is how might we help future healers unearth their ability to turn-toward the other by bringing them back to themselves?

4 The Formation of Medical "Professionals"

It's easier to train technicians than it is to train healers.
—Dennis H. Novack, Ronald M. Epstein, and Randall H. Paulsen, "Toward Creating Physician-Healers"

My somewhat extensive philosophical investigation of the clinical encounter in chapters 2 and 3 does not mean to suggest that those seeking a remedy for what ails modern medicine and medical education need to study fundamental ontology or existential phenomenology. Far from it. Heidegger himself says that "anyone can follow the path of meditative thinking in his own manner and within in his own limits.... [M]editative thinking need by no means be 'high-flown.'"[1] What the thinkers whose philosophies I have drawn on are calling for is not abstract thought experiments or rigorous analytical descriptions, but rather a consideration of our more primordial selves, a return to the fundamental aspects of being human that we all share. In telling us what patients really need is for "others to share in recognizing *with them* the frailty of the human body," Arthur Frank is calling for simplified clinical encounters, wherein disease talk is limited and clinicians are willing to face the realities of being human, recognizing that confrontation with suffering will neither paralyze nor overwhelm them.[2] Indeed, doctors might even begin to see that entering into the suffering of their patients can deepen their ways of being-in-the-world and their being-with-others. The humility that comes with recognizing that, as humans, we are all flawed and all suffer in our own ways can cultivate compassion and uncover the common bonds between us.[3]

It might be obvious that patients' suffering is intensified when clinicians and students fail to see the potential for such bonds and choose instead to distance themselves from the reality of human frailty by remaining "objective" and detached. But we cannot overlook the fact that healthcare professionals and students are, in many instances, suffering as well. Ignoring the reality of sickness and suffering and the fragility of the human condition can be exhausting, and not giving voice to these issues can distance us from ourselves. As Thomas R. Cole, Nathan S. Carlin, and Ronald A. Carson point out:

> Under today's stressful conditions of practice, physicians, nurses, allied health professionals, biomedical scientists, and students all find themselves at risk for becoming alienated or separated from the ideals that drew them to healthcare in the first place. These conditions lead to high rates of burnout, depression, impairment, and even suicide. Hence, the re-humanization of medicine involves enhancing, restoring, and attending to the humanity of students and caregivers as well as patients.[4]

Despite such apparent suffering, the culture of contemporary medicine is entrenched so deeply in calculative understandings of clinical care that the affective experience of practicing clinicians and the personal development of future clinicians are largely ignored. One of the first steps in cultivating nonindifference and helping physicians and students return to themselves is acknowledging the ways they are affected by patient care and the culture of modern medicine.

Physician Suffering, Relationship Centeredness, and Existential Reflection

In the quagmire of contemporary American medicine, where the commercial interests of a broken healthcare system intersect with paradoxical calls for both compassion and scientific detachment, the goals of medical students and clinicians alike become blurry, and the potential for real human connection gets lost amid the competing needs for efficiency and productivity. What is more, the medical education system rarely offers a space for students to explore these competing interests and clarify why it is they chose to go into medicine and what kind of interactions they want to have with their patients. And, perhaps most important, both students and physicians have few opportunities to express how the practice of medicine and their encounters with suffering, death, and meaninglessness take an emotional toll on them and why distancing themselves from the realities of suffering and mortality seems like their best and only option.

When so much emphasis is placed on "patient-centered care," when patients are reframed as "consumers" in a healthcare system ensnared in the assumptions of neoliberalism, practicing and future doctors come to believe that their encounters with patients are unilateral—that they are required only to attend to the medical needs of their patients. Though patient-centered care is needed in our broken, market-driven system in order to mitigate self-interest, one of the negative corollaries is that it can obscure the fact that the connection between doctor and patient "contains mutuality, giving and receiving between patient and provider" and that physicians and students might also suffer, sometimes intensely, because of repeated interactions with patients that are especially difficult, uncomfortable, or harried.[5] Indeed, some physicians, especially those who care for the seriously ill, respond to patients' needs with emotions that can significantly affect the care they provide, feelings of fear, frustration, and anger or of grief and powerlessness, for example; they may feel the need to rescue or "save" patients or the need to escape or separate themselves from patients who cannot be rescued.[6] Even when these feelings are intense and affect a doctor's clinical judgment, they are often left unarticulated and unexamined.[7] Unaddressed, they can lead to distress, burnout, disengagement, and, in extreme cases, suicidal ideation or even suicide.[8] In a recent study published in *Academic Medicine*, when researchers completed a national survey of over 4,000 medical students, they found that 70 percent of students had indicators for burnout, alcohol abuse or dependence, or suicidal ideation.[9] Given, for example, that the rate of alcohol dependence among these students was found to be twice that in the general population of college-educated 22- to 34-year-olds, we should consider what it is about medical education in particular that contributes to significant personal distress. In a popular *New York Times* article titled "Why Do Doctors Commit Suicide?," Dr. Pranay Sinha offers some insight:

There is a strange machismo that pervades medicine. Doctors, especially fledgling doctors like me, feel pressure to project intellectual, emotional and physical prowess beyond what we truly possess. . . . We masquerade as strong and untroubled professionals even in our darkest and most self-doubting moments. How, then, are we supposed to identify colleagues in trouble—or admit that we may need help ourselves?[10]

In light of such sentiments, there has been an influx of journal articles in the last ten to fifteen years calling for "mindful practice" and for greater self-awareness and reflection in medical care and education.[11] Most of the proponents of mindful practice believe that becoming more self-aware and more reflective about their emotions, responses, motivations, and biases can lead doctors to provide better care for their patients and to take better care of themselves.

Among those who see mindfulness and reflection as critical components of healthy medical practice are clinicians and scholars who advocate for "relationship-centered care."[12] Proponents of this approach underscore the mutuality and reciprocity of the patient-doctor relationship, the need for self-awareness, the acceptance of affect and emotion, and the fact that the work of both the doctor and the patient has moral value.[13] Unlike most approaches to patient-centered care, relationship- or *human*-centered care orients doctors toward the dynamic, affective, and interdependent nature of the clinical relationship, emphasizing what they bring to the relationship and how they are affected by their encounters with patients. Central to relationship-centered care and approaches like it is the idea that doctors' connection with others is integral to medical care and ultimately brings *meaning* to their work. It is this ability to find meaning in their work that mitigates the potential for burnout, detachment, and emotional suffering.[14]

Fortunately, the practice of medicine is rife with opportunities to engage meaningfully with others. Although confrontations with illness and frailty can be threatening to practitioners when there are no opportunities to acknowledge and process through them, these confrontations are precisely what bring meaning to medical care. Physician and educator Arno Kumagai argues that when doctors are able to be fully present with patients and bear witness to their suffering, they are able to engage in a kind of "existential reflection."[15] They enter a privileged space where they can experience "a moment of fully understanding what it means to be human."[16] Such existential reflection, Kumagai explains, is an opportunity for doctors to engage in meditative thinking as a way to slow down and break free from the calculative thinking that dominates so much of medical practice. These moments with patients are what disencumber physicians and medical students of narrow, inauthentic "they-self" understandings of care and reorient them back to the human connection that makes genuine care possible.

But the ability to slow down and engage in existential reflection is one that needs to be cultivated. Future physicians must be "primed"—for lack of a better term—to recognize such opportunities when they present themselves, and they must be comfortable enough to be fully present with their patients. Though such engagement with patients can offer opportunities to reflect on some of the most important questions about what it means to be human, physicians and medical students will fail to see these opportunities unless they are aware of and reflect on their own vulnerability, limitations, mortality, and potential for suffering. This is not to say that the twenty-something medical student should be required to—or even has the ability to—reflect on his or her inescapable finitude and inevitable death in order to be a good doctor. What that student needs, rather, is to develop the ability to recognize the fragility and unpredictability of life and to approach the reality of illness and suffering with compassion and humility, rather than impartiality, frustration, or a desire for control.

Medical Education and the Cultivation of the Self

Even though self-awareness, critical thinking, and existential reflection are prerequisites for providing meaningful, relationship-centered care and genuine healing, medical education rarely aspires to develop these qualities in students. According to physicians Dennis H. Novack, Ronald M. Epstein, and Randall H. Paulsen:

> Many aspects of medical education seem to work against the goal of creating physician-healers . . . [instead] promoting cynicism, callousness, and self-doubt. Students are stressed by the demands to acquire an overwhelming amount of knowledge and the impossibility of learning everything, the cross-examinations, and the occasional real abuse on clinical rotations, and experiences with patients' suffering and death. Like soldiers on a battlefield, students must often deal with their emotions alone, or in chance discussions with colleagues and friends. Many learn to protect themselves to survive, but at the cost of distancing themselves emotionally from patients and peers, and consequently from the greatest satisfaction of clinical care.[17]

Few medical students feel comfortable or safe enough to voice the fear, frustration, or hesitation that can come with taking care of seriously-ill patients; in fact, doing so is often framed as "unprofessional."[18] Within the modernist paradigm of medicine, students are encouraged to maintain a safe and boundaried professional stance toward patients that protects them from emotional turbulence. In other words, they are encouraged to see distancing and detachment not as human reactions to vulnerability, but rather as the expected, professional demeanor of an objective caregiver, which ultimately casts the physician in "a competent, heroic role in which fear and vulnerability do not play a part."[19] The years that students spend in medical school and residency training are some of their most intellectually, physically, and emotionally demanding ones, and they significantly affect their personal formation and acculturation into medicine; yet, much of the learning that shapes their selves during this time is tacit and relegated to the informal or hidden curriculum.[20] So, even though many espouse the ideal of instilling students with empathy, compassion, and virtue, medical education provides only fleeting moments or transitory asides for students to seriously consider these virtues.[21]

What is so desperately needed, then, is committed attention to the *maturation* of the doctor *as a person*, which includes making time and space within the curriculum for reflection, dialogue, and genuine connection with others. Nevertheless, most current medical curricula overlook the formation of the self who is becoming a doctor, relegating the acquisition of "virtue" and "ethics" to a largely ineffectual education in "professionalism."

Medical Education and the Professionalism Movement

The term "professionalism" as it is currently used is a relatively recent development. It was not until the 1980s that the American Board of Internal Medicine described dimensions of "humanism" (which included respect, compassion, and integrity), and not until the 1990s that it began using the term "professionalism"—which encompassed humanism, but also altruism, duty and service, accountability, and excellence.[22] Although there is no widely accepted definition of professionalism, according to most scholars, there is general agreement both about its central principles (excellence, humanism, accountability, and altruism), and about the purpose of adhering to these principles—to establish "the requisite trust that both sustains medicine as a moral enterprise and assures patients that their interests are always a paramount concern."[23] Thomas Inui argues that, regardless of the amount of specialized knowledge and scientific technology doctors have at their disposal, if they are not *trusted* to share values with their patients and act in accordance with those values, they cannot engage in any kind of therapeutic relationship with patients.[24] Trust, then, is a necessary precondition for caring and healing to take place. Because of the fiduciary relationship between patients and physicians, wherein patients trust that their physicians will use their knowledge for their best interest, when physicians behave unprofessionally, patients may lose their trust in them, ultimately resulting in the breakdown of not only the fiduciary but also the therapeutic relationship.

Although most of us can agree that professionalism is integral to establishing trust and providing quality patient care, medical students are often taught explicitly about professionalism only by way of principles or codes intended to guide behavior. Addressing this point in 1970, theologian Paul Ramsey observed: "These codes exhibit a professional ethic which ministers and theologians and members of other professions can only profoundly respect and admire. Still, a catechism never sufficed. Unless these principles are constantly enlivened in their application, they become dead letters."[25] More than forty years have passed since Ramsey's observation, and medical educators still find themselves wrestling with this perennial problem. Even educators who have taken a more longitudinal approach to professionalism have not escaped the trap of prescribing and assessing observable behaviors.[26]

Medical educator Janet Grant, for example, claims that, even in the absence of a widely accepted definition of the term "competency," advocates of competency frameworks abound, although, in practice, competencies are usually reduced to observable behaviors,[27] with most, if not all, such frameworks rooted in a "narrow behaviorist approach" and primarily concerned with external, managerial, or political control.[28] Unsurprisingly, in Grant's view, any competency-based framework that relies upon exhibited and assessable behaviors provides only an "impoverished view" of professionalism since the totality of what professionals do is much greater than any of the parts that can be described in terms of competency.[29] She stresses that clinical judgment is exceedingly complex and involves both intuition and experience, something that cannot be replaced by prescriptions for behavior.[30] However well competency frameworks might work in assessing observable clinical skills (performing a specific physical exam, for instance), it is extremely difficult to map such frameworks onto professionalism.

Even in more "subjective" areas such as interpersonal communication and empathy, competencies are defined "almost exclusively in checklist-, product-oriented ways (i.e., measurable, observable, and quantifiable behaviors)."[31] Thus even the more longitudinal and developmental approaches to professionalism are vulnerable to criticism, for they often continue to conceptualize professionalism as a concrete, unitary concept—something that can be attained, measured, and assessed.[32] Although it is understandable that "assessing" professionalism education might be valued by those who work within the largely outcome-based and assessment-driven practice of medicine, this approach paradoxically participates in and reinforces the kind of calculative thinking it intends to overcome. As Warren Kinghorn explains, approaching professionalism in this way reflects the "logical backbone of the modern evidence-based medicine movement," which considers replication, standardization, and the quantification of outcomes and goals more important than all other forms of valuation in medicine.[33]

As a result, professionalism—along with its codes, competencies, evaluations, and checklists—has become a rather narrow pursuit that Jack Coulehan believes is "threatened with failure because the intervention is too simple, too neat, too flimsy, and doesn't engage the problem it attempts to address."[34] As Levinas has warned, rules and codes can obscure our primordial connections and distance us from one another, and a professionalism that focuses on them can therefore get in the way of doctors' authentic connection with patients.[35] Or, as a first-year resident in internal medicine told me:

I think my biggest hang-up connecting with patients as a medical student was the emphasis on professionalism. Most aspects of my personality that I feel help me connect with people are in stark contrast to the traditional views of professionalism. I have felt empowered to take a more personal and pragmatic approach to professionalism now that I am a physician, and it's very liberating. (RI-6)

Looking back on it, this new resident suggests that his professionalism education, which was largely based on exhibiting certain behaviors, actually hindered his ability to connect with patients. As a medical student, because he had felt that aspects of his personality—joking and laughing with patients in order to form a connection, for example—were "unprofessional," he had found it difficult to personally connect with the patients he encountered. Now as a resident, with more autonomy and responsibility (for the better, it would seem), he feels liberated from his former ideas about professionalism and is able to engage with his patients in a way that, though still "professional," is more aligned with his personal identity—an identity that transcends any specific professional role.

A fourth-year medical student also expressed concern about her professionalism education, but for different reasons. She felt that medical professionalism is too often conflated with prestige: "The way we are taught about professionalism communicates the idea that a doctor's professionalism is somehow different or more important than the professionalism required for other careers. As if being a doctor makes you better than other people, and that's just not true" (MSIV-3). It seems that when abstracted from the reasons *why* it is significant—such as building trust with patients who are vulnerable, being willing to sacrifice personal comfort by confronting human suffering, acting with courage amid uncertainty, to name a few—professionalism appears to be a mere social veneer that, as the elite, doctors must accept. This student was unable to connect medical professionalism to the virtues and qualities it was intended to inspire—not surprising when professionalism is primarily defined by technical competence or prescriptive behaviors.

Medical school accrediting bodies conceptualize professionalism as a technical project that can be observed and assessed wholly separate from other domains of medical practice.[36] Most fail to see that professionalism is actually "the way that morally excellent clinicians practice."[37] As a result, most medical schools teach professionalism in a manner that perpetuates ideas about the distance and objectivity needed to provide technical care that conceals the fundamental human elements of medicine, and that alienates students and clinicians from themselves. One doctor Arthur Kleinman interviewed for his book *The Illness Narratives* explains the inadequacies of the "mask" of professionalism that pervades medical practice:

> Later, at night, you begin to think. No persona or mask then. Then it hits you: all the complexity, the threat to your sensitivity of the realities of personal tragedy and the social consequences of your actions. After midnight, the professional protection is gone. You, you feel very alone, vulnerable. The magnitude of the moral effects of your decisions and actions become upsetting images, intruding thoughts that keep you awake or, worse still, become dreams, nightmares. That is the hour of truth for the clinician. For most of us who struggle to be authentic in our work it is bad enough. But for those who hide their humanity behind professional and institutional barriers, who can't handle the human side of sickness, it must be awful. No one prepares you for this, this assault on your sense of being—a much more troubling and difficult-to-shake feeling than the self-questioning about the limits of our professional competency.[38]

The limitations and inadequacies of medical professionalism and professionalism education have significant personal consequences for doctors, medical students, and patients alike. Frederic Hafferty argues that, if we are going to advocate for a professionalism based on the transformation of medical students and practitioners at the level of "core value and self-identity," then we must call for a fundamentally different educational program, one that goes well beyond confronting professionalism at the level of attitudes and behavior.[39] He calls on us to ask what we expect of medical students: "Do we expect them to *learn* about professionalism—*appreciate* key professionalism principles—*behave* in professionally appropriate ways? Or do we expect them to *identify* with the precepts of professionalism, *be* or *become* professionals, and make these precepts part of their core identity?"[40] Simply adding more rule- or competency-based approaches will not address the conflict between tacit and explicit values, speak to issues of "core identity," or change in any significant way the dominant culture of medicine.

Professional Identity Formation In light of such critiques, some scholars have advocated for developmental models that conceptualize professionalism as a process or journey, a continual striving toward principles and virtues, rather than merely the display of specific attributes.[41] Though some might claim that it does not *really* matter what physicians believe as long as they *act* professionally, the ambiguities and uncertainty of the clinical experience—which require practical reason, wisdom, and intuition—require a "professional presence that is best grounded in who one *is* rather than what one *does*."[42] As such, clinicians and educators have begun to move beyond the static term "professionalism" and toward a discussion of "professional identity formation." Often influenced by the work of Inui and Hafferty, scholars within the movement typically see professional identity formation as the foundational and transformational process medical students experience during their transition from laypersons to physicians.[43] These scholars conceive of the transformation as "an integrative developmental process that involves the establishment of core values, moral principles, and self-awareness."[44] The emphasis here on transformation is particularly important because it alludes to the idea that professional identity formation is integral to—or perhaps even synonymous with—the medical student's journey of *becoming* a doctor. The notion of "becoming" is central to professional identity formation because it emphasizes the idea that medical education is not simply a type of training or the acquisition of new technical skills, but rather a process of socialization—the "melding of knowledge and skills with an altered sense of self."[45] Inui suggests that such identity formation should include reflection, increased knowledge of the self and of the field, and "constant attention" to one's inner life and one's life in action.[46]

Although a clear step in the right direction, the professional identity formation movement is not without its shortcomings. The assessment of students' professional identity formation is still largely contingent on domains, subdomains, objectives, and competencies.[47] This presents two conceptual problems: (1) "competencies" implies that mastery or completion of certain aspects of professional identity is possible and expected, which works against the idea of journeying or becoming; and (2) distinguishing between "personal" identity—the "inner self"—and "professional" identity can be confusing. In my view, encouraging a "turning-toward the other" and fostering the courage to confront vulnerability and intense human suffering require developing not just students' professional identities, but their whole selves as well (a point discussed in greater detail below).

So, even though developmental approaches to professionalism claim that the formation of students' professional identities involves much more than *behaving* professionally in the clinical setting, taken together, these approaches are limited by their failure to address personal suffering and struggles or the anxiety produced by the realities of human vulnerability and mortality—realities encountered time and again in medical practice. What is more, it seems that proponents of the professional identity formation movement have presupposed the necessity of virtue development, mentorship, and the moral integration of the self without fully developing what these ideas entail. To me, a clearer understanding of the virtue ethics of Aristotle (and also of Alasdair MacIntyre) would serve both to bolster the claims of the movement and to provide the nuanced understandings of care and altruism we need to reorient our focus toward a pedagogy that emphasizes authentic engagement with the other, moral clarity, and integration of the self.

Professionalism and Virtue Ethics Emphasizing the development or "becoming" of the individual, though not unique to professional identity formation, is an important addition to the professionalism movement. There is noticeable congruency among descriptions of contemporary medical professionalism, primarily because ideas about being a *virtuous person* usually serve as their foundation.[48] This suggests to me that most conceptualizations of professionalism that call for something more than behaviors, skills, or attitudes take as their philosophical grounding Aristotelian virtue ethics.[49]

Generally, virtue ethics emphasizes not only the "right actions" of moral agents but also their *being*, the character that both influences and is cultivated by the agents' engaged activity in the world. Thus the question such ethics takes as central is, What does it mean to be "the right sort of person?"[50] Like philosophers such as Levinas and like feminist scholars, virtue ethicists within the field of medicine point to the failure of general, universal principles or rules to attend to the specifics of "the unique nature of each human being," and they maintain that the good or morally virtuous physician does not rely *only* on principles but takes into account the specifics of individual cases and makes decisions based on the best interest of individual patients.[51] Although virtue ethics may not point directly to a specific "right" answer in every ethical dilemma, it encourages the development of the characters of doctors by asking them to consider the virtues necessary for the excellent practice of medicine.

Particularly helpful when thinking about the practice of medicine, Alasdair MacIntyre's virtue ethics lies squarely in the Aristotelian tradition, yet he argues that virtues ultimately find their definition within the particularities of specific practices, defining "practice" as any coherent and complex social activity in which internal goods are realized in the process of achieving standards of excellence within the particular practice.[52] Especially important are the "internal goods" of that practice, which are different from its external, tangible goods. Internal goods can be achieved only through virtuous participation within the practice itself, goods such as learning to listen well, finding a sense of meaning and purpose, refining critical thinking, and so forth. Virtues and engaging in virtuous activities, then, help us to acquire these internal goods.[53] Although a practice like that of medicine requires the exercise of technical skills, it is intrinsically about much more than a set of skills. It includes the entire conception of ends and goods that those skills aim for and enrich. Thus any practice that values the pursuit of *external goods* over all else would first suffer an attrition and attenuation of the notion of virtues, followed by near total abandonment of the virtues themselves, though "simulacra might abound."[54]

The internal goods of medicine and the virtues (or dispositions) that allow practitioners to achieve those internal goods are determined by the end, aim, or telos of the practice of medicine. According to Edmund

Pellegrino, who looks to the Hippocratic oath for guidance, the end or aim to which medicine is directed is "the good of the patient."[55] This good is not limited to cure, he points out, since not all patients can be cured. The good of the patient is the good and right decision for *this* particular patient, which may mean to care for, comfort, be present with, or alleviate the suffering of the patient. In this sense, healing is more than curing, for healing still can occur even when a patient is dying.[56] To be *good* doctors, then, practitioners must regularly and predictably embody certain dispositions that allow them to do their work well.[57] For William May, the virtues of doctors include, at minimum, a measure of charity and good faith in dealing with others, humility before their power and knowledge; the discipline to seek wisdom rather than "showing off"; the integrity not to pretend to have more certainty than they have; and enough bravery to act when they must, even in the face of uncertainty.[58] Although *behaving* professionally might be part of being virtuous, it is certainly not the whole of it. That is to say, however necessary it may be, professionalism education is insufficient for the cultivation of virtuous healers: the character or moral excellence of physicians is distinctly different from their technical skills and cannot be produced or assessed in the same way.[59] Many medical novices have to first concentrate on honing technical skills that might later become second nature, thereby allowing the time and energy for other virtues to flourish.[60] But virtuous novices, whether trainees or practicing doctors, recognize *why* developing their technical skills matters at all—which is to care well for the patients they encounter—and also to discern how to employ these skills and personally respond to the persons before them. Doing so requires practical, reflective, and moral discernment, or phronesis. In the *Nicomachean Ethics*, Aristotle argues that phronesis, which he says is associated with "action" and "things human," is different from the other intellectual virtues including *technē* (technical skill), *sophia* (philosophical wisdom), *nous* (intuitive reason), and *episteme* (scientific knowledge).[61] The function of phronesis, unlike that of technical skills, is not to "produce" anything, but rather to direct human action in a particular way in order to achieve the internal goods consistent with the end of a particular, concrete practice.[62] As Hans-Georg Gadamer points out, phronesis is needed when we are responding to a person in a specific situation; we do not acquire this kind of knowledge beforehand and then deploy it later, as we would "an objective skill, a *technē*."[63] Rather, we always already find ourselves in a situation where we must act, which requires in-the-moment deliberation that considers both the means and ends of actions.[64]

Determining what a specific situation calls for, both clinically and interpersonally or morally, requires that doctors discern the medically and morally salient features of a situation that require a response.[65] Only after recognizing these features are they able to determine the right end of action in that situation and then make a wise choice. But Aristotle makes it clear that it is not possible to have such discernment without being a good person, and it is not possible to be a good or virtuous person if one lacks moral and practical discernment.[66] The wise doctor, however, can be counted on by students, colleagues, and patients to be not only truthful, hardworking, and fair, but also compassionate, skilled, and kind—a doctor someone would trust with a loved one during the crisis of that person's life.[67] Physicians of practical wisdom do not *need* prescriptive codes or guidelines to tell them how to act virtuously.[68] They are able to discern *for themselves* (though still in relationship and dialogue with others) what is the best, most virtuous action to take in the given situation at hand.

Because phronesis is the ability to discern and then decide the right action for *particular* circumstances embedded within the situation in which we find ourselves (as opposed to theoretical quandaries), Aristotle makes it very clear that it is experience and activity in the world that allow us to develop phronesis. Doctors' ability to recognize what needs doing in a real-life situation is developed and honed over time through their actual practical work.[69] An important caveat, however, is that such practical experience cannot cultivate phronesis without the guidance and mentorship of someone who is wiser and more experienced than the learner. In order to know the good of medicine and what it means to care well for patients, students must have good teachers or mentors to help them discern what the good is.[70] That is to say, medical students learn what is most clinically or morally salient in a situation—and how to respond to that situation—through watching and practicing alongside their mentors.[71] Just as students learn from their more experienced mentors the correct way to palpate the abdomen—where to place their hands, what they should feel for, how to percuss, what to listen for—so they also learn from their mentors how they should respond to patients, what questions to ask, what words to pay attention to, how to decipher what "matters" and what does not. Because our assumptions (about medicine, for instance, or about what we "owe" to others more generally) influence what we see as relevant or as requiring a response, the particular assumptions guiding a mentor's perspective can either challenge or cement the learner's own assumptions. The virtuous mentor, for example, who responds to the moral, emotional, or interpersonal dimensions of the clinical situation can attune students to these issues, communicating to them that doctors are in fact called to address their patients' emotional or existential suffering.

Through their experiences with virtuous mentors, students can critically reflect upon and (re)negotiate the presumptions guiding their interpretations of the situations in which they find themselves. Virtuous mentors, then, do not simply "tell" students how to respond to patients in any procedural way, but help sensitize students to the circumstances that require action by actively engaging with students—by expressing to them how they personally see the situation and how they feel about it, highlighting the relevant considerations, concepts, and emotions embedded in the situation at hand. The hope is that with enough time and habitual practice alongside experienced mentors who have lived complex lives and have "witnessed and judged not abstractly and at a safe distance but up close," students' sentiments, emotions, and practical reason can be guided and refined as they grow toward becoming virtuous physicians.[72]

It is for this reason that Coulehan believes the first requirement for a necessary and significant change in current medical professionalism education is to dramatically increase the number of clinicians who are able to "role-model professional virtue at every stage of medical education."[73] As novice apprentices, students can observe the importance of attending to practical moral considerations and to the human particulars of cases, but, absent opportunities to emulate and engage with mentors adept in the exercise of phronesis, they will lack the experience necessary for cultivating the habit of reflective deliberation. And even with such mentors, medical students and practitioners are not immune to the undermining influences of their larger institutions, which are often concerned with external goods and structured in terms of status and power. Though it is true that the external goods institutions seek may be necessary to sustain the practices that they support (profits of hospitals being necessary for patient care, for instance), the ideals and internal goods of practice remain vulnerable to the materialism and competiveness of institutions. Thus the ideal formation of the student-physician can be undermined by an institution that values efficiency and productivity over engaged and empathic patient care. And given that academic medical institutions are fairly reluctant to view themselves as sites of personal or moral transformation, the development or attrition of virtue, left unaddressed at the level of the formal curriculum, is addressed instead at the individual level by mentors interacting with their students (e.g., "This is how we *really* do things around here"). As a result, many students "struggle profoundly" to understand the disconnect between the explicit values of professionalism they are taught in the classroom and the implicit values communicated through some of their experiences with faculty mentors on the wards.[74]

When Mentors Behave Badly

Because mentorship is so critical to the identity formation of medical students and residents and their development of phronesis and clinical reasoning, when we think about who they are becoming, particular attention should be paid to the interpersonal interactions with their mentors that convey what it means to be a doctor.[75] And if it is true that some students and residents are left feeling confused, belittled, and impoverished by these interactions, then perhaps we should be worried about the kinds of doctors and future mentors the medical education system is creating. In 1990, in response to two of the first studies that highlighted medical student abuse inflicted by faculty and house staff, clinician and educator Jerald Kay published an editorial in the *Journal of the American Medical Association*.[76] Kay suggested that students' "brief, albeit painfully intense" experiences with their mentors could often "undercut [their] sense of self-worth . . . and contribute to a lowering of [their] ideals about their teachers and medicine itself" and that, when they did, these experiences were best characterized as "traumatic deidealizations."[77] The "cumulative trauma" that medical students endured was trauma to the human psyche caused by "day-to-day unempathic responses" and by participating in the "toxicity of a learning milieu that fails to recognize student mistreatment or considers student abuse inconsequential."[78]

In 2014, medical educator and editor in chief David Sklar reviewed articles on student and resident mistreatment that had appeared in the pages of *Academic Medicine* over the years.[79] Describing this mistreatment as intentional or unintentional behavior that disrespects the dignity of others and unreasonably interferes with learning (e.g., sexual harassment, discrimination, public humiliation, psychological or physical punishment), Sklar underscored the fact that such mistreatment was still a very real and very common problem in medicine.[80] In fact, a 2014 study of twenty-four American medical schools indicated that 64 percent of medical students reported a least one instance of mistreatment by faculty and 76 percent reported being mistreated by residents.[81] And in a 2016 article, physicians William Bynum and Brenessa Lindeman reported that "disrespectful behavior masquerading as 'necessary' teaching methods remains common, and the belief that 'you remember what is yelled at you' permeates many learning environments."[82] Such reports suggest that medical student mistreatment is part of the "fabric of our institutional environments" and a problem that requires "innovative thinking for its solution."[83]

What is most troubling about the mistreatment of medical students and residents is that it comes at the hands of their mentors. And this is why the concept of "deidealization" is so critical. The mistreatment by these mentors violates residents' and students' expectations of the practice of medicine and what it means to be a doctor. But it is important to recognize that deidealizing mentorship can be subtle. Many of the students with whom I spoke would not admit to being overtly "mistreated" or "abused" by their clinical mentors, though some of them did share instances (particularly in the operating room) that I certainly would consider overt mistreatment. Still, all of them seemed to sense a significant disparity between what they expected the practice of medicine would be like and the reality of being on the wards, and all of them recounted instances where the behavior of their mentors defied their ideas and assumptions about what it meant to be a doctor. As a third-year medical student told me, "More often than not, my attendings and residents are condescending and infantilizing, to both students and patients" (MSIII-7).

This is not the only student who used the word "infantilizing" to describe the attitude of mentors on clinical rotations. Students I talked to said they felt like they spent most of their time in the hospital "shadowing" residents and attendings, "trying to stay out of the way," and desperately attempting not to "look bad" on rounds. As another third-year explained:

As students, we roll into the hospital before the sun and start prerounding. There are so many patients and so little time, and the ultimate goal of the morning becomes not looking foolish when it's time for rounds. I'm too often left with the terrible dilemma of either cutting patient interactions short or spending quality time with all of them and then being underprepared for rounds and looking bad in front of my attending. (MSIII-6)

For this student, the clinical years of medical school felt more like a time to impress clinical mentors and stay out of trouble than to care well for patients. For him and other students, it sometimes felt as though they ought to act professionally for the sake of their grades rather than for the sake of establishing trust with patients, a byproduct of the competitive and sometimes hostile learning environment in which they found themselves. Even though research shows adult learning, especially in clinical education, requires that students be treated with respect and granted relative autonomy—that is, "supportive autonomy" grounded in dialogue, listening, and nonantagonistic question asking—this kind of learning does not always occur on the wards.[84] In fact, Thomas Beckman and Mark Lee have found that clinical teachers "rarely use the adult learning principles of encouraging dialogue, asking questions, and giving meaningful feedback."[85] With the result that many if not most students are hesitant to speak up or ask questions for fear of looking "stupid" or unprepared, and most of their energy is spent impressing mentors who may not embody the qualities of a virtuous physician themselves. As Kinghorn bleakly puts it:

> It is unreasonable to expect that students and residents will develop the excellences of professionalism if those excellences are not valued by and embodied in their teachers. The most important thing that an institution can do, if it values professionalism, is to recruit, support, and retain teachers of moral and clinical excellence. If this is not done, every other professionalism initiative or program is likely to fail. . . . [S]tudents are fed moral platitudes in their preclinical medical curriculum and then are sent out to the wards where their real moral medical education begins. The problem is that this education is more often than not an education in vice rather than moral excellence, as students internalize and then replicate the unprofessional attitudes and practices of their residents and attendings.[86]

It should be said, however, that despite this tendency, there are excellent clinical mentors in medical education who are committed to their patients and their students and who are dedicated to cultivating future healers.[87] But, more often than not, students who struggle to embody virtuous qualities do so most often *in spite of* their less than admirable mentors. Recently, a third-year medical student told me about an experience he had with a young pediatric patient and her mother. The medical team he belonged to was frustrated with the mother, believing that she refused to be "compliant" with her daughter's medication regimen, which was leading to the daughter's unremitting seizures. This student felt frustrated, too, until he met and spoke with the mother and daughter:

> And then something happened. I sat down and talked to the mom at six in the morning before I was overwhelmed with note-writing, learning issues, physical exam points, and listened to her. It was so simple but so enlightening. It gave me all the confidence I needed on rounds that day to actually make a difference. I didn't need to know the answer to all the questions on rounds, but I could speak up because I felt like I knew the patient's story and concerns. If anyone would have just listened to the mom, they would have known why she was changing the medicine and what was actually going on and how much she was struggling inside with all that was happening with her daughter.... We get so bogged down with expectations that we forget who we are representing on rounds and who we need to be worried about. Yeah, maybe it will mean I look like a fool sometimes on rounds and won't know the answers, but this mom has a daughter who is seizing thirty times an hour. I can take the humiliation if it means letting me have some time to sit down and hear my patients. (MSIII-8)

This student's account of his realization—when he saw how crucial the story of the patient and family was to providing good medical care—is encouraging. "Morally sound clinical care," Ronald Carson explains, "begins and ends with the patient's experience. Every ordinary encounter between a patient and a physician necessarily begins with the patient's story, which is an invitation to a conversation."[88] And yet this student came to this realization, at least from his perspective, at the expense of potentially looking "like a fool" on rounds since taking the time to hear the mother's story took away from his time for "note-writing, learning issues, and physical exam points," the "real stuff" of medicine that he ought to be doing in order to impress his residents and attendings. It is rather distressing that this student risked humiliation by taking the time to sit down with patients to hear their story, even when doing so could lead to better clinical care, as it did in this instance.

So, even when clinical mentors do not mistreat students outright, by suggesting to them—whether explicitly or implicitly through their own actions—that clinical practice requires emotional detachment from patients and their families and the ability to simply stick to the "facts," they can derail the students' development as healers. Statements of the need for clinical detachment undermine the idea that clinical education is necessarily a moral education that involves the whole person who is called to care for others in need.[89]

Development of the Virtuous—Whole—Person The notion of "whole person" is critical to medical education, especially if the system does, in fact, change students at the deep level of core values and identity, for better or worse. Although it can be met with resistance, especially by those directly affected, it is my view that training in and the practice of medicine cannot be confined to what medical students and practitioners *do*, something that can be contained and separated from who they *are* outside the clinic.

Speaking to this point, MacIntyre suggests that, though they are defined in terms of practices, virtues are exercised *not only* within these practices.[90] The virtue of constancy or integrity of a person, for example, must include some knowledge of the person's whole life, not merely knowledge of the decisions that person makes in a particular role or within a particular practice. Virtues, then, cannot be conceived of as synonymous with professional skills because genuine virtues manifest in situations beyond particular practices, and anyone "who genuinely possesses a virtue can be expected to manifest it in very different types of situation(s)."[91] Furthermore, when a sharp distinction is made between individuals themselves and the roles they play, the "unity of human life" remains hidden.[92] For MacIntyre, the unity of the self resides within the unity of the narrative embodied in its life, a narrative that links birth, life, and death. When we interpret and evaluate our actions within distinct contexts rather than within our whole life narratives, our lives begin to look like unconnected episodes, and our selves are dispersed into the prescribed roles we play.[93]

To be sure, this does not mean that physicians and medical students need to "behave professionally" in every situation, in every relationship, and in every context, simply because they are or will be doctors. Indeed, the integration of the self is not about behavior—or restricting behavior—at all. It is, rather, about doctors' cultivating and living by deep values that guide their decisions inside and outside the clinic. Psychiatrist and educator Robert Coles wonders if it is right to separate our personal or private lives from our working lives.[94] He concludes that a "person's work is part of a person's life, and the two combined as lifework must be seen as constantly responsive to the moral decisions that we never stop making, day in and day out."[95] On the other hand, the workplace may actually work *against* personal growth, precisely because it fosters the polarization and compartmentalization of personal and private life.[96] This is, in part, a result of our reluctance to accept the working environment as something that shapes who we are, an environment in which we cannot separate our personal from our working selves—even though the workplace is just another "long-term human context," such as community, family, or marriage, "which, like it or not becomes a culture for a person's growth."[97]

Ethicist and medical humanist David Barnard claims that, though some distinction between the personal and the professional is necessary in medical practice, a strict distinction between them seems to deny that physicians are affected by their personal encounters with other human beings.[98] For Barnard, we are beings who seek love and meaning in the face of suffering and death, and the clinical encounter is a meeting between two such human beings.[99] Doctors are thus called to acknowledge the existential questions that inevitably arise in clinical encounters, lest they become estranged from their own being.[100] Kumagai makes a similar argument:

> At least as commonly defined, the concept of professionalism implies a dichotomy between professional and personal, public and private selves. In other words, one can be a real professional on the job all the while he or she is terribly unethical in private. *Phronesis*, on the other hand, involves the person as a unified whole, what Heidegger would call a "Being-in-the-World," and the dichotomy between private and professional, personal and public, belief and action doesn't apply.[101]

It is for this reason that redirecting medical education away from professionalism as prescribed behavior and toward the cultivation of the whole person who is becoming a doctor is so critical. Ignoring the human experiences in medicine that affect how doctors and medical students see themselves and understand the world works against the cultivation of empathy, compassion, and connection. It is in moving our focus away from the doctor as a technical problem solver that we begin to appreciate the doctor as a person who is also striving for meaning, purpose, and contentment in this life. When we begin to understand that the clinical encounter is a meeting of two persons who both seek to find meaning, we can see that both have the potential to gain new insights and to be heard and known. But, in contemporary medicine and medical ethics, emphasis is placed almost exclusively on the patient's need to be heard and recognized in the clinical encounter, and understandably so. Too often, patients' stories are lost in medicine's dominant discourse that reduces authentic dialogue to narrow question-asking and note-taking. Yet, what is overlooked is that the physician is also transformed in this encounter and receives something in this meeting with the other. That is to say, doctors come to know themselves and *become* themselves through the other they encounter.

When we can recognize that, in responding to suffering, the doctor also receives something from the encounter, our understanding of professionalism changes. We come to see that professionalism is not simply a conglomeration of competencies or observable traits, but rather a *way of being*, a lived posture of openness to and gratitude for the other, a deep appreciation for the patient—which comes from a recognition of the mutual giving and receiving that takes place in the clinical encounter. It is no wonder that, viewed as a science that responds efficiently and effectively to functional loss, medicine places such emphasis on objectivity and technical efficiency, the two things required to make this kind of scientific work possible. Yet, as Carson explains: "Medical practice, . . . contrary to the view of it as applied science, is experiential, relational, and hermeneutical through and through."[102] It is this experiential, relational, and hermeneutical nature of medicine that calls for a different or *meditative* way of thinking, one that does not reduce patients to the biological workings of their bodies or medicine to a set of technical skills, but that allows for authentic moments of ambiguity, uncertainty, grief, connection, and awe. Yet how can we cultivate this kind of meditative thinking among doctors in training? How can we encourage this way of thinking that not only imbues the mainstream medical approach with different ways of knowing and understanding, but also cultivates a comportment of openness, authenticity, and gratitude?

Attempting to Form "Good Doctors": The Distraction of Assessment

As part of the larger culture of medicine, medical education in many ways follows a path paved with the ideals of objectivity, clarity, and efficiency—and professionalism training is no exception. Because medical practitioners and educators are so deeply entrenched in this way of seeing and doing things, anything that does not fit neatly into a rubric or cannot be measured or quantified becomes suspect, for it appears to fall outside the culture of modern medicine specifically and contemporary Western thought more generally. As a result, the narrowly predefined behaviors of medical professionalism significantly delimit clinicians' engagement with their patients. Frank explains that, as a patient, "I do not want my questions answered; I want my experiences shared. But the stress and multiple demands on physicians and nurses too often push such sharing outside the boundaries

The Formation of Medical "Professionals"

of 'professional' activity."[103] Moving away from a narrow conception of professional activities and toward the cultivation of an expansive virtuous self open to connecting with others is impeded by both the admission requirements for and the grading system within medical school, as well as by the requirements for residency and future job placement. According to May, even though these "well-enough known" elements of medical education are "much criticized," paradoxically, they remain "impervious to criticism" and continue to prioritize technical and quantifiable skills as before.[104] They do so because the practical and moral warrants for the ideals of technical performance and measureable outcomes are seldom considered seriously. Rather, it simply is assumed that the best—and perhaps the only—way to assess medical professionalism is through rubrics, predefined competencies, objective assessments, and measurable outcomes. Indeed, assumptions about teaching and evaluating professionalism are yet another instantiation of the calculative thinking that has come to dominate Western medicine.

In that regard, the students I spoke with stated that they were often evaluated by faculty members with whom they spent very little time and who rarely, if ever, saw them interact with patients. Instead, students were assessed primarily for their ability to provide accurate and succinct case presentations and to answer correctly the questions directed to them by faculty and residents on rounds. Students felt that the faculty did not know them well enough to evaluate their ability to become "good doctors," nor did these students receive consistent, timely, or useful feedback either from faculty or from patients, peers, nurses, social workers, or anyone else they encountered on their rounds that would help them improve. Instead, the behaviors of these students were assessed and graded by "objective" scales that lacked the nuance or sensitivity to assess their personal formation and integration.

Calls for objective assessment tools to measure students' professionalism abound, suggesting that there might exist some way to "make certain" that students have mastered their professionalism competencies. It is as if verifying that students exhibit professional behavior—based on relatively shallow indicators and benchmarks—is more important than actually fostering professionalism within the students at a deep and personal level.

Could it be that we might place less emphasis on "objective" assessment and evaluation of medical students if we trusted the process of medical education, if we knew that students were receiving quality mentorship from skilled, virtuous, and compassionate physicians? Is it possible that that the narrow focus on professionalism assessments obscures the larger issue: students are *not* receiving the kind of mentorship that might help them grow into the doctors we want them to be—and the doctors *they* want to be? If it is actually the case that students rarely interact meaningfully with quality clinical mentors, no evaluation tools—no matter how "accurate"—are going to remedy the problem we face in medical education. The current evaluation process, which assesses how well students perform under pressure in front of faculty during rounds, may in fact be exacerbating the problem. As Jack Coulehan and Peter Williams point out, the rigor, intensity, and abusiveness of medical training tends to undermine professionalism and to produce instead a self-interested sense of entitlement to prestige, high compensation, and social influence—all in clear violation of the expressed tenets of professionalism.[105]

It is troubling to learn that the evaluation processes intended to ensure that we are educating good doctors might be doing just the opposite. But it is perhaps more troubling to learn that many medical students do not even realize that the behavior they believe will get them a good evaluation is directly contrary to the espoused virtues of professionalism. In what Coulehan and Williams call "non-reflective professionalism," students and physicians consciously espouse traditional medical values, while remaining unaware that much of their behavior is based on beliefs that contradict these values.[106] Because the explicit commitment in medicine to empathy and compassion is often overridden by the tacit commitment to an ethic of detachment or the epistemological virtue of objectivity, students and doctors most often "reconcile" these conflicting commitments by believing that the best way to manifest explicit values is to embrace tacit values.[107] Those who engage in such nonreflective professionalism tend to confuse self-interest with the best interest of patients, convincing themselves that the medical culture of efficiency and detachment does indeed serve the deepest needs of patients. A student confronted with this conflict in medical values might genuinely believe that the best way to show compassion is to remain clinically detached or to substitute technical interventions for personal engagement. And such a belief would be reinforced by our contemporary Western culture, which places such a high value on calculative thinking.

The existence of nonreflective professionalism points yet again to the need for reflection and dialogue in medical education. Like those who see professionalism as something more than the behaviors practitioners exhibit while engaged in a specific role, Inui calls on educators to help medical students "re-integrate personhood and professionalism," which can, in part, be achieved through reflection and open and honest discussion about how they think and feel as individuals about matters of value, morality, limitations, and the like.[108] Encouraging students to reflect on their experiences can help them make sense of troubling events and give voice to the inconsistencies and value conflicts within medical practice that are so often ignored. Rather than simply telling students what it means to be professional or attempting to control their behavior through prescriptive codes and rules, educators need to shift their attention to the students as persons; they need to encourage students to ask themselves why they chose to become doctors in the first place, what kind of doctors they want to be, what they think will bring a sense of meaning and purpose to their lives, and what it means to care for others well. Educators need to, as Heidegger might say, "leap ahead" of students in order to help them discover *for themselves* what it means to be good doctors. This kind of engagement with students "does not so much leap in for the Other as leap ahead of him in his existential potentiality-for-Being, not in order to take away his 'care' but rather to give it back to him authentically as such for the first time. This kind of solicitude pertains essentially to authentic care . . . it helps the Other to become transparent to himself *in* his care and become *free* for it."[109] Rather than "leaping in" and teaching codes or rules, medical educators can encourage students to uncover *for themselves* who they want to be in their life of medicine.

The practice of medicine is filled with moments imbued with questions about life, death, suffering, and even joy, and "leaping in" for students by implicitly communicating that the best way to approach such moment is by remaining "professional" and detached can take away students' potential for authentic patient care. However, by taking time to reflect on their experiences during training, students can become active participants in their development.[110] What we need, then, is a pedagogical approach that awakens students to the existential realities of medical practice and encourages self-reflection and authentic engagement with others. We need to encourage a "professionalism" that is expansive enough to allow students, residents, and doctors, in Frank's words, "to share in" the experiences of patients. We need to help students authentically encounter others and to find their own voices, especially considering that "when in the presence of human suffering, the language of medicine is often silent."[111]

Even though engaging with others, relying on social support, and expressing emotion have been shown to help students respond in ways that promote their adaptation, reduce their anxiety and depression, and improve their well-being, medical students seldom reflect on their training experiences.[112] And even though some U.S. medical schools have successfully incorporated reflective writing into their formal curricula, throughout most of their clinical experiences, students and residents are often not given the opportunity to openly express feelings evoked by even the most traumatic experiences.[113] After considering the lack of discussion following patient deaths, Katharine Treadway explains:

> Because we cannot comfortably express these feelings, sometimes we put them away forever or feel incompetent and overwhelmed when we do try to express them. Perhaps if we could discuss this part of our practice lives as easily as we discuss a diagnostic dilemma or the proper management of a complex case, we might create a culture that supports and nourishes us as we try to come to terms with experiences that are part of our daily lives.[114]

What would it look like for students, residents, and faculty to "comfortably express" emotion and discuss the difficult, profound, and beautiful parts of medical practice? What does reflection look like in medical education?

The term "reflection" suggests a "turning back" of our attention to ourselves or our experiences. In the context of medical education, many of those who advocate for this turning back usually consider reflection to be an undeniably worthy and beneficial endeavor. But however undeniable the need for greater reflection in medical practice and training, some medical educators have rightly pointed out that this emphasis on personal reflection ought to be considered critically.[115] Particularly in the rational, technical, objective world of Western medicine, personal reflection can readily degenerate into an individualistic, narcissistic, problem-solving pursuit that perpetuates notions of personal power and autonomy. To keep that from happening, medical students engaging in reflective dialogue or writing should be encouraged to be critical of the institutional and political frameworks of medicine as it is practiced, as well as the presuppositions they hold about themselves and others.[116]

With personal reflection, we consider not only our experiences, reactions, and feelings, but also the conditions and discourses that shape our identities and constitute our norms. Although reflective dialogue with others can occur anywhere, including on the wards, personal reflection should occur in spaces where students can freely express their critical, affective, or concerned thoughts and experiences.[117] Such reflection can contribute to the "development of personal values and an orientation toward oneself, others, and the world . . . an *understanding*, which may be defined as a deep and abiding engagement with the human aspects of illness and medical care."[118]

Although such spaces for personal reflection can be carved out intentionally in the medical school curriculum in the form of workshops, courses, or small group discussions, they need not be defined by a specific locale or label. They can be wherever students feel it necessary to take the time to acknowledge and reflect upon the human dimensions of medicine.[119] This is not to say that students are unable to reflect privately on their own, through personal writing or creative self-expression, for instance. Indeed, reading and writing can prompt reflection, and this process is closely associated with the activity of reflective dialogue.[120] But reflection can be made richer when carried out in a group or facilitated by a mentor—that is, when participants are able share their reflections and identify shared experiences and common fears or triumphs (a point to be pursued in chapter 5).[121]

To push against the modernist biomedical paradigm that dominates medicine and create a space where genuine reflection can occur, Jonanna Shapiro believes we need role models who are reflective themselves, who "express vulnerability, share mistakes, incorporate not-knowing; who are aware of and transparent about their emotional reactions to patients . . . and most importantly, who acknowledge common bonds of humanity with their patients."[122] Students are generally unaware that they develop their identities primarily through their interactions with mentors, who should reflect on and remain cognizant of the influential role they play in students' development.[123] And this point needs to be made explicit to students and faculty alike. Indeed, if we want students to become more reflective about who they are becoming during medical school, encouraging reflective practice among clinical mentors is critical and will require additional faculty training and development.[124]

Undoubtedly, asking students to become more reflective, especially if it requires them to write, will be met with some resistance. The crowded medical school curriculum and the pressures to perform well on tests and impress faculty with their clinical acumen tend to make students feel as if there is no time to "slow down" and reflect. Yet it is important to remember that reflection can occur at any time and in any place and need not require significant additions to the medical curriculum.[125] That said, in teaching medical students and facilitating reflective sessions, I have found students are grateful for a space to decompress and hungry to reflect on clinical experiences that seem to be something happening *to* them rather than something they are freely participating in. A third-year medical student and friend of mine, for instance, posted to his Facebook page an experience he had with a clinical mentor earlier that day:

"He has cancer," and then I took a pause.
    I am tender. Can I say that or will I be disciplined? "I am tender," I told the man who lectured me. Ah! He could smell, see, and hear my declaration. . . . "You are here to learn the opposite," he told me in an annoyingly roundabout way. Ah! Of course, that makes perfect sense. Tenderness is an adjective we, the objective bodies in charge of the crossroads of illness, have limited to solely convey the physical pain of the other. I am sorry but I've forgotten that I must now and always speak in a way that reflects my training (or status?) in our society. . . . The man and those like him, they probably once were tender, and then the crisis happened. I must talk about defense mechanisms that we all quite personally understand are necessary to remain stable. In one piece and in one place, neither here or there, I reside where I am stable and synonymously safe. In regards to protection, a shield should be somewhat effective if appropriately selected. Oh no, though! I refuse to accept that one shield, forged in the culture of effectiveness and emotional austerity, is or should be mine. I am tender, and I am very okay. Death is as old as the stars; celestial in its own right. Let's respect and be humble in its presence.[126]

Inui warns us that, as students move through their experience in medical school, they also move "from being open-hearted and empathetic to being emotionally well defended, from idealistic to cynical about medicine, medical practice, and the life of medicine."[127] This is an important reminder for those of us who are concerned about the cultivation and formation of medical students; it reminds us that it is often the case that students come to medical school with tenderness and openheartedness and a capacity for empathic care, only to experience a diminution and attrition in all of these, due in part to their experiences on the wards and in larger part to their encounters with mentors. A fourth-year medical student told me that her first experiences on the wards were jarring and "disenchanting" because she was "too idealistic and naive," believing that she would be there "to make meaningful connections with people," only to find out "that was definitely not the case" after repeated encounters with "overworked attendings who were mean to residents and stressed-out residents who yelled at students" (MSIV-I). Perhaps we should spend less time and effort inculcating students with the express principles of "professional" medical care to maintain the status quo of a harried system, and more in drawing out and nurturing capacities that the students *already possess*. When professionalism is considered in the context of virtue and the integration of the whole person, we can embark upon a new educational pathway that centers on personal moral clarity, authentic engagement, and reflection—one that encourages, not diminishes, openheartedness.

Physician (Re)Formation

A clinical encounter is not a value-free scientific endeavor, but rather a therapeutic engagement of doctor and patient—two people who are, in some deep sense, constituted by each other. It is a meeting in which, if they allow it, both can broaden their personal horizons and be transformed by a shared sense of human vulnerability and suffering. Perhaps, in the end, professionalism is not about behaviors, attitudes, or even competencies, but is instead the capacity of doctors to value their patients for creating opportunities for the existential reflection and mutual transformation that can occur within any therapeutic relationship and to be grateful that these patients have come to them for help.

The doctor mentioned in the prologue of this book reminds us that we have "a deep, deep problem in this country with physician formation." The "insidious" process of his own formation, he says, led to personal burnout and required that he be "loved back" into compassionate care for others. It is my view that part of being "loved back" requires that medical students and physicians become reconnected with one another, with their patients, and with themselves—a process that can begin once they give voice to the human suffering, and even the great joy, that comes with taking care of the sick.[128] It requires that medical students and healthcare professionals acknowledge they are affected by their encounters with patients and that objectivity and calculative thinking go only so far.

The next and final chapter looks at how we might foster connection and reflection within medical and premedical education, particularly emphasizing the role of the medical humanities. It argues that the capacity for compassion, empathy, critical thinking, and humility can be cultivated, but that it will require a new pedagogical culture, one that acknowledges and embraces human suffering and recognizes that it is our encounters with suffering—whether through narrative accounts or personal experiences—that teach us, (re)connect us, and remind us what it truly means to be human.

5 The Journey Back to Oneself: Reimagining Medical Education

It strikes me that medicine should be *the* field where a poetic imagination might flourish. The constant presence of suffering, pain, loss, birth, struggle, and death—these all-too-human experiences and events—requires a poet's grasp of language and understanding.
—Arno K. Kumagai, "On the Way to Reflection"

Developmental approaches to professionalism that value ideas about the journey of becoming a doctor are making considerable strides in medical education. But these approaches are limited by their not taking seriously the fact that medical education significantly contributes to the personal and moral formation of the whole self—a self formed, in part, by the existential anxiety produced in the face of our shared vulnerability and mortality. Because current medical epistemology and pedagogy have their foundation within calculative frameworks that are a result of our desire to flee from this existential anxiety, we need to draw attention to the formative process of medical training and to work toward creating a pedagogical culture that fosters more expansive notions of care, awakens students to the reality of shared human suffering, and encourages reflection and authentic engagement with others.

Creating this kind of change is a tall order, to be sure, but we can take steps that will at least get us closer to a more responsible education of our future healers provided we no longer approach physician formation in the passive, didactic, memorize-and-regurgitate fashion that has come to define so much of medical education. Instead, following Kierkegaard and his Socratic ideal of "indirect communication," we need to bring students back to questions about what it means to be human, to live well, and to care for others—questions they will have to answer for themselves through reflection, self-awareness, and engagement with others.[1] For Kierkegaard, such a process can never take place through didacticism or objective modes of discourse, for such modalities rarely lead to personal insight about our unique perspectives, why we have adopted such perspectives, and what strengths and limitations they create for us.[2] Thus we might say that medical educators and mentors are called to meet students where they are—cognitively, morally, personally—and then to "leap ahead" of them, encouraging them to question their assumptions, or to imagine what it might be like to be someone who is sick, scared, or facing the end of life—revealing to them new ways of seeing, thinking about, and knowing the world and medicine, illness, and care in particular.

As Heidegger reminds us, "There are two kinds of thinking, each justified and needed in its own way."[3] Although calculative thinking has its place in medicine and medical education, a pedagogical culture that supports the personal and moral development of students—and cares for them well—must be infused with meditative thinking and an openness to mystery, uncertainty, and humility in the face of the other who is ill or suffering. Such a culture may help reveal that, because medical knowledge is always situated within the particular lifeworld of the patient, calculative and meditative thinking are intertwined in medicine in complex ways.[4] Any observation or understanding of a patient's "dis-ease" is always an interpretation that requires attention to the patient's story—a realization that can help dissolve the dichotomy between "hard" and "soft" knowledge, between clinical objectivity and empathy, and between biomedicine and the humanities.[5] Helping students recognize that intuition, storytelling, and human connection are intrinsic aspects of the clinical encounter might convince them that a pedagogy that fosters meditative thinking will help make them not only nicer, more compassionate doctors, but also better clinicians and diagnosticians.

Because healing requires authentic engagement, one of the goals of medical education (along with teaching requisite scientific and clinical knowledge) should be to cultivate an authentic understanding of care and healing, which requires students to break free from pervasively narrow perceptions of medicine as fixing, curing, and restoring.[6] Although, from a Heideggerian perspective, authentic being only comes after a resolute return to the world following its total collapse, this, of course, does not mean that medical educators should seek to provoke attacks of anxiety and crises of identity among their students. This would, after all, constitute a "leaping in" for students, "taking over" or "dominating" their journey toward authentic engagement with the world.[7] It does mean, however, that students must slow down and recognize the human elements of medicine, reflect on who they are becoming and want to be, and question the assumptions and values of the systems in which they are participating. I am convinced that incorporating the medical humanities into medical education in an intentional, integrated, and sustained way is what will bring meditative thinking back to medicine and students back to themselves and to others. The medical humanities, with their emphasis on teaching by indirection, pedagogies of suffering, critical reflection, and cultivation of the moral imagination, are precisely what is needed to jostle medicine and medical education out of their narrow epistemological frameworks.

What Are the Medical Humanities?

Although they have been on the scene for almost half a century, there is still little agreement about the aims and scope of the medical humanities or how we might define them.[8] Most would agree, however, that they gather together the wisdom and insight of many disciplines—from literature, philosophy, religion, history, and art to bioethics, visual and disability studies, and the social sciences—in order to foster a richer understanding of the human experience of illness, health, dis/ability, identity, gender, embodiment, and healthcare.[9] Their continued presence in medical schools underscores the fact that medicine gives rise to existential questions about the meaning of life and death and that, at bottom, we humans are the ones medicine serves; without people in need, medicine and healthcare would cease to exist.[10]

Recently, there has been a push in the academic world to change the name of the field to the "health humanities" to emphasize its inclusion of all healthcare professionals.[11] Although I understand—and advocate for—the need to engage with and embrace the contributions of healthcare professionals who may feel marginalized by the term "*medical* humanities," I also believe that we should question the normative meanings of and seek to understand why the terms "medicine" and "medical" are so narrow and exclusive and work toward broadening what they mean and include. That is to say, rather than changing its name, we should instead work toward enriching and nuancing the field and actively seeking opportunities to engage with all professionals within the arena of human health. I am convinced that, when the medical humanities are done well, they embrace diversity and intersectionality, are critical of power, do not rely on canonical knowledge, and are concerned with the "individual and cultural experiences of illness and disability and with the social/structural/political impediments to health and healing,"[12] every bit as much as the "health humanities" might. It is for these reasons, and because so much of the present work draws on medical education and residency training, that I feel comfortable using the term "medical humanities" when proposing pedagogical reforms in medical education.

By helping medical students and practitioners understand their role within broader social, historical, cultural, and emotional contexts, the medical humanities encourage them to *act* in response to their new self-knowledge.[13] Thomas Cole, Nathan Carlin, and Ronald Carson define the "medical humanities" as an "inter- or multidisciplinary field that explores contexts, experiences, and critical and conceptual issues in medicine and healthcare, while supporting professional identity formation."[14] In this sense, the medical humanities are about both thinking through issues related to medicine and healthcare *and* educating future caregivers. Far from having a narrow understanding of medical education and professional identity formation, the authors focus on the ability of the medical humanities to cultivate doctors as persons, "to form individuals who take charge of their own minds, who are free from narrow and unreflective forms of thought, who are compassionate . . . to evoke the humanity *of* students."[15] Informed by the meaning of the Latin *humanitas*—"human feeling"—the medical humanities uphold the educational ideal of combining human feeling with liberal learning and engaged action in the world.[16] Their point, then, is not to encourage healthcare professionals to refine their sensibilities or develop a "civilizing veneer" through the study of classic texts or works of art.[17] It is, rather, to cultivate virtuous caregivers who participate in engaged action in the world—compassionate healers who also think deeply and critically about their relationship to others, to the systems in which they participate, and to the social and cultural context in which they find themselves.[18] In other words, the medical humanities intend to cultivate phronesis, which, as we have noted, is oriented ultimately toward good and virtuous *action in the world*. Although biomedical theory and technical skills are critical to the practice of medicine, the medical humanities, by drawing students back to the non- or pretheoretical *experience* of medicine, remind them to consider its "for-the-sake-of-which."[19] That is to say, the medical humanities can help students and doctors alike consider *why* it is both important and necessary to memorize scientific and clinical information, to refine and employ their technical skills, and to embrace professionalism. Their intent is to help them see that the knowledge and skills they have acquired are for the sake of others—to care for others well and to alleviate their suffering to the greatest extent possible.

In contrast to this view of the medical humanities—a view I believe in and stand by—is that of Jeffrey Bishop, as expressed in his 2008 article "Rejecting Medical Humanism."[20] Though he aims his critique largely at Rita Charon's narrative medicine movement, Bishop contends that medical humanism, as he calls the field, is simply perpetuating a Western metaphysics grounded in efficiency. With their methodological focus on the patient's story and the development of the requisite skills to elicit this story, medical humanism and narrative medicine are being used to get patients "to do what we need them to do."[21] As Bishop puts it:

Medical humanism, like all other humanisms, promises intimacy, but is really about control. . . . Thus, the narrative overlay becomes the tool by which the doctor can sway a patient, to make him or her feel better, to create a therapeutic relationship; indeed, narrative sensibility becomes a therapy itself. The usefulness of humanism is precisely about efficient control of the bodies—the animality—of the body politic, even while humanism thinks of itself as being about emancipating and liberating.[22]

As sweeping a generalization as it may be, Bishop's criticism is important to consider. Though the medical humanities and narrative approaches to the clinical encounter have served to elicit patients' stories, we should take time to consider the motivation behind their doing so. Is the point to understand more fully the complex situatedness of patients as whole persons in order to care for them well, or is it to manipulate patients into "compliance"? Moreover, do narrative approaches create the idea that patients are simply passive texts to be "read" by doctors? In their 1992 article, Nancy King and Ann Folwell Stanford—who are sympathetic to the notion of hearing the patient's story—caution that a monologic, one-sided reading of patients as static texts can "simply become paternalism in modern dress," considering that some physicians may overread or impose personal interpretations onto patients without corroborating their stories with them.[23] And writing in 1994, Anne Hudson Jones warns about the potentially reductive nature of the analogy of patients as texts.[24] So, although Bishop raises valid points, these points had received much consideration from those in the medical humanities, even before he raised them. Indeed, the medical humanities have always taken a critical stance toward medicine and healthcare—perhaps all the more so with the increasing presence of the social sciences and political theory.[25] Issues concerning paternalism, biopolitics, health disparities, and inequalities related to gender, race, ability, and class have been and remain a central concern among medical humanists. Indeed, one would be hard pressed to find a medical humanist who sees the humanities as a handmaiden to reductionistic medicine or who supports the epistemological and metaphysical assumptions guiding contemporary medicine and medical education.

Thus, however they may differ on specific points, medical humanists agree that an exposure to literature, philosophy, history, religious studies, gender studies, the arts, social sciences, and the like is intended neither to manipulate patients nor to make students and doctors appear refined and cultured. The point of studying the history of medicine, for example, is not to glorify the triumphs of scientists and doctors of the past, but rather to draw attention to egregious violations in human subjects research or question the taken-for-granted progress narrative to which most students unknowingly subscribe, in order to show that "unchanging" scientific medical truths are rooted in cultural beliefs and specific, sometimes troubling historical contexts. Exploring such issues not only engenders humility among medical professionals and helps students uncover their own biases, but it also illuminates the social nature of medical discovery and the human relationships that constitute the core of medical practice.[26] Thus medical humanists might ask their students, How have our understandings and explanations of disease and pathophysiology, as well as our beliefs and practices around death and dying, shifted over the past century? How have our ideas about what it means to be human changed over time? What role has public health historically played in medicine? What does this mean for nations who lack necessary healthcare resources, and what role can physicians play in community and global health? Likewise, those informed by philosophy or social theory might ask them how is the body viewed in medicine? Is it a passive object to be assessed by physician-observers? How does gender, culture, or sexuality inscribe themselves onto the body and affect a patient's understanding of illness and medical care? Why is it important to consider embodiment when caring for the sick? Is an individual's health or illness determined only by genetics and behaviors? In what ways do cultural ideas about health, illness, and pathology carry normative assumptions, invoke moral judgments, express prejudice, or even bolster pharmaceutical sales?[27] And if health and illness are significantly determined by social and economic factors, then is access to healthcare a fundamental human right?

These are the just some of the questions that medical humanists might ask to help students determine *for themselves* what it means to be "healthy" or "ill" in our world and how our understandings of illness and medicine—even with all of our seemingly objective scientific knowledge—are historically and socially contingent. Their being able to ask such questions is, for me, what makes the medical humanities uniquely necessary. Medical humanists pose these questions not just to medical students and practitioners, but also to researchers and administrators, indeed, to all those providing healthcare. It is for this reason that the medical humanities are an inherently educational project. If the point of the medical humanities is to create a medical culture that cares well for patients and their families—or perhaps more broadly, to open medicine and society to more expansive notions of health, illness, suffering, and care—then the formation of this culture depends almost entirely on educating those who participate and learn in it. The medical humanities are thus an *engaged* field, one that sees interacting with, teaching, and working alongside healthcare professionals, patients, caregivers, and students as essential to its larger project.

The Medical Humanities and the Moral Imagination

The medical humanities are thus not only an engaged field, but also a very diverse one. There is, however, one thing that unites the disparate disciplines within the medical humanities—whether history or the arts or critical theory or literature—and that is their ability to capture, engage, and educate the moral imagination. Because each discipline engages the moral imagination differently, there are those in the field, especially those with degrees in the medical humanities like myself who, acting as interdisciplinarians, bring various approaches from multiple disciplines to bear on complex questions in medicine in order to educate healers' moral imaginations.[28] Describing the moral imagination as the emotional and intellectual capacity to imagine what it might be like to be in the situation of someone else, Carson goes on to explain:

One of our principal tasks as teachers in the medical humanities is to take our students where we find them, with their own mother tongues of morality, and—with the help of texts and ways of thinking drawn from our disciplines—to help them clarify their moral outlooks, become aware and respectful of other intelligences and sensibilities, and become fluent in their moral thinking.[29]

Offered new ways of seeing the world and cultivating their moral imaginations through literature, poetry, and narrative accounts that express the human experience of medicine and illness, students might begin to recognize their own potential for suffering. Imagination and wonder have the power to jostle them out of their typical ways of thinking and perceiving and take them someplace else—toward understanding, for example, what it might be like to be in the situation of someone who is in need of care.[30] Educating the moral imagination can help a student grow into the kind of doctor patients need—one who, as Carson says, "knows how to listen for the storyline and hear the heartbeat of [patients'] lives."[31]

Although the moral imagination can enable medical students and doctors to enter into authentic therapeutic encounters with their patients,[32] the risk with encouraging them to engage their moral imaginations is that they may suppose they know precisely what their patients feel when, in reality, they do not. That said, the risk may be far greater when they *don't* engage their moral imaginations. As a fourth-year medical student told me:

The other day, the doctors on my team were acting really indignant about a patient who couldn't or didn't want to get up and walk after her surgery, saying that if they were her, they would definitely get up and walk if their doctor asked them to. And I said to myself, "How do you know what you would do if you were a patient? You've never been in this lady's place. You don't know what it's like to be her right now, how much pain she might be in." I feel like all of them need some humility when they talk about patients. (MSIV-7)

Emmanuel Levinas reminds us that we can only ever *approach* the experience of the other before us.[33] As the fourth-year medical student rightly pointed out, what doctors need in order to empathize with patients is humility—not assuming they know the experience of the other, but learning more about the other and imagining what it might be like to be that other, someone who is irreducibly other than themselves. Shekinah Elmore calls this ability the "empathic imagination."[34] Though she recognizes that, as a future doctor, she "can only imagine" what it will be like to be someone else, she maintains that "maybe the 'only' is not so important if the imagining is taken seriously"—in other words, perhaps empathy is possible if we really believe in the power of imagination and wonder and if we believe that patients have just as much to teach students as professors and clinical mentors do.[35] "The mechanism for heartbreak and loss," she says, might not ever be learned in a classroom, but "to varying degrees, we all know loss. We must hold fast to it, thinking about how something very similar runs through the veins of each patient that we see."[36] Although we must hold on to the fact that other persons' experiences exist independently from our own, imagining what it might be like to be frightened, lonely, weak, or in pain can temporarily transport us out of our own experience and into that of another.

The question that remains, however, is whether and how we can educate the moral imagination or cultivate the kind of humility that is necessary to engage it. I would agree with Carson that fostering new ways of interpreting the world and better understanding others' lived experiences can, indeed, be taught—not didactically but by indirection, the way we learn from art, literature, and poetry—through exposure to stories of suffering and strength.[37] So much of a medical student's time is spent attending lectures or watching them online, memorizing information, and learning the "facts" of biomedicine. Teaching by indirection, which is quite different in both content and form, can feel foreign and uncomfortable to students, especially to those who see such teaching as irrelevant to the task at hand—namely, learning "scientific" medicine. But, as most students eventually discover in the course of their training, current medical pedagogy does not prepare them for the all-too-human encounters that constitute the practice of medicine. Rarely are students asked to consider how much they share with their patients. And yet it is possible to uncover and cultivate an empathetic connection in students—provided we conceive of the educational project of medical school as something other than didactic instruction. Education, from the Latin *educere*, meaning "to lead out," is not about inculcation or indoctrination, but, as Heidegger might say, about "leaping ahead" of students in order to lead out the whole selves of who they are becoming in their lives of service to others.[38] Indeed, the countless encounters its students have with human vulnerability make medical school, in many ways, the ideal place for the liberal education of the whole self to occur.[39] We need to remember, however, that cultivating students' clinical and moral discernment occurs not through manipulating their beliefs and emotions, but only through supporting their personal development—by engaging their own critical capacities and by recognizing and accepting that they will make mistakes as they discover, for themselves, what it means to be good doctors.

One of the ways medical students are led out from themselves and toward others is through tutored exposure to stories—whether firsthand to patients' personal stories or to patients' stories as told in literature, narrative, and other artistic or interactive mediums. The notion of *tutored* exposure is important because, as mentioned earlier, the imagination is powerful and can indeed be misleading.[40] That said, intentional and reflective engagement with others' stories—stories about doctors, patients, love, loss, pain, hope, resilience, or death—can and does speak to students powerfully and compellingly. Philosopher Stephen Toulmin explains that, in the humanities, "our understanding reflects on and refines our feeling of how life is lived, how things go right or wrong, well or badly: we reread works of literature to sharpen and refine our understanding of these things, in the light of our personal experience."[41] The humanities turn us toward concrete experiences, illuminating questions about what it means to live well alongside others and exposing us to new ways of seeing and interpreting the world around us. When exposed to new stories outside biomedicine's master narrative, students can become more sensitive to the nuanced moral, interpersonal, and clinical particularities of the situations in which they find themselves. This, Arthur Frank explains, is because people don't just listen to stories; they "think with them" and get "caught up" in them.[42] Stories can "get under people's skin" and affect what they think, know, and perceive—they teach people what to look for and what to ignore, "what to value and what to hold in contempt."[43] Thus Frank claims in *The Wounded Storyteller*: "What makes an illness story good is the act of witness that says, implicitly or explicitly, 'I will tell you not what you want to hear but what I know to be true because I have lived it. This truth will trouble you, but in the end, you cannot be free without it, because you know it already; your body knows it already.'"[44] This is what he means by a "pedagogy of suffering"—the idea that those who are or have been ill can serve as teachers to those who care for them.[45] For Frank, both face-to-face encounters with the people who are ill or dying and stories about them can be transformative. Bearing witness and responding to the testimony of their patients opens up the possibility for personal transformation of medical students and doctors: they are made aware of their own fragility and brokenness and begin to see that suffering is part of what it means to be human.[46] That is to say, encounters with others' stories—"second-person" experiences of the world—can offer students knowledge both of suffering, pain, and vulnerability and of the moments of beauty and gratitude that can arise out of their midst.

A pedagogy that emphasizes perspective taking and genuine engagement with others' experiences, emotions, and ideas can enhance students' empathy, expand their worldviews, and contribute to their tacit knowledge about people, illness, and what it means to be a doctor.[47] When someone takes the time to see and hear the other, the separate horizons of the two merge or fuse with each other, resulting in an expansion of each person's particular way of seeing things. It is this fusion of horizons, which Hans-Georg Gadamer claims can happen in all human relationships, that leads to a richer knowledge of ways of being in the world. Frank reminds us that our horizons are never fixed and can be expanded and fused with others' horizons if we remain open to others' stories or ways of seeing the world.[48] As students engage in authentic meetings with others, as they enter into their patients' stories, they are granted access to the patients' own interpretive horizons, which may challenge the students' worldviews, or at least broaden their horizons in order to take in the stories of the patients.[49] This "fusion of horizons" can even transcend the exchange between two persons and the situation at hand. According to Gadamer, what occurs in an authentic encounter can, in fact, lead to a shared understanding of the human experience.[50] This is what Rita Charon means when she says that "authentic engagement" between doctors and patients can be transformative, ultimately affirming our commonalities as human beings.[51]

Engagement with the Other: Death and Dying as an Example If it is true that students' "authentic" engagement with patients—listening to them, limiting disease talk, allowing themselves to be and feel with patients—can be transformative, then we should be concerned by how little this point is stressed during medical school. The students I interviewed suggested that spending quality time with patients is rarely emphasized, and most felt pressured to limit their interactions with patients because of perceived time constraints and the need to quickly glean medical facts in order to report this information back to their teams. Although the systemic financial problems and pressures of our healthcare system are very real, they are not the only reason why students' interactions with patients are defined more by "efficiency" and protocols than by authenticity. As some of the best doctors will say, engaging with patients meaningfully can occur even in brief encounters—but the potential for such engagement is undermined by the way doctors are trained, even in the context of caring for the most vulnerable patients. Many students and residents report feeling woefully unprepared when it comes to caring for and communicating with dying patients—this despite the end-of-life training requirements set by both the Liaison Committee for Medical Education (LCME) and the Accrediting Council for Graduate Medical Education (ACGME).[52] Indeed, because most of the required end-of-life training is didactic, and because clinical training in hospice and palliative care with actual patients is usually not required, many students graduate from medical school with limited exposure to dying patients, and some with none at all.[53] Thus death and dying in medical education are conspicuous by their absence.[54]

Like most of the curricular deficits in medical education that are most formative for students, the development of students' perception of death and dying is usually left to the hidden curriculum.[55] Unfortunately, medicine's tacit assumptions about suffering and death are significantly influenced by larger cultural attitudes—most notably, by our desire to flee from such realities. Within a medical culture dominated by ideas about restoration and cure, too often students witness attending physicians and residents who "are struggling with their own feelings of uncertainty and vulnerability, for themselves and their patients, and fail to communicate such feelings to students who are learning from them."[56] As discussed earlier, death on the wards is usually not addressed in any substantive way, and students are left on their own to process through patients' deaths. In fact, "The Status of Medical Education in End-of-Life Care," published in 2003, reported that 39 percent of residents felt "not very well" or "not at all" prepared to talk with dying patients about their thoughts or feelings about dying, and more than half felt unprepared to instruct medical students in end-of-life care.[57] As a result, many residents provided little or no feedback when students did interact with dying patients, and some residents chose not to assign dying patients to students at all, asserting that such cases were "too complex" or presented too few meaningful learning opportunities.[58]

A 2011 article published in the United Kingdom suggests that residents' hesitations about end-of-life care and education, according to the residents themselves, are a result of both inadequate training in undergraduate medical education and poor instruction from senior doctors during their residency training.[59] Thus one study participant stated, "I think at medical school we learn a lot about trying to get people better, but not so much about what to do when they don't."[60] Another explained, "To be honest . . . I think we get distracted by so many other things, like just memorizing disease and pathologies and treatments, that I think I overlooked [care for the dying]."[61] Participants also suggested that hospital culture in general discourages learning about death and dying.[62] The first-year residents in the study indicated that most of their mentors did not engage in end-of-life care and spent little time teaching it to new residents. Moreover, all of the participants reported that death was a "taboo" subject in the hospital, and some suggested that many older physicians "continued to focus on cure," insisting on treatment for patients, even when this had been shown to be futile.[63] As one participant noted, "I guess it's the whole concept that if someone dies it's a failure."[64] When talking about his older mentors, another participant stated that "they come around and say: 'Right, can't do anything about this, going to die, palliative care.' [So] we just sort of called palliative care and it was their job."[65]

Although the behavior of such mentors might indicate a general discomfort with addressing end-of-life issues, it might also reflect the influence of the dominant paradigm of Western medicine, which tends to isolate the two "spheres" of curative and palliative care. In many ways, the kind of care offered by hospice and palliative teams is still perceived as something wholly separate from the dominant curative sphere of modern medicine.[66] This dominant way of thinking perpetuates normalized assumptions about what kind of suffering falls under the purview of mainstream medicine, and those who do not see themselves as palliative care clinicians "may begin to believe that basic symptom management and psychosocial support are not their responsibility, and care may become further fragmented."[67] Rather than caring for each patient as a whole person, doctors, residents, and students attend to only the fixable and tangible issues that are amenable to "medical" intervention.

Although some medical schools have attempted to incorporate palliative care into their required curriculum, teaching medical students that palliative care is the work of all physicians has yet to become part of mainstream medical education.[68] What is more, as the studies above suggest, the current didactic instruction in palliative and hospice care is simply not enough: students need personal experience both with dying patients and with mentors and role models who provide quality end-of-life care. In fact, it has been shown that having such experiences can reduce both clinicians' apprehension about communicating with those at the end of life and their own anxiety in the face of death.[69] As David Weissman and colleagues point out, "the single greatest opportunity" for improving end-of-life care is changing how it is taught on rounds.[70]

Spending time with dying patients allows these patients to teach students what their dying means to *them* and how they have or have not made sense of their suffering and offers students the unique opportunity to see and respond to the more subjective, experiential, and nonmedicalized side of care for the dying. Teaching students to engage with patients and hear their stories, to learn what their lived experiences are like, and to reflect on what it might be like to be in their situations can transform their ideas about dying and how they, as doctors, should care for those at the end of life. When Barbara Head and colleagues evaluated a new required palliative care course for third-year medical students at the University of Louisville, their findings suggested as much. In addition to learning about quality medical treatment for the dying, students indicated in their written reflections that their experiences helped them understand the lived experiences of patients and families, showed them what it means to be a doctor, and taught them about themselves—their own limitations and potential, how they might become "better" physicians, and ways of personally coping with death.[71] Reflecting on the course, one student remarked: "It's easy to wander in and out of patient's rooms without really ever stopping to think about how I am wandering in and out of another human being's life. When I stop to think about it, I feel completely undeserving."[72] Another student "came to understand [the patient] more. To me, he became a person and no longer a patient to try and fix," while a different student remarked, "It made me remember why I had initially wanted to pursue medicine."[73]

Personal encounters with death and dying can change our way of seeing the world and ourselves in that world. And research indicates that students *want* to know when they are going to learn more about death—outside the typical "breaking bad news" lectures—and about how to cope with emotions and talk to patients about end-of-life issues; they believe experiences with death "may allow them to grow as individuals and doctors."[74] "Protecting" students from dying patients or seeing these patients as cases that offer too few learning opportunities for students serves the best interests of no one—students will continue to miss out on potentially transformative experiences, and patients will continue to receive care from doctors who believe that caring for the dying is not part of medicine.

It is important to note, however, that engaging intentionally with patients who are suffering or dying is not enough; students must be afforded the opportunity to reflect on these experiences, with mentors and with one another. Some experiences on the wards can be uncomfortable and even troubling for students not familiar with death and dying, and these students need the space to reflect openly about such experiences. When my colleagues and I established a hospice and palliative care program at the University of Texas Medical Branch at Galveston to train students as hospice volunteers (after hearing from healthcare students from all schools across our campus about the significant lack of palliative care experiences), organizing monthly dialogue sessions was one of our top priorities. Because we asked students to step outside their roles as healthcare professionals in order to simply "be present" with patients—something they do not usually do during their training—some students felt uneasy when they couldn't engage in a "medical doing something" or when they were unable to change the patients' circumstance. Moreover, although we prepared our students for what they might expect when a patient was "actively dying," we knew this experience could be traumatic. We therefore made ourselves available for any students who needed or wanted to talk about their experiences, and we also discussed as a group how to develop the capacity to be a compassionate presence for patients, even during an experience that could be difficult, painful, or distressing. Without the mentorship and opportunities for reflection we provided, some students would have had a hard time making sense of things, or worse, might have experienced feelings of trauma and isolation that could reinforce their perceived need for distance and detachment.

But might such intense experiences with suffering and dying be too much to bear for some students? Might these experiences expose them to too much too soon? One student, for example, who took the palliative care course at the University of Louisville "was afraid to see people so weak and helpless. I was scared to see an 'actively dying' patient.... Some lessons you learn aren't great or profound. They're ugly, nasty, and painfully real. The encounter was terribly upsetting for me."[75] The majority of students who attend medical school do so right out of their undergraduate years, and many of these young students have not yet witnessed intense suffering or death firsthand. And even for seasoned doctors who have witnessed much suffering, such personal encounters might be too difficult for them to reflect upon with sustained attention.

Charon argues that this is the very reason the medical humanities—and literature and narrative studies in particular—were so appealing when they came on scene in the 1960s and 1970s. Those in medicine, she claimed, were looking for something that could frame crises of loss and illness that were "otherwise too hot to handle."[76] Fiction, poetry, narrative, and historical accounts provided "fireproof handholds," allowing doctors and students to touch illness and suffering without being annihilated themselves. Because representations of illness can mediate human suffering and allow us to experience it at "the remove of imagination," they can help students and doctors engage authentically and empathetically with suffering instead of turning away in self-protection.[77] And once doctors and students experience such things imaginatively, they can experience the actual suffering of their patients with empathy and compassion—rather than fear or indifference—during their encounters with them.[78]

Whether it is before they ever see their first patient or during their clinical years of training, using literature, narrative, film, poetry, photography, and art to facilitate reflection and dialogue engages students' moral imaginations and safely guides them back to the human elements of suffering from which so many would rather flee. Because the lived experience of illness is so easily covered over by what students perceive to be the real substance of medicine—namely, the facts and information they are tested on and held accountable for—teaching by indirection with artistic representation can open students up to new horizons of understanding, revealing to them what it might be like to live with a serious illness or injury.

Authentic Engagement through Artistic and Narrative Representation
Incorporating art and narrative into medical training to foster care that is more empathic and holistic seems intuitively desirable to many educators.

But what is it about artistic or narrative representations that gives rise to a deeper understanding of medicine, illness, or suffering? As Cole, Carlin, and Carson point out, the arts can offer answers to questions about the personal and particular[79]—questions that can't be answered with traditional (didactic) lectures, but that require exploration and conversation. What is it like to be a disillusioned medical student or a stressed-out resident? What is it like to live with a chronic illness? What does it mean to be alienated or marginalized? What would it be like not to have access to healthcare when you need it most? Engagement with the arts and the kind of teaching by indirection they offer, on the other hand, can reveal new truths to students, opening them up to new ways of thinking and seeing.[80]

Art requires us to slow down and consider what we see, and in that seeing, we are confronted with a new understanding. As William May explains: "The work of art, whether literary or plastic, is both a knowing and a doing: It offers a knowledgeable access to the world, but it also brings into being a new world that was not there before."[81] A piece of literature, for example, can temporarily transport us into the inner life of another—while we still remain ourselves—expanding our understanding of what it might be like to be someone else in a way that may be unavailable to us in real life.[82] Whether literature, painting, sculpture, film, or poetry, a work of art can reveal another person or another way of life, bringing into relief a different time and place or saying something about our own culture and history. And when it does, we experience, as Heidegger would say, an "opening-up" of our worlds.[83] Artistic expressions offer us truth as uncovering (alethia); they uncover a new lifeworld, engage our imagination, and expose us to a bearable kind of ambiguity. When we engage with a work of art, when we wonder about the person in the story or what is depicted in the painting, for example, we wonder not only at the aesthetics of the work, but about what is being expressed. In this wondering, our typical horizons of understanding are expanded, and what is revealed in the work reconfigures our relation to being. Heidegger describes such a revelation as "the bringing forth of a being such as never was before and will never come to be again."[84] Put simply, art can help us understand what it means to be human in ways that facts, statistics, and objective descriptions simply can't.

To me, it is the ability of the arts and humanities to express the lived, embodied, phenomenological experience of illness and suffering (of both patients and healers) that offers the greatest gift to medicine and medical education. Indeed, the arts—especially literature, poetry, and narrative—can serve as their own pedagogy of suffering, fostering compassion and empathetic engagement with others. Although it is true, as Arno Kumagai and others argue, that it is *empathy* that allows us to "tap into someone else's narrative—his or her way of understanding the world,"[85] as I see it, hearing another's narrative can itself lead to empathy and a sense of what it might be like to be in that person's place.

Engagement through Representation: Literature and Narrative as an Example Although literary accounts cannot replace firsthand experiences with flesh-and-blood patients and their families, I do believe that authentic engagement with written texts can function as a kind of pedagogy of suffering, teaching students about the lived experience of illness. What is more, teaching with stories can show students that professionalism is not about disembodied skills, codes, or even behavior, but about identity and character. Mikhail Bakhtin emphasizes the value of stories—in particular "great novels," such as those by Dostoevsky and Tolstoy—and how they can express the complexity of lived dilemmas, the dynamism of human relationships, and the multiplicity of voices and perspectives that go into decision making.[86] Novels, Bakhtin maintains, lead to much richer discussions about morality and ethics than the examples offered by some philosophers, which might be too schematic and detail sparse to account for authentic ethical dilemmas.[87]

This same richness is what allows stories to express the phenomenological experience of illness, injury, treatment, recovery, trauma, resiliency, suffering, and death. Although all narratives, including the unwritten and informal stories we live by every day, often smooth over the tattered edges of our complex lives, many of them still capture and express the profundities of the human condition in ways that facts, descriptions, and statistics cannot. Such stories, however, can be difficult to hear in the medical world, not only because they point to issues of suffering, embodiment, or vulnerability that most of us would rather not think about, but also because the biomedical, "scientific" narrative, perceived to be the most true, right, and accurate, tends to override all other narratives in contemporary medicine.[88] Nevertheless, patients are beginning to rethink themselves, their identities, their roles, and their relations to others, and, Frank argues, they are reclaiming the capacity to tell their stories in medicine.[89] Narratives of illness told by "wounded storytellers" have gained popularity in recent years, and patients have started to write and publish personal stories that run counter to prescriptive and narrow biomedical renditions of the illness experience.

Pushing against reductionistic understandings of illness, these stories engage us and, in the words of Anne Hunsaker Hawkins, "offer us cautionary parables of what it would be like if our ordinary life-in-the-world suddenly collapsed."[90] They draw us toward suffering others and bring us nearer to their experiences. Texts like Frank's own personal narrative of illness, which I have made liberal use of throughout *Afflicted*, reveal to us what it might be like to have a diagnosis crash into our lives and shatter our worlds, and they speak to the changes in our bodies and our being that might bring us face-to-face with our mortality. The same holds true for Simone de Beauvoir's masterful narrative *A Very Easy Death*, which vividly recounts the last weeks of her mother's decline and eventual death from stomach cancer.[91] Although the narrative takes place during the 1960s, when medical paternalism and overutilization of treatment at the end of life were far more common and conspicuous than they are now (especially in France, where the narrative takes place), Beauvoir grapples with issues that are still relevant for patients, practitioners, and students today: futile treatment, truth telling in medicine, the patient-doctor relationship, the embodied experience of illness and dying, and the challenges of caring for a dying parent. Beauvoir's engaging style and candor help readers empathize with her mother and her and provide an insider's view into patient care at the end of life. She is particularly adept at expressing the phenomenological experience of both illness and caregiving. Drawing her readers to the issue of embodiment, for instance, Beauvoir tells of when her mother asked in earnest: "Tell me, have I a right side?"[92] Beauvoir explains that "the broken thigh, the operation-wound, the dressings, the tubes, the infusions—all that happened on the left side," and wonders if this is why the right side of her mother's body "no longer seemed to exist" to her.[93] In this moment, we can see how her mother's whole being and identity have been usurped by her medical care. Her body has become hyperreal, and her lifeworld is now defined by treatment and technological intervention. For Beauvoir, too, the world around her has come to be defined by her care for her dying mother, even while walking alone through the streets: "Scents, furs, lingerie, jewels: the sumptuous arrogance of a world in which death had no place: but it was there, lurking behind this façade, in the grey secrecy of nursing-homes, hospitals, and sick-rooms. And for me that was now the only truth."[94] Beauvoir, in fact, declares that her whole world has "shrunk to the size of [her mother's] room," succinctly capturing the world-altering experience of caring for a loved one who is dying.[95]

Shorter patient narratives, such as online essays and blog posts, can also compellingly express the complex dynamics of life that shape subjectivities and inform patient decision making. In her post "Why I Make Terrible Decisions, or, Poverty Thoughts," Linda Tirado points out the barriers to accessing "free" healthcare:

> "Free" only exists for rich people. It's great that there's a bowl of condoms at my school, but most poor people will never set foot on a college campus. We don't belong there. There's a clinic? Great! There's still a co-pay. We're not going. Besides, all they'll tell you at the clinic is that you need to see a specialist, which seriously? Might as well be located on Mars for how accessible it is. "Low-cost" and "sliding scale" sounds like "money you have to spend" to me, and they can't actually help you anyway.[96]

Tirado goes on to describe the "unhealthy" decisions she makes that provide her with fleeting moments of pleasure in a life defined by the unrelenting stress of poverty:

> I smoke. It's expensive. It's also the best option. You see, I am always, always exhausted. It's a stimulant. When I am too tired to walk one more step, I can smoke and go for another hour. When I am enraged and beaten down and incapable of accomplishing one more thing, I can smoke and I feel a little better, just for a minute. It is the only relaxation I am allowed. It is not a good decision, but it is the only one that I have access to. It is the only thing I have found that keeps me from collapsing or exploding.[97]

Presenting students with honest narratives that challenge their presumptions about "noncompliance" and "personal responsibility" offers the opportunity to engage them in conversations about the sociopolitical forces and structural violence that radically condition the lives of some of the patients they will encounter in their life in medicine. These stories—more than any statistics—are what will begin to shift their entrenched perspectives about poverty and the social determinants of health.

Doctors' Stories Along with narrative accounts from patients and loved ones that uncover the lived experience of illness, it is important for students to engage with works that speak to healers' experiences—the joys, frustrations, and feelings of hurt, ambivalence, or fear that can come with caring for the sick. Physician Jack Coulehan argues that stories by and about doctors are central to the task of cultivating medical trainees who are humble and virtuous, for they "teach us more about virtuous traits than we could ever learn by definitions, rules, guidelines, or algorithms for virtuous behavior."[98] In his poem "Iatrogenic," for instance, physician and poet Rafael Campo captures how a student or clinician, by merging horizons with a patient, might come to realize what they both share as two mortal beings—a realization, however, that leads to feelings of both connection and pain:

You say, "I do this to myself. Outside,
my other patients wait. Maybe snow falls;
we're all just waiting for our deaths to come,
we're all just hoping it won't hurt too much.
You say, "It makes it seem less lonely here."
I study them, as if the deep red cuts
were only wounds, as if they didn't hurt
so much. The way you hold your upturned arms,
the cuts seem aimed at your unshaven face.
Outside, my other patients wait their turns.
I run gloved fingertips along their course,
as if I could touch pain itself, as if
by touching pain I might alleviate
my own despair. You say, "It's snowing, Doc."
The snow, instead of howling, soundlessly
comes down. I think you think it's beautiful
I say, "This isn't all about the snow,
is it?" The way you hold your upturned arms,
I think about embracing you, but don't.
I think, "We do this to ourselves." I think
the falling snow explains itself to us,
blinding, faceless, and so deeply wounding.[99]

The speaker, in remaining open to the patient, in acknowledging the patient's brokenness—both physical and existential—is transformed. In seeing the patient's physical wounds, the doctor's own woundedness—the kind that comes with being thrown into a world filled with blind and faceless suffering—comes into view. This willingness to see and share in the patient's suffering is what it means to be vulnerable. Indeed, "vulnerable" comes from the Latin *vulnerabilis*, meaning "wounding." It is doctors allowing themselves to be wounded by their patients' suffering that draws them in, revealing what it might be like to be the patient before them, reminding them of their own potential for suffering. In allowing themselves to approach suffering and feel pain, it is not that doctors are so deeply wounded it renders them helpless; rather, virtuous doctors endure a superficial flesh wound, a small graze that allows the patient's story to get under their skin.

Although the perception that emotional connection and vulnerability only "cloud" a physician's judgment persists, this perception obscures the fact that attending to the particularities of the moment is as much a matter of emotional awareness as it is a matter of cognitive understanding.[100] It is because of our emotional vulnerabilities that we are able to discern relevant features of a situation that risk going unnoticed when we strive to see the situation dispassionately.[101] We must feel something of what the other feels and thus "see with the heart" in order to truly acknowledge the other's distress and respond appropriately.[102] Of course, doctors must form the right sorts of emotional responses to their patients, learning over time and through experience how to "feel with" their patients, mindful of what is best for both themselves and patients. Pediatric palliative care doctor Amy-Lee Bredlau writes about the inevitable pain that comes with caring for patients, pain that can be neither ignored nor "bottled up" inside: rather than ignoring it, "I let the pain wash through me, and I let it leave. I think of the children I've cared for . . . I think of them often. I hurt for them and their suffering, but I don't put the pain anywhere, I let it wash through me and go wherever it goes."[103]

If they remain open to them, the personal stories that future physicians witness can affect them deeply and speak truth to their lives. In remaining open to these stories, perhaps future healers will come away with some understanding of what it might be like to hear terrible news or lose their identity in the face of illness—an understanding that will help them enter into patients' experiences rather than turn away from them in the name of clinical objectivity or efficiency. But even tutored exposure to stories told in literature, narrative, and poetry can "change the way people think and live their lives."[104] When students read these stories closely and carefully, whether before they see their first patients or during their clerkships, they can begin to notice the unexpected, which can "shake up [their] preconceived notions" and attune them to new meanings and ways of being[105]—a skill, I would argue, not unlike the "phronetic" ability to discern what is most clinically and morally salient in specific patient encounters, rather than simply seeing what one expects to see. Such stories can expand students' understanding of what it means to be a patient with a serious illness, a daughter with a sick mother, or a doctor trying to care for both of them well.

An exposure to the stories in literature and narrative can also provide learners with the language and skills to reflect on their own feelings and emotions, thereby helping "to heal the nascent healer."[106] It is important for students to take the time to reflect on these stories. To do so, they might engage in formal reflective writing, which, by interrupting their automatic, taken-for-granted thoughts and assumptions, can help them begin to process the profound experiences with the human condition uniquely available to them as doctors in training.[107] Both producing and reading reflective writing requires a kind of meditative thinking, where truth is uncovered, revealed, and cocreated, rather than discerned as objective, observable facts. The movement or freedom within this thinking allows for ambiguity, contradiction, and multiple interpretations: narrating and reflecting on their own experiences might change the stories students tell or help them gain access to other cultural scripts outside contemporary medicine or even come to know themselves differently.[108] According to Johanna Shapiro, Deborah Kasman, and Audrey Shafer:

As a part of their socialization process, medical students learn specialized vocabularies, prescribed cognitive frameworks, and routine patterns of action that value authority and certainty. Reflective writing requires learners to break free from familiar orienting points, typically relied upon to interpret and make sense of medical events, and approach these same events in new, sometimes foreign ways. Through writing, learners think about other people's situations, including patients', and contemplate their own reactions in relation to those situations from a subjective, personal, and indefinite vantage point.[109]

It is the "breaking free" provided by reflective writing that seems particularly important for medical students who so often become mired down in and disoriented by the constrictive "cognitive frameworks" and "routine patterns" of medical culture. Reflecting on how experiences with patients cause them to react or feel allows students to think outside the prescriptive and limiting language of medicine that all too often renders profound experiences inconsequential and thus can help the students authentically dwell within the affective experience of patient care. Personal accounts told in the "reflective mode" offer an alternative and usually affective and embodied rendition of events, one that can "protest against dehumanizing aspects of ward culture."[110] In contrast to the "mimetic mode" of the larger medical culture, the reflective mode both requires and cultivates a kind of meditative thinking that can bring depth and intensity to traditional medical accounts that are so often dominated by calculative thinking. Because of this, reflective writing assignments can encourage medical students to "discover or recover dimensions of imaginative thinking" as they express themselves.[111] Some even argue that reflective writing can serve a therapeutic function, helping students to reorganize stressful or traumatic events, such as experiencing a patient's death for the first time, and to process through their emotional reactions.[112] It can also offer students an opportunity to express their moral distress when the realities of medicine defy their expectations or when they struggle to offer compassionate care in a medical system that is all too often economically unfair and socially unjust.

What is more, reflective writing can bring attention to the process of socialization itself, attuning students to the ways they are being formed by the culture of medicine and medical education. Writing about personal experiences can bring elements of the hidden curriculum into focus; they can draw attention to—and perhaps even rally against—implicit and injurious modes of professional identity formation. In reflecting on such experiences, students can embrace their own values and emotions, while also challenging or rejecting what they find problematic within the normative culture of medicine.[113] Here, however, we should keep in mind that the formation of doctors does not always proceed in a linear or predictable fashion. The trajectory from medical student to junior resident to senior resident to "fully formed" doctor is a complex process of constructing, abandoning, and reconstructing identities as those involved struggle to incorporate the new expectations that come with their new identities.[114] Fourth-year medical students transitioning to new interns, for example, might find it difficult to reconcile their identities as both learners and as legitimate members of healthcare teams who engage in critical decision making. Reflective writing and the meditative thinking required for it can capture the complex process of negotiating multiple identities in these transition periods by allowing the identities to dwell alongside one another without contradiction, and may perhaps eventually lead to their integration and a unified sense of self. Learning to become more comfortable with ambiguity and complexity, whether related to identities specifically or to the practice of medicine more generally, is a difficult endeavor. Yet giving medical students the opportunity to think and write reflectively about their personal experiences may open up the space for them to succeed in this endeavor, especially when it may be the only real opportunity they have to do so in a professional and academic world so defined by the discursive regime of modern medicine.

Reflecting Together Because reflections are, as Heidegger would suggest, always already interpretations of events as opposed to accounts of an objective or verifiable reality, sharing these reflections in dialogue with others can generate new understandings of these fluid and pliable experiences. When shared and discussed with others, narratives that are painful, confusing, or incomplete can be nuanced into more generative narratives that facilitate perspective shifts and personal growth. Students' horizons of understanding can shift or broaden as they encounter the horizons of others who offer alternative perspectives or interpretations of events, something critically important for students who are learning what it means to be healers. For, as Kumagai points out, when reflection lacks a social component and is not shared with others, it runs the risk of "being limited to feeling" instead of leading to change or growth.[115]

In the exchange of personal narratives, even when it does not lead to the construction of a new narrative, others can offer empathetic witnessing and authentic listening that can lead to validation of a student's perspective and an opportunity for the student to process through difficult emotions. Medical students who have participated in small groups say that they have come to see their classmates' narratives "in a new light after listening to the written stories," even if they had previously heard those stories in other settings.[116] What is more, when students recognize that their own reactions to experiences in the clinic are not unlike the reactions of their classmates, they begin to feel more connected to them, creating a sense of solidarity and a space for honesty and reflection.[117] In their analysis of a course that asks medical students to create reflective projects about clinical experiences, for example, Lloyd Rucker and Johanna Shapiro reported that, though at first hesitant to create such projects, by the end of the course, students found the process offered them insight into their experiences and helped them see they were not alone in their "anxiety, confusion, and even despair."[118] One of them remarked that when students talk about things on the wards, they "don't talk about them like we're doing now. We're showing sides of ourselves that we've kept hidden 'til now."[119] Attentive listening to others' stories can foster bonds between students, help them become more mindful and present, and lead to feelings of reciprocity and mutuality that defy the traditional hierarchical order of medicine.[120]

The Medical Humanities and Premedical Education Whether it is through reflective writing, the creation of poetry or art, or dialogue with peers and mentors, it is essential that we provide medical students a space where they can slow down and reflect on questions about who they feel themselves becoming, who they want to be, and how they might be changed by their encounters with those around them—that is, of course, if we are genuinely interested in helping them become reflective, deep-thinking healers. One might argue that future healers should reflect on such questions much earlier in their journey to become doctors. Indeed, many would agree that the formative process of their journey starts during their undergraduate years as premedical students. As Jeffrey Gross and colleagues contend, "students must realize that the undergraduate premedical experience is not just a means to enter medical school; it is also an experience that is shaping their character."[121] And yet if, as one undergraduate recently told me, "most premeds just volunteer to get their names on everything and add lines to their résumé," then Gross and colleagues might be right to conclude that, by the time many students get to medical school, they have learned to *demonstrate* character as "a shortcut to developing it."[122] Like medical school, premedical education can be rigorous and fiercely competitive. In his 2016 blog post "It's Time to Retire Premed," Harvard medical student Nathaniel Morris explains that "we want doctors who can work in teams and who put patients' interests first. Yet our current pre-med system bears little relationship to the practice of medicine and encourages students to focus on their own success above all else."[123] As a result, many students avoid courses that challenge their assumptions or that orient them toward new ways of thinking when such courses aren't required for a premedical degree or when poor performance in them might threaten their grade point average.[124]

Although I admit this kind of student behavior is discouraging, I agree with former editor in chief of *Academic Medicine* Steven Kanter when he says that "we must stop complaining about the problematic choices made by premedical students and start fixing the system that is fostering such choices" which requires us to articulate a pedagogical philosophy for premedical education—a philosophy that should

> state that a premedical education must go beyond preparing a student to do well on an admission test and in the courses he or she will take in medical school, and must prepare the student to develop into an independent and creative thinker, with a strong moral compass and a commitment to social justice. It should call for premedical education to include courses that help students cultivate their intellects and sensibilities in ways that will help them function optimally in an environment characterized by change and uncertainty.[125]

If we are to change how undergraduates are introduced to and shaped by the culture of healthcare and healthcare education, it is critical that we think about and then clearly articulate a philosophy for prehealthcare education. Students must no longer be seen as passive receptacles for passed-along knowledge. Students, teachers, and clinical mentors need to develop real relationships, have real conversations, and offer one another the chance to speak and learn and grow. This kind of education is patient; it is reflective and intentional; for it to flourish, we need to provide spaces for critical discussion and contemplation.[126] Feminist author and activist bell hooks reminds us that the classroom should be an exciting place and that such excitement should be cocreated with our students—students whose presence and voices are valued.[127] Getting students engaged and excited about what we teach requires us to be humble and to recognize that, as educators, we learn from our students and that we, too, can change and grow from our experiences in the classroom.[128] And though such educational experiences rarely are acknowledged and rewarded in the managed and audited culture of the neoliberal university, they bring real meaning and value to both teachers and learners. In emphasizing the "slow" educational process more than quantifiable outcomes, educators can begin to break down traditional hierarchies between themselves and students, reconnect students to the social import of their current and future work, and reveal the emancipatory potential of education.[129]

Even though they require students to slow down and consider the texture of patients' lives, these kinds of pedagogical changes can easily be introduced within established premed or medical curricula. In teaching my undergraduate students, I have found ways to incorporate narrative understanding and personal reflection wherever possible. Each day at the start of my classes, for example, I ask my students (most of whom are prehealthcare majors) to write a short, informal reflection about the day's assigned readings, encouraging them to express their own interpretations—what the readings mean to them, how they might challenge or reaffirm their assumptions, biases, or beliefs, and what frustrated, confused, or delighted them. Such reflection helps students crystallize their perspectives and engenders richer dialogue for the remainder of the class. What is more, presenting a mix of theoretical, critical, and philosophical pieces alongside narratives and poems written by patients, caregivers, and healthcare professionals expresses to students the embodied, lived experience of illness, suffering, and death in a way that primary philosophical pieces or critical social theory alone may not. The centrality of narrative is made all the clearer when, midway through the semester, students are asked to identify someone they know (perhaps themselves) with a serious, chronic, or terminal illness who is willing to share his or her story. With the express permission of this person, students then write an illness narrative that illustrates this person's struggles, triumphs, and fears, which they then share with the rest of the class. Such assignments require an element of vulnerability—and bravery—in the classroom, on the part of students and educator alike. The hope is that such experiences will open students up to new ways of seeing and knowing and that they will begin to imagine what it might be like to live a life that may be so different from their own.

Although I recognize that my classroom and office are not intended to be spaces for therapy sessions, and I am careful to maintain appropriate boundaries with undergraduates, medical students, and residents, I also know that asking them to reflect on who they are becoming and who they want to be requires me to be equally reflective and vulnerable. Delese Wear and Joseph Zarconi remind us that "mentoring for fearlessness" in healthcare education—encouraging students to be reflective and critical of the forces that shape them—requires that mentors speak openly to students about their own successes and failures and that they not be afraid to use words like "compassion" and "kindness."[130] Attempting to promote real transformation and growth among at least some of our students requires us to break down the hierarchy and let go of the privileged dominance of the clinician or professor in educational spaces.

If they are perceived as worthwhile, mentoring for fearlessness and encouraging reflective practice, imagination, and wonder can easily become part of healthcare and medical education, especially if educators and students come to see reflection as complementary, rather than extraneous, to scientific thinking and clinical care. My hope is that exposing students to stories of suffering and strength and providing them with opportunities to reflect on such experiences will help them become students who are attuned to the lived experience of illness and suffering, who understand the social determinants of health, who think critically about the systems in which they participate, and who might identify themselves as leaders in social justice and advocates for health for all.

Although I certainly believe that the cultivation of the self ought to begin early on in students' journey to become doctors, we need to remember that addressing the deficits in undergraduate education and medical school admission policies will not, by itself, change the reality that medical school and residency affect who learners become in substantive ways.[131] It is tempting to conclude that, by the time students reach medical school, their moral compasses are already set near the direction that will guide them for the rest of their lives. But, as an environment laden with intense confrontations with human fragility and mortality, medical school rarely leaves students' personal and moral outlooks unscathed.[132] Throughout our lives, our interactions and experiences with others affect how we make sense of the world as we see it and who we are in that world; our personal development is not something that stops once we have reached some arbitrarily defined moment of maturation. And, despite the dominant enculturation that begins even before they are accepted to medical school, there are students who start their medical training with open—or at least, not completely closed—hearts, only to leave with feelings of frustration and cynicism and a narrow understanding of care. To prevent this from happening, we must recognize that students and residents are affected by their intense encounters with human fragility and mortality during their training, and we must encourage them to reflect on how such experiences affect them, rather than letting these encounters passively and all too often detrimentally shape the kind of doctors they will become.

Making Curricular Inroads Falling outside the major epistemological framework of medical (and premedical) education, the medical humanities are particularly well suited for cultivating meditative thinking and creative modes of learning; yet this is also why they have struggled to find a central place in medical school curricula. Although over the past decade or so, the Liaison Committee on Medical Education (LCME) has stated that medical schools must provide educational opportunities for learning about end-of-life care, medical ethics, "societal problems," healthcare disparities, and communication skills, it has set forth few specifications about how such educational goals should be met. And because there is no mention of the "medical humanities" in either the LCME standards[133] or the residency training standards of the Accrediting Council for Graduate Medical Education (ACGME), whether and how medical humanities courses are incorporated into medical school curricula vary widely, remaining largely on the periphery of curricula in some schools.[134] This is in part a result of the perennial problem faced by medical humanists: proving the efficacy of our pedagogy.[135] As shown above, the major work of the medical humanities is to foster reflection, imagination, personal and moral clarity, and a greater, more expansive understanding of what it means to be human—all of which can be quite difficult to assess or measure, especially when using narrow quantitative standards or metrics. In light of this, studies have suggested that the "outcomes" of humanities courses might best be assessed using more qualitative methodologies, and some researchers have done so through focus groups or by analyzing student narratives after the completion of a course or program.[136] These researchers have found that courses in the medical humanities are indeed "effective," with students' self-reports pointing to development of greater self-awareness, personal growth, and care for themselves, of critical thinking and social skills, of greater understanding of the larger context of medicine, and of greater empathy and compassion, as well as appreciation for a sense of community and connection.[137]

Such studies are helpful for illuminating what the medical humanities do for students, but one might wonder whether their findings are even intelligible in the world of academic medicine, where calls for rubrics and observable competencies abound. Jacob Ousager and Helle Johannessen, for example, argue that the medical humanities' lack of "empirical evidence" and "measurable learning outcomes" will prevent them from gaining and holding a firm position in medical education.[138] "After all," they say, "the present trend of evidence-based learning ... requires that the study of the humanities, like any other curricular activity within medical education, should in principle be able to justify its existence with evidence of its effectiveness."[139] Although I recognize the need for the medical humanities to demonstrate their value in terms that are meaningful to stakeholders and decision makers in academic medicine, by measuring the intrinsic value of the medical humanities in the same way as that of the rest of medical education, we run the risk of falling victim to "they-self" notions of "success" that only further embed us into closed, calculative understandings of being-in-the-world. If the medical humanities are intended to challenge the epistemological assumptions of mainstream medicine, then measuring them against criteria born of this epistemology misses the mark entirely.

This is not to say, however, that medical humanists can't present persuasive reasons for why the humanities are critical to medical education. Indeed, we can do so in rhetorically effective ways with more qualitative studies and by learning to speak the language of academic medicine. For instance, we might make the case for a pedagogy that encourages the cultivation of the self by identifying the personal qualities we intend to engender in future doctors and then mapping these qualities onto LCME or ACGME standards or onto the list of competencies of a particular medical school.[140] That said, when it comes to "proving" the efficacy of the medical humanities, we may never be able to offer the kind of quantitative results that the system demands. Indeed, in trying to measure outcomes using calculative standards of success, we risk measuring the wrong things—namely, demonstrable behaviors that may or may not emanate from deeper values and that serve as reductionistic surrogates for character. Or, as Kumagai argues, an emphasis on "observable outcomes, standardization, and externally imposed criteria" threatens to reduce the profound human interactions inherent in the act of healing into "overly simplified checklists [and] stereotyped, fragmented behaviors."[141] Granting that such an approach may be "accurate," he goes on to ask: "Is it *authentic*? That is, does it truly document the evolution of a learner into a professional being-in-the-world?"[142]

Though calculative standards cannot fully reflect the educational goals or "outcomes" of the medical humanities, this does not mean there is no way to assess students' growth toward becoming healers. Indeed, a pedagogy that embraces more tacit ways of knowing and that teaches through stories, reflection, and art can more readily access and assess students' formative processes than most other pedagogical approaches. Reflective work, such as narratives and essays, for instance, can display the development of certain virtues, such as remaining open, being willing to listen to and become absorbed in a patient's story, managing uncertainty and ambiguity, and pushing against prescriptive and restrictive ways of knowing. Reading a student's detailed narrative account allows a mentor to understand the student's way of being-in-the-world-with-others, as opposed to the student's adherence to codes or ability to exhibit observable "professional" behavior as prescribed by an ethic of detachment.[143]

Reflective work—including closely reading texts, writing essays, journal entries, or short stories, keeping a "parallel chart," and creating artwork or film that explores the lived experience of medicine—can cultivate meditative thinking, encouraging shifts in perspective and personal growth.[144] This kind of "assessment" is *formative* rather than summative: instead of an accounting *of* learning at the end of a rotation or semester that allows for little to no in-the-moment guidance and feedback, a formative assessment is an accounting *for* learning, allowing educators and mentors to "impart information, instill values, and inspire excellence and ongoing learning" throughout educational experiences.[145] It is not easy to create and facilitate this kind of pedagogy; supporting personal growth and accounting for it require that educators *engage* with students—that they pose difficult questions, listen intently, and initiate honest dialogue. Moreover, mentors must take time to offer students specific and meaningful feedback. Whether through formal evaluations on the wards or in response to students' work outside the clinical setting, it is essential that mentors recognize that their feedback contributes to students' development. Feedback should be seen as an opportunity to engage in conversation with students, to commend them for their accomplishments, to address areas in need of improvement, and to help students question assumptions—both their own and those of contemporary Western medicine more generally.

Creating Culture Change through Relationship

It is no secret that incorporating the medical humanities into medical education has been met with resistance, from administrators, faculty, and students alike. Because reading literature and engaging in reflective writing, for instance, are perceived to be so different from, and perhaps even extraneous to, traditional medical education, some see the medical humanities as unnecessary, gratuitous, and even self-indulgent.[146] And some students find being asked to reflect on personal values or emotional reactions to patient care too intrusive—an important criticism to keep in mind when creating spaces for reflection that feel safe to students.[147] Moreover, the ambiguity, existence of multiple truths, and lack of clear, concise, "right" answers in the medical humanities—something that makes them a powerful corrective to biomedical reductionism—can also arouse anxiety in students who feel more comfortable with knowledge that seems certain and verifiable.[148]

But perhaps the biggest challenge when it comes to getting students to engage seriously with the medical humanities is changing their perceptions of the humanities in general, perceptions largely shaped by the hidden curriculum of medical education. Because it is difficult to assess in the ways academic medicine deems valuable, students are seldom held accountable for engaging with the humanities—questions about the lived experience of illness, social justice, or virtue ethics do not (and perhaps cannot) appear on the tests or exams that "really matter." David Jones and colleagues explain that students

> approach the knowledge taught to them with one eye firmly on the bottom line: is this knowledge relevant for their future as practitioners (or more immediately, on the Board exams)? Students have an uncanny ability to parse the curriculum and divine what parts of their coursework will be more or less represented on their medical boards and other assessments, regardless of what their professors say. They quickly figure out the "hidden curriculum" of what is and is not necessary to pass courses, survive on the wards, and get through their licensing exams.[149]

In other words, many students view material they won't be tested on as simply irrelevant to their education. As unfortunate as this reality is, it is hard to blame students when messages about what is most important to their training are subtly (and sometimes not so subtly) communicated to them time and again: their grades are primarily determined by multiple-choice tests that cannot reflect the nuance of the questions posed by the humanities, very little time is spent offering meaningful feedback on patient interactions, humanities courses are mostly optional, and students feel enormous pressure to perform well on medical board exams, which almost exclusively focus on scientific or clinical knowledge.

It is for this reason that establishing close, respectful, and respected relationships with deans and administrators is crucial for educators in the medical humanities since systemic transformation often depends on the individuals who make up the system.[150] Collaborating with those who make decisions about the medical curriculum and demonstrating to them the value of the humanities in medical education is the first step in eventually changing students' perceptions. If the humanities, as a result of collaborative relationships with administration and faculty, are subsequently integrated into the medical curriculum in a substantial way—and students are held accountable for the knowledge the humanities offer—then these students might begin to view the humanities as essential to their understanding of medicine. Though it is true that most medical schools have neither explicit requirements nor the requisite funding to incorporate the medical humanities into their curricula and that efforts need be made to catalyze change among accrediting bodies such as the LCME, with the support of deans and administrators, individual schools can do much to move in that direction.[151] But encouraging administrators to make these changes will require the help of students, residents, faculty, and still others who recognize that the wisdom of the medical humanities is fundamental to the everyday practice of medicine in the fullest sense. "The idea, of course," say Jack Coulehan and Peter Williams, "is to infiltrate the culture by co-opting residents and attending physicians—first obtaining their goodwill, then fanning goodwill into enthusiasm."[152] Doing so can lead to curricular changes for medical students and may also help to blur the line drawn between scientific medicine and the "softer" domains of patient care.[153]

But even if faculty and administrators show enthusiasm for the medical humanities, incorporating them into medical school curricula will take time and concerted effort. Treating the medical humanities as a post hoc addition or disconnected addendum to the traditional curriculum will leave the larger medical culture essentially unchanged. Indeed, having the medical humanist "parachute in" for abbreviated didactic lessons taught in the fashion of the traditional curriculum will do little to change either the epistemology or the pedagogy of medicine. Rather, the humanities must be incorporated as a central part of the curriculum throughout all four years of medical training in a way that encourages open dialogue and reflection about how that training forms who students are becoming—something a fourth-year medical student wished had been the case for her. "It's been my relationships with graduate students in the medical humanities," she told me, "and the conversations I have had with them that have really helped change my ideas about medical care and being a doctor. Everyone needs to have that kind of constant conversation" (MSIV-10).

In my experience, engaging in such sustained conversations and developing real relationships with students have brought about the most significant changes in students' ideas about what it means to be a doctor. Though also important, lectures or small group sessions will not facilitate the same kind of change. To be sure, Heidegger says that meditative thinking in general "requires a greater effort" than calculative thinking and that it must "be able to bide its time."[154] But this does not mean that opportunities for meditative thinking must be carved out as designated spaces in the medical curriculum. Rather, reflecting and thinking meditatively need to become an embedded practice sustained through everyday engagement with the world. If students interact with mentors who take a moment to acknowledge a patient's death or who express their own moral distress about practicing within an imperfect system, then they may also come to feel that reflection is simply part of medical care. Moreover, these same mentors can encourage active reflection, asking students directly—both in the classroom and on the wards—to consider what it means to help others and care well for them. What, as doctors, do they "owe" patients in need? What specialties most suit their particular personalities and which will bring them the deepest satisfaction based on the values they have clarified for themselves? We need to acknowledge and reward the dedication of these mentors to their students, and we also need to publicly express our commitment to quality mentorship in medical education.

Along with this, we should work to identify the elements of current medical school curricula that naturally lend themselves to reflection, narrative understanding, and meditative thinking. Many medical schools, for instance, have adopted problem-based learning (PBL) curricula, where students in small groups facilitated by faculty members work together to diagnose a patient problem, usually in the form of a case vignette, and to create a clinical treatment plan. If these vignettes were presented with richer narrative detail than the standard vignettes—offering more information about the patients, the socioeconomic conditions of their lives, or the way their medical problems affect their everyday ways of being—or if small-group facilitators encouraged students to wonder about the patients' life circumstance or the historical contingencies of certain disease categories, students might become more attuned to the lived experience of patients they encounter on their clinical rotations. Because problem-based learning is "a vehicle for the development of clinical problem-solving skills," helping students recognize early on in their work with PBL vignettes that a patient's lifeworld does, in fact, affect how clinical decisions are made may lead to changes in clinical care later on with real, flesh-and-blood patients.[155]

Such pedagogical changes can be easily introduced since they make few demands on established curricula and "depend only on the engagement of the faculty and the interests of each cohort and students."[156] If educators and students come to see meditative thinking and reflection as complementary, rather than extraneous, to clinical care, these practices can become part of medical education, enhancing rather than detracting from scientific or clinical training.

Yet, even if reflective practice does not in fact take up much time, the notion of its being too time intensive for the fast-paced world of medicine should give us pause. The very fact that medicine has been reduced to rushed, depersonalized interactions between doctors and patients limited by the pressures of hospital regulations and healthcare economics points to the need for doctors and medical students alike to express the subjective experience of patient care that "defies this depersonalization."[157] Reducing clinical interactions to perfunctory exchanges undermines the human connection and prevents physicians and patients from recognizing the profundity of illness and care. Taking the time to see and respond to the all-too-human moments of medicine is what reminds us why we need one another in the first place. It is for this reason, among others, that physician-writer Kate Scannell believes that "writing and speaking about doctoring can save your life."[158]

This is not to say that the medical humanities offer a panacea for all the ills of medical training. It is too simple to argue that the epistemology of medicine always undercuts authenticity, whereas the epistemology guiding the humanities always fosters authentic, virtuous engagement with others.[159] Both calculative and meditative thinking are required for alleviating suffering, a point that has become more and more clear to me as I have spent time teaching and supporting residents at a busy community hospital. I now recognize that developing a technical skill that promotes healing can be just as virtuous and necessary as being a compassionate witness to another's suffering. Too often, however, the subjective experience of patient care and the mutual dependency of doctor and patient are buried and forgotten in a hospital culture that valorizes medical interventions, technical expertise, and productivity. The ability of the medical humanities to voice the embodied, lived experience of illness and suffering, to foster introspection and reflection, to reorient worldviews, and to cultivate the moral imagination can work toward opening up physicians and future physicians to more authentic ways of being-with-others.

Asking for fundamental change in the culture of academic medicine is asking quite a lot. But society has asked even more of our doctors. In many ways, the world of medicine is a microcosm of life—a concentration of the all-too-human elements of being alive: birth, death, illness, suffering, isolation, fear, love, uncertainty. Nearly everyone who cares for the sick crosses the threshold into the space where human mortality and vulnerability—and the feelings of helplessness associated with them—come to the fore. So, whether we intend to or not and whether we like it or not, society has asked healthcare practitioners to carry a very heavy burden. And, unfortunately, we all too often fail to prepare them adequately for the task. It falls to us, then, to infuse medical education with other ways of knowing, thinking, and relating, and to create spaces for physicians and physicians in training to learn about and reflect upon the distress and pain that can arise when caring for patients and their families. Calling for medicine to be grounded in humility and a broader understanding of care is not, however, an unsympathetic critique or a demand for caregivers to simply "do more" or "do better." Rather, it is a plea for all of us to begin to truly support our present and future healers and to care for them well.

Epilogue

The opposite of love is not hate, it's indifference
—Elie Wiesel

Not long ago, an anesthesiologist and critical care specialist told me that, without love, he and his team members could not possibly sustain themselves in their field. It was the love he had for his patients and his willingness to witness their suffering during a very frightening time in their lives that brought meaning and purpose to his life as a physician. Although this doctor might simply have been humoring me, the token medical humanist with impossible ideals, his willingness to use the word "love" to describe his interactions with patients and their families, and the ease with which he said it over and over again, seemed genuine—and more like courage than flattery.

Advice about loving patients probably doesn't go very far in spaces where maintaining emotional distance is viewed as a professional virtue, but "love" may be exactly the word we need to use when we talk about medicine and medical education. Loving well means caring for others, even when it is hard and even when we want to turn away. Loving others means *seeing* them, recognizing their suffering, and helping them know that both they and their experiences matter. Because we so often encounter others in our inauthentic mode of being, which produces fear and trembling in the face of suffering and death, it is much easier to turn from the persons before us. But loving them requires us to turn toward them, even when they suffer in ways that remind us that we, too, can suffer and will die. When doctors are called to respond to and alleviate suffering, they are called to recognize that suffering, even when it is ugly and distressing, even when it is terrifying.

If Emmanuel Levinas is right and responding to one another is what makes us more fully human, then doctors, in responding to their patients, are indeed engaging in loving acts, both for the patients and for themselves. As Levinas says: "Practically, this goodness, this nonindifference to the death of the other, this kindness, is precisely the very perfection of love."[1] Most of us, however, have lived long enough to know that loving others—especially those who are difficult or sick or angry—is hard. Asking busy, stressed, and tired doctors to love their patients can seem excessive. And yet there are doctors who do turn toward their patients with genuine concern and care and who recognize that doing so connects them to what makes life most meaningful, to what makes us human. Recognizing another and truly seeing that person is something a medical kiosk or supercomputer will never be able to do. It is what happens between two human beings who are open to each other, who are able to see the other's struggle to live well in this world, to see the other's need, and to respond to it with an earnest desire to alleviate the suffering we all share.

We need to see medicine for what it is, as encounters between people—doctors and patients—intended to bring healing in the broadest sense of the word. So much of medicine, even diagnosing and treating, depends on unquantifiable human qualities, such as clinical intuition, personal discernment, and the ability to recognize what is needed most in the specific situation at hand. Caring for others requires much more than technical skill and clinical knowledge, which fall short when determining what is best for patients whose needs have been shaped by rich and complex lives. This is why any kind of handbook that views patient-physician communication as a mere exchange of information and offers prescriptive ways for breaking bad news will do very little to improve the kind of care offered to patients. But because novice learners will need guidance when it comes to broaching difficult issues with patients, they would do well to follow the lead of Atul Gawande when it comes to speaking about death and dying:

> It's a hard conversation to have. But there's actually an incredibly simple way to broach the subject. It just needs these simple words: I'm worried. You're saying, I'm worried about what I'm seeing going on. It doesn't say, I'm certain you're going to die next week, because we're not certain exactly what's going to happen. But it puts the worry on the table, and then it also says that we can talk about those best cases and worst cases here.[2]

Conversations that leave room for uncertainty, express genuine concern, and give patients and family members the opportunity to listen and respond can occur, if doctors are courageous enough to express their worry.

Epilogue

Even though genuine conversation and engagement can occur in the clinic, some might argue that what patients *really* need most is not compassionate listeners, but expertly trained technicians who can perform the tasks at hand well. Admittedly, there are moments when it is tempting to think that is so. Coincidentally, as I write this, my father is recovering from open-heart surgery—an invasive procedure that terrified me and made me believe for a moment that what my father needed most was an expert technician, regardless of whether he or she was a "good person." But only for a moment. When the man who would eventually place his hands inside my father's open chest walked into the hospital room, he seemed very competent, to be sure. He was a busy and experienced cardiac surgeon with thousands of successful cases to his credit. When he explained the procedure to us, he was clear and thorough, outlining the risks and benefits of the surgery. He was professional. He was an expert. And yet, there was something else about him—how he patiently listened as we told him what we feared, the way he touched my father's legs and chest to show him where incisions would be made, how he spoke with both confidence and humility, the way he acknowledged the change in my father's face when he heard about potential complications—that expressed an ineffable, but crucial quality transcending expertise. Something about *who he was* told us we could trust him, that he cared whether my dad lived or died, and that he would do his very best for a man he had only just met.

It was something I have always known, something I have told my students over and over, but, in this moment, it became real to me for the first time: trust is needed for healing to take place—and this trust has its foundation in something more than technical skill.[3] We trusted this surgeon not simply because he was competent and well trained, but because he also seemed to care; and, without this trust, my father and our family would have gone into the surgery more hesitantly and fearfully. Looking back on this encounter causes me to marvel even more at the sentiment I so frequently hear: that people would rather have a doctor who is skilled than one who is compassionate. I wonder why so many feel the need to see this as a dichotomy, as a matter of "either-or." Can't a doctor be like my father's surgeon and have both skill and compassion? Indeed, isn't it *necessary* for a doctor to have both? Isn't this the foundation of trust between caregivers and patients? And if it is, then much more is at stake when we think about the ways we educate our future caregivers. Ensuring that they learn to communicate effectively and professionally, though necessary, is not enough. We need to be concerned about the kind of people they are becoming, especially because their training has such a profound effect on their development.

However strange it may sound, healing medical education will require the kind of love Levinas points to. It will require us to encourage students to examine their "existential qualms" about illness and death, as Danielle Ofri puts it,[4] and to show them that because we all share the potential to suffer, there is very little that separates doctors from patients, aside from the specifics of the moment. Drawing students and practitioners back into compassionate care—care for both themselves and others—will require real relationship. It will require them to recognize that caring for patients is difficult and sometimes painful, especially in our fragmented healthcare system, and that sometimes they need the support of their colleagues and peers. This is especially true for students, who may be witnessing suffering and death for the very first time. Telling a patient that he or she is going to die is hard, especially when the patient and family don't want to hear it, and witnessing another's world collapse can shake one's own existential footing. Students need help navigating the perplexing and sometimes chaotic world of medicine. Like patients, students need to *be seen*, they need their suffering acknowledged, and they need someone to listen as they struggle to make sense of this peculiar and incredible journey they have embarked upon.

Students' and residents' journeys to become doctors are made all the more treacherous by the sociopolitical and economic forces that shape modern medicine. Our fee-for-service model that contributes to the commodification and corporatization of medical care reduces doctors to "providers" and patients to "consumers," dictating the time doctors can spend with patients and how many patients they must see in a day, and inevitably diminishing the kind of care students and doctors can offer. The problems of commercialization and capitalism are not specific to medicine and are deeply embedded in the vast geopolitical landscape of our world, making them extremely difficult to address. And I would argue that the encroachment of capitalism into medicine is yet another instance of our tendency to flee in the face of vulnerability. Diminishing our relationships to market exchanges and limiting our responsibilities to one another by conceiving of them only as contractual obligations can—just like calculative approaches to medicine—serve to disburden us of our responsibility to really see each other and the ways we suffer.

Caring well for students and practitioners in this environment requires us to see that it is not individuals who are deficient but the systems they work in and the narratives they live by. This is why any attempts to address the recent call from the ACGME to promote "wellness" or "resiliency" among residents will be futile if they fail to seriously consider the systems and institutions that engender stress and burnout or make it difficult for residents to find meaning in their work. Placing the onus on residents—and on students and clinicians, as well—to be resilient and to stay well without acknowledging an institution's *obligation* to create a healthy and supportive culture may give rise to "resilient" clinicians who have only learned to survive within a dehumanizing system, allowing institutions to evade responsibility for promoting wellness.

The educational environments in which our residents and students, both medical and premedical, find themselves are powerful indeed. Just recently, I gave a guest lecture to a group of premedical students. At the end of class, one student said that, though she understood that patients suffered in complex ways, it was just not possible for doctors to address this suffering because they were not trained to do so, the clinical encounter was much too short, and other people, like nurses and social workers, were better equipped to handle it. Although much of what she said may be true, her comment made it painfully clear to me that, even before getting to medical school, students are thinking and learning under master narratives that narrowly circumscribe their notion of what doctors do or even what they *might do* if conditions were to change. Immersed in these narratives, they find it hard to conceive of the doctor as someone other than a biomedical expert. When students come to see calculative and reductionistic understandings of health and illness as having cornered the market on truth, or believe that test scores are representative of success and failure, or perceive economic pressures in healthcare to be unrelenting, or see fixing and curing as the hallmarks of the good doctor, then it is hard for them to imagine otherwise. When students' perspectives of medicine are formed by narrow understandings of what it means to be human and what it means to care well for others, the task of broadening their notions of health, illness, and care seems daunting.

Daunting, yes, but not impossible. Though it will take time, commitment, and resources to significantly shift the culture of medical education in this direction, there are small changes to be made right now. We know students don't need more facts or figures or rubrics. They need to be encouraged to imagine what it might be like to be sick or scared or in need of help. They need exposure to new narratives that free them for new ways of being-in-the-world. And they need mentors who encourage imagination and wonder, who *see* them, and who are committed to helping these future doctors become future healers.

I needed the closeness with the patients as much as or even more than they needed mine.
—Dr. Richard Selzer (1928–2016)

Notes

Prologue

1. E-mail from physician, February 28, 2014; name withheld to protect privacy.

2. As quoted in Arthur Kleinman, *The Illness Narratives: Suffering, Healing, and the Human Condition* (New York: Basic Books, 1988), 215; emphasis in original.

Introduction

1. Peter S. Cahn, "Seven Dirty Words: Hot-Button Language That Undermines Interprofessional Education and Practice," *Academic Medicine: Journal of the Association of American Medical Colleges*. (e-publication online ahead of print, November 1, 2016). https://insights.ovid.com/pubmed?pmid=27805953/.

2. Eric J. Cassell, "The Nature of Suffering and the Goals of Medicine," *New England Journal of Medicine* 306, no. 11 (1982): 640.

3. Ibid.

4. In the context of medicine and doctoring, we might limit the term "existential suffering" to the particular existential suffering brought on by or accompanying illness, injury, or medical treatment. Because of the almost irresistible momentum in contemporary Western medicine to medicalize many forms of suffering, we should be wary about attempts to "diagnose" and "treat" the existential suffering or anxiety that comes with simply being human. That said, doctors who are committed to healing should, at the very least, acknowledge the existential suffering specifically brought on by illness or injury.

5. David Barnard, "Love and Death: Existential Dimensions of Physicians' Difficulties with Moral Problems," *Journal of Medicine and Philosophy* 13, no. 4 (1988): 395, 396. Barnard's conception of existential suffering by patients facing terminal illness is similar to what Lynn Jansen and Daniel Sulmasy call "agent-narrative suffering" from loss of independence, feelings of despair or loneliness, and the like, which

results in (usually terminal) patients' inability to maintain important social connections or narrative coherence in their lives. This kind of suffering is contrasted with "neuro-cognitive suffering" from pain, shortness of breath, or other distressing physical symptoms directly related to the underlying the pathology or disease of the patients. See Lynn A. Jansen and Daniel P. Sulmasy, "Proportionality, Terminal Suffering and the Restorative Goals of Medicine," *Theoretical Medicine and Bioethics* 23, nos. 4–5 (2002): 321–337.

6. Ronald A. Carson, Chester R. Burns, and Thomas R. Cole, "Introduction," in *Practicing the Medical Humanities: Engaging Physicians and Patients*, ed. Ronald A. Carson, Chester R. Burns, and Thomas R. Cole (Hagerstown, MD: University Publishing Group, 2003), 1. For more on the history and development of the medical humanities, see Ronald A. Carson, "Engaged Humanities: Moral Work in the Precincts of Medicine," *Perspectives in Biology and Medicine* 50, no. 3 (2007): 321–333.

7. Daniel M. Fox, "Who We Are: The Political Origins of the Medical Humanities," *Theoretical Medicine* 6, no. 3 (1985): 329, 331.

8. See, for example, Bruce W. Newton, Laurie Barber, James Clardy, Elton Cleveland, and Patricia O'Sullivan, "Is There Hardening of the Heart during Medical School?" *Academic Medicine: Journal of the Association of American Medical Colleges* 83, no. 3 (2008): 244–249.

9. Sherwin B. Nuland, *How We Die: Reflections on Life's Final Chapter* (New York: Vintage Books, 1995), 247; see also Kathryn Montgomery, *How Doctors Think: Clinical Judgment and the Practice of Medicine* (New York: Oxford University Press, 2005).

10. Gert Olthuis and Wim Dekkers, "Medical Education, Palliative Care and Moral Attitude: Some Objectives and Future Perspectives," *Medical Education* 37, no. 10 (2003): 929.

11. See, for example, Andrew H. Brainard and Heather C. Brislen, "Viewpoint: Learning Professionalism; A View from the Trenches," *Academic Medicine: Journal of the Association of American Medical Colleges* 82, no. 11 (2007): 1010–1014; Frederic Hafferty, "Professionalism and the Socialization of Medical Students," in *Teaching Medical Professionalism*, ed. Richard L. Cruess, Sylvia R. Cruess, and Yvonne Steinert (New York: Cambridge University Press, 2009), 53–70; and Thomas S. Inui, *A Flag in the Wind: Educating for Medical Professionalism* (Washington, DC: Association of American Medical Colleges, 2003).

12. Inui, *A Flag in the Wind*, 16.

13. Montgomery, *How Doctors Think*, 36.

14. Ibid., 172. An interesting distinction is made in the German between the natural sciences (*Naturwissenschaften*), of which pure biomedicine can be considered a member, and the human sciences (*Geisteswissenschaften*), which are often associated

with studies in the humanities, such as history, philosophy, and religion. But, as will become clearer later in this work, I advocate a harmonization of the natural and human sciences within a broader approach to medical practice and training that embodies the methods and wisdom of both. For more on *Naturwissenschaften* and *Geisteswissenschaften* in the context of medicine, see Fredrik Svenaeus, "Hermeneutics of Medicine in the Wake of Gadamer: The Issue of *Phronesis*," *Theoretical Medicine and Bioethics* 24, no. 5 (2003): 412.

15. Jeffrey P. Bishop, *The Anticipatory Corpse: Medicine, Power, and the Care of the Dying* (Notre Dame: University of Notre Dame Press, 2011), 303.

16. Linda Wiener and Ramsey Eric Ramsey, *Leaving Us to Wonder: An Essay On The Questions Science Can't Ask* (Albany: State University of New York Press, 2005), 79. I am using "science" or "the sciences" throughout *Afflicted* to refer to the natural sciences. See note 14.

17. Martin Heidegger, "Memorial Address," in *Discourse on Thinking*, trans. John M. Anderson and E. Hans Freund (New York: Harper & Row, 1969), 56; emphasis in original. This speech was given in 1955 in Heidegger's birthplace, Messkirch, Germany, in celebration of the 175th birthday of composer Conradin Kreutzer.

18. Wiener and Ramsey, *Leaving Us to Wonder*, 83.

19. Edmund D. Pellegrino, "The Internal Morality of Clinical Medicine: A Paradigm for the Ethics of the Helping and Healing Professions," *Journal of Medicine and Philosophy* 26, no. 6 (2001): 559–579.

20. In her study "Walking a Mile in Their Patients' Shoes: Empathy and Othering in Medical Students' Education," *Philosophy, Ethics, and Humanities in Medicine* 3, item no. 10 (2008), Johanna Shapiro makes the argument that deep-seated modernist beliefs create barriers to empathy in medicine. She references Jacques-Marie-Émile Lacan's psycho-structural I/Other split, which tends to mark difference more significantly than similarity, along with Western fears of contamination and decay as some of the implicit philosophical and cultural beliefs that can reinforce othering, distance, and self-preservation among medical students and physicians.

21. Montgomery, *How Doctors Think*, 175.

22. Michele Carter and Sally Robinson, "A Narrative Approach to the Clinical Reasoning Process in Pediatric Intensive Care: The Story of Matthew," *Journal of Medical Humanities* 22, no. 3 (2001): 188.

23. Ibid.

24. For more on gallows humor, see Nicole M. Piemonte, "Last Laughs: Gallows Humor and Medical Education," *Journal* of Medical Humanities 36, no. 4 (December 2015): 375–390.

25. Walter F. Baile, Robert Buckman, Renato Lenzi, Gary Glober, Estela A. Beale, and Andrzej P. Kudelka, "SPIKES—A Six-Step Protocol for Delivering Bad News: Application to the Patient with Cancer," *Oncologist* 5, no. 4 (2000): 302–311.

26. As Alan Bleakley points out in *Medical Humanities and Medical Education: How the Medical Humanities Can Shape Better Doctors*. (New York: Routledge, 2015), 9: "Thirty years worth of developing communication skills in undergraduate medicine—largely through simulation, as a quasi-scientific laboratory-tested training—has not addressed . . . medical error [and] poor practices in clinical teamwork and patient consultations."

27. Arthur W. Frank, *The Renewal of Generosity: Illness, Medicine, and How to Live* (Chicago: University of Chicago Press, 2004), 20.

28. Ronald A. Carson, "Educating the Moral Imagination," in *Practicing the Medical Humanities*, ed. Carson, Burns, and Cole, 26.

29. Ibid.

30. Patrick Gardiner, *Kierkegaard* (New York: Oxford University Press, 1997), 38.

31. bell hooks, *Teaching to Transgress: Education as a Practice of Freedom* (New York: Routledge, 1994), 12, 15.

32. Susan Sherwin, *No Longer Patient: Feminist Ethics and Health Care* (Philadelphia: Temple University Press, 1992).

33. Bleakley, *Medical Humanities and Medical Education*, 2.

34. See Heidegger, "Memorial Address," 47.

35. Donald Schön uses the term "technical rationality" to describe the dominant worldview in the West that grew out of the Enlightenment, according to which human progress could be achieved by harnessing the methods and achievements of science and technology. Schön tells us that, by the late nineteenth and early twentieth centuries, professionals, including physicians, began to be seen as "vehicles for the application of the new sciences to the achievement of human progress," and medicine was "refashioned in the new image of a science-based technique for the preservation of health." See Donald A. Schön, *The Reflective Practitioner: How Professionals Think in Action* (New York: Basic Books, 1983), 31. For more on the historical rise of technical rationality, see also Max Weber, "Science as a Vocation," in *From Max Weber: Essays in Sociology*, ed. and trans. H. H. Gerth and C. Wright Mills (New York: Oxford University Press, 1946), 129–156.

36. Martin Heidegger, *Being and Time*, trans. John Macquarrie and Edward Robinson (New York: Harper & Row, 1962), 186.

37. Richard B. Gunderman and Steven L. Kanter, "Perspective: 'How to Fix the Premedical Curriculum' Revisited," *Academic Medicine: Journal of the Association of American Medical Colleges* 83, no. 12 (December 2008): 1161.

38. All recordings and transcripts were de-identified. Codes were assigned to transcripts in lieu of names in order to ensure anonymity. Thus, for example, "MSIV-1" was assigned to transcript 1 of comments by an unnamed fourth-year medical student.

39. Frank, *The Renewal of Generosity*, 145.

40. Ibid., 146.

Chapter 1

1. Warren A. Kinghorn, "Medical Education as Moral Formation: An Aristotelian Account of Medical Professionalism," *Perspectives in Biology and Medicine* 53, no. 1 (2010): 88.

2. Woody Caan, "A Testing Time for Ethical Standards," *BMJ* 330, no. 7506 (2005): 1510.

3. Newton et al., "Is there a Hardening of the Heart during Medical School?"; Mohammadreza Hojat, Michael J. Vergare, Kaye Maxwell, George Brainard, Steven K. Herrine, Gerald A. Isenberg, et al., "The Devil Is in the Third Year: A Longitudinal Study of Erosion of Empathy in Medical School," *Academic Medicine: Journal of the Association of American Medical Colleges* 84, no. 9 (2009): 1182–1191; Melanie Neumann, Friedrich Edelhäuser, Diethard Tauschel, Martin R. Fischer, Markus Wirtz, Christiane Woopen, et al., "Empathy Decline and Its Reasons: A Systematic Review of Studies with Medical Students and Residents" *Academic Medicine: Journal of the Association of American Medical Colleges* 86, no. 8 (2011): 996–1009; Chris Feudtner, Dimitri A. Christakis, and Nicholas A. Christakis, "Do Clinical Clerks Suffer Ethical Erosion? Students' Perceptions of Their Ethical Environment and Personal Development," *Academic Medicine: Journal of the Association of American Medical Colleges* 69, no. 8 (1994): 670–679.

4. According to William F. May, *The Physician's Covenant: Images of the Healer in Medical Ethics*, 2nd ed. (Louisville: Westminster John Knox Press, 2000), 98: "The criteria for admission to medical school, the grading system that prevails there, the system for the placement of graduates in residencies, and eventual job references—all these hurdles and pressure points combine to emphasize the preeminent place of technical performance in the formation and career of the professional." For more on premedical education and medical school admission processes, see Lewis Thomas, "Notes of a Biology-Watcher. How to Fix the Premedical Curriculum," *New England Journal of Medicine* 298, no. 21 (1978): 1180–1181; and Gunderman and Kanter, "Perspective."

5. Johanna Shapiro, Jack Coulehan, Delese Wear, and Martha Montello, "Medical Humanities and Their Discontents: Definitions, Critiques, and Implications," *Academic Medicine: Journal of the Association of American Medical Colleges* 84, no. 2 (2009): 194.

6. Gunderman and Kanter, "Perspective," 1161.

7. See Shapiro, "Walking a Mile in Their Patients' Shoes," 13.

8. Gunderman and Kanter, "Perspective," 1160–1161.

9. We might ask further if the notion of a "calling" still exists within a cultural milieu that so fervently endorses the value of efficiency, productivity, and technical thinking. As Max Weber argues in his 1917 lecture "Science as a Vocation," 152, science (and medical science) cannot answer questions concerning how to be. Rather than being a calling, "science today is a 'vocation' organized in special disciplines in the service of self-clarification and knowledge of interrelated facts."

10. Gunderman and Kanter, "Perspective," 1160.

11. Shapiro et al., "Medical Humanities and Their Discontents," 193.

12. Ibid.

13. Undergraduate "prehealthcare" education will be discussed in greater detail in chapter 4.

14. Kinghorn, "Medical Education as Moral Formation," 88.

15. Hafferty, "Professionalism and the Socialization of Medical Students."

16. Ibid., 60.

17. Ibid., 54, 59.

18. Ibid., 63; emphasis in original.

19. Ibid., 64; emphasis in original.

20. Montgomery, *How Doctors Think*, 167.

21. Ibid., 6.

22. Paul Komesaroff, "The Many Faces of the Clinic: A Levinasian View," in *Handbook of Phenomenology and Medicine*, ed. S. Kay Toombs (Dordrecht: Kluwer Academic, 2001), 317. The idea of the physician as detached observer of the body-object perpetuates an antiquated subject/object dualism.

23. Montgomery, *How Doctors Think*, 6, 173.

24. Lorraine J. Daston and Peter Galison, *Objectivity* (New York: Zone Books, 2010), 41–42.

25. Ibid., 53. As Daston and Galison point out, the concept of objectivity in science is only one of several "epistemic virtues" and is "younger" than the scientific notions of precision and "Truth." Moreover, the history of objectivity is only a subset of the history of epistemology and is not synonymous with certainty or accuracy (indeed,

an "objective" representation of something is not always accurate or precise). Our contemporary understanding of objectivity (since the mid-nineteenth century) is that of a scientific approach that attempts to "filter out the noise that undermines certainty" (17). "Objectivity" can have various meanings, and Daston and Galison argue that too few scholars take the time to precisely define what they mean by term. In *Afflicted*, I take "objectivity" to mean a particular attitude or stance taken toward medical practice and patient care. In medicine, an objective attitude or stance overlaps with methodology; it is believed that if one approaches the patient with a stance of detached objectivity, then this approach will yield certain and verifiable information, allowing one to make the "correct" clinical decision.

26. Ester Carolina Apesoa-Varano and Charles S. Varano, *Conflicted Health Care: Professionalism and Caring in an Urban Hospital* (Nashville: Vanderbilt University Press, 2014).

27. Ibid., 22.

28. Ibid., 158, 196.

29. Bishop, *The Anticipatory Corpse*, 20.

30. Ibid., 20. For more on Aristotle's Four Causes, see Andrea Falcon, "Aristotle on Causality," *Stanford Encyclopedia of Philosophy*, ed. Edward N. Zalta, Spring 2015, http://plato.stanford.edu/archives/spr2014/entries/aristotle-causality/.

31. Ibid., 21.

32. Ibid., 302. See also Michel Foucault, *The Birth of the Clinic: An Archaeology of Medical Perception*, A. M. Sheridan Smith, trans. (New York: Vintage Books, 1975).

33. Bishop, *The Anticipatory Corpse*, 303.

34. Cassell, "The Nature of Suffering," 640.

35. Ibid. Chapter 2 discusses what exactly this "remainder" is.

36. Edmund Pellegrino, "The Caring Ethic: The Relation of Physician to Patient," in *Physician and Philosopher: The Philosophical Foundation of Medicine*, ed. Roger J. Bulger, John P. McGovern, and Daniel P. Sulmasy (Charlottesville, VA: Carden Jennings, 2001), 167; emphasis in original.

37. Timothy E. Quill and Amy P. Abernethy, "Generalist plus Specialist Palliative Care—Creating a More Sustainable Model," *New England Journal of Medicine* 368, no. 13 (2013): 1173–1174.

38. See S. Kay Toombs, *The Meaning of Illness: A Phenomenological Account of the Different Perspectives of Physician and Patients* (Boston: Kluwer Academic, 1993).

39. Arthur W. Frank, *The Wounded Storyteller: Body, Illness, and Ethics* (Chicago: University of Chicago Press, 1997).

40. Ibid., 7.

41. Ibid., 88.

42. Ibid., 84.

43. Nuland, *How We Die*, 253.

44. Ibid.

45. Ibid., 247.

46. Ibid.

47. Ibid., 249.

48. Anonymous, "I Never Understood the Loss of Empathy during Medical Training... Until Now," *KevinMD.com* (blog), posted September 2, 2014, http://www.kevinmd.com/blog/2014/09/never-understood-loss-empathy-medical-training-now.html.

49. Ibid. Here, "rubric" refers to a document that lists explicit expectations and criteria for an assignment, task, or activity, usually describing levels of quality from excellent to poor.

50. Katharine Treadway, "Perspective: The Code," *New England Journal of Medicine* 357, no. 13 (2007): 1274.

51. May, *The Physician's Covenant*, 103.

52. Shekinah Elmore, "A Piece of My Mind. The Good Doctor," *JAMA* 306, no. 14 (2011): 1525–1526.

53. Ibid., 1525.

54. Ibid.

55. Ibid.

56. Ibid.

57. Ibid.

58. Ibid.

59. Susan D. Block and Andrew J. Billings, "Learning from the Dying," *New England Journal of Medicine* 2, no. 1 (2005): 1315.

60. Reidar Pedersen, "Empathy Development in Medical Education—A Critical Review," *Medical Teacher* 32, no. 7 (2010): 598.

61. Ibid., 600.

62. Wiener and Ramsey, *Leaving Us to Wonder*, 121.

63. Shapiro et al., "Medical Humanities and Their Discontents," 194; emphasis in original.

64. Ibid.

65. Wiener and Ramsey, *Leaving Us to Wonder*, 121.

66. Ibid., 15.

67. Kevin Aho, *Heidegger's Neglect of the Body* (New York: State University of New York Press, 2010), 16–18.

68. Ibid., 17.

69. Michael J. Inwood, *Heidegger* (New York: Oxford University Press, 1997), 10. See also, Martin Heidegger, "What Is Metaphysics?" in *Existentialism from Dostoevsky to Sartre*, ed. and trans. Walter Kaufmann (New York: New American Library, 1975), 242–279.

70. Charles B. Guignon, *Heidegger and the Problem of Knowledge* (Cambridge, MA: Hackett, 1983). "Dasein," meaning "to be there" or "to exist" is the term Heidegger employs to describe both the human and the type of being the human has. Dasein is not a "thing," but the possible ways of being. See Inwood, *Heidegger*, 18, 19.

71. Heidegger, *Being and Time*, 77.

72. Guignon, *Heidegger and the Problem of Knowledge*, 15.

73. William James Bartles, "The Status of Epistemology in the Thought of Martin Heidegger (Knowledge, Art, Phenomenology)" (Ph.D. diss., Rice University, 1985), 43–56.

74. Heidegger, *Being and Time*, 75; emphasis in original. As Heidegger says in "What Is Metaphysics?," 269: "Metaphysics . . . thinks of Being only by representing beings as beings. It means all beings as a whole, although it speaks of Being. It refers to Being and means beings as beings. From its beginning to its completion, the propositions of metaphysics have been strangely involved in a persistent confusion of beings and Being. This confusion, to be sure, must be considered an event and not a mere mistake. It cannot by any means be charged to a mere negligence of thought or a carelessness of expression. Owing to this persistent confusion, the claim that metaphysics poses the question of Being lands us in utter error."

75. Bartles, "The Status of Epistemology in the Thought of Martin Heidegger," 73.

76. Heidegger, *Being and Time*, 73.

77. Guignon, *Heidegger and the Problem of Knowledge*, 13–14; see also Inwood, *Heidegger*, 41: "We end up by taking such a sentence as 'Snow is white,' which occurs more commonly in logic textbooks than in down-to-earth talk, as a paradigm of significant discourse. Such assertions are seen as the locus of truth. They are true if, and only if, they correspond to the facts or to some such entity in the world."

78. Guignon, *Heidegger and the Problem of Knowledge*, 21–23.

79. Ibid., 23.

80. Ibid., 30.

81. Ibid., 16.

82. Ibid.

83. Charles Taylor, *Philosophical Arguments* (Cambridge, MA: Harvard University Press, 1995), 3.

84. Inwood, *Heidegger*, 55. This is also true for phenomenologist Maurice Merleau-Ponty, who says: "If we want to subject science itself to rigorous scrutiny and arrive at a precise assessment of its meaning and scope, we must begin by reawakening the basic experience of the world of which science is the second-order expression." See Maurice Merleau-Ponty, *Phenomenology of Perception* (New York: Routledge, 2002), ix.

85. Susann M. Laverty, "Hermeneutic Phenomenology and Phenomenology: A Comparison of Historical and Methodological Considerations," *International Journal of Qualitative Methods* 2, no. 3 (2003): 24. See also Heidegger, *Being and Time*, sections 31 and 32, 182–195.

86. Martin Heidegger, *Zollikon Seminars: Protocols, Conversations, Letters*, ed. Medard Boss, trans. Franz Mayr and Richard Askay (Evanston: Northwestern University Press, 2001), 4.

87. Wiener and Ramsey, *Leaving Us to Wonder*, 5.

88. Ibid., 6.

89. Charles Taylor, *Philosophy and the Human Sciences*, vol. 2 of *Philosophical Papers* (New York: Cambridge University Press, 1985), 3.

90. Ibid.

91. Martin Heidegger, "The Question Concerning Technology," in *The Question Concerning Technology, and Other Essays*, trans. William Lovitt (New York: Harper & Row, 1977), 3–35. See also Inwood, *Heidegger*, 42; Daniel O. Dahlstrom, *The Heidegger Dictionary*, (New York: Bloomsbury Academic, 2013), 10–12.

92. Inwood, *Heidegger*, 44.

93. Ibid., 69.

94. According to Dahlstrom, *The Heidegger Dictionary*, 37: "A metonym for 'Dasein,' 'being-in-the-world' signifies the holistic or unified phenomenon in terms of which Heidegger explicates Dasein's worldhood, who Dasein is . . . and the ways it is in the

world." In *Being and Time*, 231, Heidegger claims that Dasein is the only being for whom its being is an issue.

95. Inwood, *Heidegger*, 43.

96. Ibid., 56.

97. Inwood, *Heidegger*, 44.

98. Heidegger, "Memorial Address."

99. Ibid., 46. Philosopher Bernard Williams, in *Philosophy as a Humanistic Discipline*, ed. A. W. Moore (Princeton: Princeton University Press, 2008), 182, claims that this way of thinking has come to dominate much of Western philosophy, mostly in the analytic tradition. He refers to this as "scientism," which he defines as "a misunderstanding of the relations between philosophy and the natural sciences, which tends to assimilate philosophy to the aims, or at least the manners, of the sciences." Williams thinks this occurs because science appears to possess an "intellectual authority" that philosophers would like to share in, but this approach is deeply misguided because most philosophical investigations are entirely unlike those of the natural sciences and can never be abstracted from their historical and cultural foundations (188–189).

100. William Bynum, "Why Physicians Need to Be More Than Automated Medical Kiosks," *Academic Medicine: Journal of the Association of American Medical Colleges* 89, no. 2 (2014): 214.

101. Heidegger, "Memorial Address" 54.

102. Wiener and Ramsey, *Leaving Us to Wonder*, 79; see also Heidegger, "The Question Concerning Technology," 21.

103. Wiener and Ramsey, *Leaving Us to Wonder*, 84; see also Heidegger, "The Question Concerning Technology."

104. Guignon, *Heidegger and the Problem of Knowledge*, 16.

105. Heidegger, "The Question Concerning Technology," 24; Wiener and Ramsey, *Leaving Us to Wonder*, 79.

106. See Heidegger, "The Question Concerning Technology"; see also Kevin Aho, "Why Heidegger Is Not an Existentialist: Interpreting Authenticity and Historicity in *Being and Time*," *Florida Philosophical Review* 3, no. 1 (2003), 15.

107. See Hans-Georg Gadamer, *The Enigma of Health: The Art of Healing in a Scientific Age*, trans. Jason Gaiger and Nicholas Walker (Stanford: Stanford University Press, 1996), 6.

108. Wiener and Ramsey, *Leaving Us to Wonder*, 79.

109. Ibid., 81; Heidegger, *Being and Time*, 73–75.

110. Wiener and Ramsey, *Leaving Us to Wonder*, 79.

111. Heidegger, "Memorial Address," 50. It is important to note, however, that Heidegger's larger critique of philosophy and epistemology extends further back than the critique that emerged during the Enlightenment.

112. Bishop, *The Anticipatory Corpse*, 38-39. Foucault's investigation spans approximately the years 1770–1830.

113. Foucault, *The Birth of the Clinic*, 88-106.

114. Bishop, *The Anticipatory Corpse*, 39.

115. Ibid.; Foucault, *The Birth of the Clinic*, 187, 195.

116. Foucault, *The Birth of the Clinic*, 195.

117. Ibid., 162.

118. Bishop, *The Anticipatory Corpse*, 91.

119. Mark J. Kissler, Ben Saxton, Ricardo Nuila, and Dorene F. Balmer, "Professional Formation in the Gross Anatomy Lab and Narrative Medicine: An Exploration," *Academic Medicine: Journal of the Association of American Medical Colleges* 91, no. 6 (2016): 774.

120. Ibid.

121. Cassell, *The Nature of Suffering*, 641. Almost ninety years ago, physician Francis Peabody suggested the importance of uncovering "what is the matter" with the patient in order to help alleviate suffering. See Francis W. Peabody, "The Care of the Patient," *Journal of the American Medical Association* 88, no.12 (1927): 877–882.

122. See Toombs, *The Meaning of Illness*, 115.

123. Nuland, *How We Die*, 258–259.

124. Guignon, *Heidegger and the Problem of Knowledge*, 19.

125. In his "Memorial Address," 55, Heidegger states that "the meaning pervading technology hides itself." See also Heidegger, "The Question Concerning Technology," 14.

126. Heidegger, "Memorial Address," 50.

127. Taylor, *Philosophy and the Human Sciences*, 4.

128. Ibid., 6.

129. Lauren F. Friedman, "IBM's Watson Supercomputer May Soon Be the Best Doctor in the World," *Business Insider*, April 22, 2014, http://www.businessinsider.com/ibms-watson-may-soon-be-the-best-doctor-in-the-world-2014-4.

130. Andrew McAffee, as quoted in ibid. See also McAffee's blog at http://andrewmcafee.org/.

131. As Taylor points out in *Philosophical Arguments*, 6: "The plausibility of the computer as a model of thinking comes partly from the fact that it is a machine, hence living 'proof' that materialism can accommodate explanations in terms of intelligent performance; but partly, too, it comes from the widespread faith that our intelligent performances are ultimately to be understood in terms of formal operations."

132. Heidegger, "Memorial Address," 51.

133. Wiener and Ramsey, *Leaving Us to Wonder*, 80.

134. Heidegger, "Memorial Address," 50.

135. Cassell, "The Nature of Suffering," 644.

Chapter 2

1. See Patricia J. Huntington, "Heidegger's Reading of Kierkegaard Revisited: From Ontological Abstraction to Ethical Concretion," in *Kierkegaard in Post/Modernity*, ed. Martin J. Matuštík and Merold Westphal (Bloomington: Indiana University Press, 1995), 43–65. It should be noted that Huntington considers the appearance of Kierkegaard's ideas in *Being and Time* not as an extension of Kierkegaard's thought, but as a "significant transmutation" of his ideas that strip them of their ethical import (44).

2. Gardiner, *Kierkegaard*, 2.

3. Ibid., 36.

4. Søren Kierkegaard, *Concluding Unscientific Postscript to Philosophical Fragments*, vol. 1, trans. Howard V. Hong and Edna H. Hong (Princeton: Princeton University Press, 1992), 313.

5. Ibid., 302.

6. Ibid., 308.

7. Ibid., 242.

8. In response to the argument that Kierkegaard is primarily a religious thinker and not "really" a philosopher, Merold Westphal and Martin J. Matuštík write: "Insofar as this view stems from the assumption that to be taken seriously a philosopher must either be secular or abstract from his or her religious identity, it can be dismissed as a prejudice rooted in very dubious Enlightenment conceptions of the autonomy of human thought." See Merold Westphal and Martin J. Matuštík, "Introduction," in *Kierkegaard in Post/Modernity*, ed. Matuštík and Westphal, vii.

9. Friedrich Wilhelm Nietzsche, *On the Genealogy of Morals*, trans. Walter Arnold Kaufmann and R. J. Hollingdale (New York: Vintage Books, 1989), third essay, section 24, 152; emphasis in original. Nietzsche is quoting himself here verbatim from an

aphorism headed "How we, too, are still pious" from *The Gay Science*, trans. Walter Arnold Kaufmann (New York: Vintage, 1974), book 5, section 344, 281, where he argues that "science also rests on a faith; there is simply no science 'without presuppositions.'" He further develops this idea in his discussion of "the ascetic ideal" in *On the Genealogy of Morals*, 149–155, where he makes the claim that the search for truth does not set out from nowhere—from a detached, presuppositionless stance—but necessarily from somewhere. That "somewhere" for science, and for rationalistic thinking generally, is the "faith" that what is true is that which is discoverable by scientific means and methods, and that what is not discoverable by such means is not true. In other words, Nietzsche argues that it is merely an illusion to believe it possible to abstain altogether from convictions and presuppositions in the search for truth, whether in science or morality.

10. See Nietzsche, *On the Genealogy of Morals*, third essay, section 24, 148–152; Wiener and Ramsey, *Leaving Us to Wonder*, 66, 68.

11. Nietzsche, *On the Genealogy of Morals*, third essay, section 24, 151; emphasis in original.

12. Wiener and Ramsey, *Leaving Us to Wonder*, 68.

13. Nietzsche, *On the Genealogy of Morals*, third essay, section 12, 119; emphasis in original.

14. Cassell, "The Nature of Suffering," 640. As Charles Guignon explains in *Heidegger and the Problem of Knowledge*, 37: "The Cartesian tradition has postulated the existence of only two types of substance, mind and matter, and the dream of unified science has been to reduce all explanations to the physical."

15. Theodor W. Adorno, *Negative Dialectics*, 2nd ed., trans. E. B. Ashton (New York: Bloomsbury Academic, 1981), 5.

16. Gardiner, *Kierkegaard*, 35.

17. Bishop, *The Anticipatory Corpse*, 294.

18. Though neither Kierkegaard nor Nietzsche is considered a phenomenologist, according to Wiener and Ramsey, *Leaving Us to Wonder*, 76, "Nietzsche is thus a forerunner of twentieth century phenomenological philosophy that attempts to . . . give us insight into our original experience of the world and the connection of this experience to scientific knowledge."

19. Toombs, *The Meaning of Illness*, 86.

20. Fredrik Svenaeus, "Illness as Unhomelike Being-in-the-World: Heidegger and the Phenomenology of Medicine," *Medicine, Health Care and Philosophy* 14, no. 3 (2011): 333–343.

21. Laverty, "Hermeneutic Phenomenology and Phenomenology."

22. Dermot Moran, *Introduction to Phenomenology* (New York: Routledge, 2000), 3.

23. Merleau-Ponty, *Phenomenology of Perception*, vii; see also Moran, *Introduction to Phenomenology*, xiii.

24. Paul B. Armstrong, "Phenomenology," in *The Johns Hopkins Guide to Literary Theory and Criticism*, ed. Michael Groden and Martin Kreisworth (Baltimore: Johns Hopkins University Press, 1994), 562. Near the end of his career, Edmund Husserl coined the term "lifeworld" (*Lebenswelt*) and identified it as the central theme of phenomenology. See Merleau-Ponty, *Phenomenology as Perception*, vii.

25. Moran, *Introduction to Phenomenology*, xiii, 9; Laverty, "Hermeneutic Phenomenology and Phenomenology," 4.

26. Moran, *Introduction to Phenomenology*, 11.

27. Fredrik Svenaeus, *The Hermeneutics of Medicine and the Phenomenology of Health: Steps Toward a Philosophy of Medical Practice* (Dordrecht: Kluwer, 2001), 76.

28. Ibid.

29. Moran, *Introduction to Phenomenology*, 3.

30. Ibid., 13.

31. Ibid., 16. Phenomenology (the study of everyday experience) is a methodology that Heidegger draws on to explain his "fundamental ontology," which was discussed in chapter 1 and will be discussed later in this chapter. A phenomenological inquiry into fundamental ontology involves an exploration into the foundational being of human beings—that is, what it means "to be" in the first place. See Dahlstrom, *The Heidegger Dictionary*, 147.

32. Moran, *Introduction to Phenomenology*, 16; See also "Hermeneutic Phenomenology," *Phenomenology Online*, http://www.phenomenologyonline.com/inquiry/orientations-in-phenomenology/hermeneutical-phenomenology/.

33. Tilottama Rojan, "Hermeneutics," in *The Johns Hopkins Guide to Literary Theory and Criticism*, ed. Groden and Kreisworth, 375.

34. Some scholars have drawn a distinction between "phenomenology" and "hermeneutic phenomenology," claiming that phenomenology is concerned primarily with describing lived experience, whereas hermeneutic phenomenology studies the "interpretive structures" of lived experience. But, considering that nearly all present-day phenomenologists stress the situatedness of human experience and its effect on interpretation, this distinction between the two traditions no longer seems useful. Thus Toombs, for example, though not explicitly referring to her phenomenological account of illness as "hermeneutic," emphasizes that a person's perception or "global field of meaning" is inevitably "social, historical, economic, political, and so on," and "the meaning of a particular object cannot be separated from the global

field of meaning of the individual's world." See Toombs, *The Meaning of Illness*, 5; see also Moran, *Introduction to Phenomenology*, 197; and Laverty, "Hermeneutic Phenomenology and Phenomenology."

35. Jeff Malpas, "Hans-Georg Gadamer," *Stanford Encyclopedia of Philosophy*, ed. Edward N. Zalta, Winter 2014, http://plato.stanford.edu/archives/win2014/entries/gadamer.

36. Moran, *Introduction to Phenomenology*, 231.

37. Ibid.

38. Toombs, *The Meaning of Illness*, 23.

39. Merleau-Ponty, *Phenomenology of Perception*. First published in 1945, this work was not translated into English until 1962.

40. David Woodruff Smith, "Phenomenology," *Stanford Encyclopedia of Philosophy*, ed. Zalta, Fall 2011, http://plato.stanford.edu/archives/fall2011/entries/phenomenology/.

41. Merleau-Ponty, *Phenomenology of Perception*, 95; see also Kevin Aho, "The Missing Dialogue between Heidegger and Merleau-Ponty: On the Importance of the Zollikon Seminars," *Body & Society* 11, no. 2 (2005): 8.

42. Aho, "The Missing Dialogue between Heidegger and Merleau-Ponty," 1. Although Heidegger's fundamental ontology explicated in *Being and Time* makes it possible for Merleau-Ponty's description of bodily perception—which assumes Dasein's prereflective understanding of being-in-the-world—Merleau-Ponty (as well as Jean-Paul Sartre) was critical of Heidegger for paying too little attention to the body and embodiment in *Being and Time*. Aho sees Heidegger's later philosophy in his Zollikon seminars as "strikingly similar" to Merleau-Ponty's, yet he defends Heidegger's apparent neglect of the body in *Being and Time*, arguing that Heidegger's fundamental ontology was intended to describe the meaning of Dasein as the clearing or space of meaning that makes bodily perception possible in the first place. Aho's argument in this article is that Dasein is "already there, prior to bodily perception"; therefore, phenomenological accounts of the body, though crucially important, are nevertheless regional, ontic investigations (1, 16, 20). See also Inwood, *Heidegger*, 24: "Dasein as Heidegger describes it, essentially requires a body of a certain sort, and is not a soul or an ego that might conceivably exist in a disembodied state or in a body quite different from the typical human body."

43. Heidegger, *Zollikon Seminars*, 86.

44. Ibid., 86–87. "Ecstatic" is used here in the sense of the Greek *ekstasis*—a standing outside or beside oneself. This refers to our ability, for example, to "be near" a friend to whom we are writing a letter, even when this friend is miles away physically, or to project ourselves "near" the door after hearing a knock, even before we walk toward it.

45. See Aho, "The Missing Dialogue between Heidegger and Merleau-Ponty," 16. "Everydayness" as used here should not be confused with Heidegger's specific use of "everydayness" in *Being and Time*, 422, which designates existing that is primarily determined by the "they-self" or culturally prescribed ways of being. Here I am referring simply to the everyday tasks or movements we engage in routinely.

46. Heidegger, *Zollikon Seminars*, 84.

47. Gadamer, *The Enigma of Health*, 42.

48. Ibid., 73.

49. Ibid., 42.

50. Sandra Butler and Barbara Rosenblum, *Cancer in Two Voices* (Duluth: Spinsters Ink, 1996), 138.

51. Ibid., 136.

52. Susan Sontag, *Illness as Metaphor* and *AIDS and Its Metaphors* (New York: Picador USA, 2001), 3.

53. Svenaeus, "Illness as Unhomelike Being-in-the World," 339.

54. See Kevin Aho, "Medicalizing Mental Health: A Phenomenological Alternative," *Journal of Medical Humanities* 29, no. 4 (2008): 248.

55. Svenaeus, "Illness as Unhomelike Being-in-the-World," 335.

56. Heidegger, *Being and Time*, 174.

57. Svenaeus, "Illness as Unhomelike Being-in-the World," 333.

58. Ibid., 335.

59. Arthur W. Frank, *At the Will of the Body: Reflections on Illness* (New York: Houghton Mifflin, 1991), 6.

60. Ibid.

61. Ibid., 8.

62. Svenaeus, "Illness as Unhomelike Being-in-the-World," 336.

63. Toombs, *The Meaning of Illness*, 115; Svenaeus, "Illness as Unhomelike Being-in-the World," 338. Svenaeus notes the possibility of remaining within a homelike state—or perhaps re-creating a different homelike state—despite being ill. He also points out that there are those who experience feelings of unhomelikeness and yet have no detectable biological disease. Indeed, experiences of both homelikeness and unhomelikeness are essential parts of being-in-the-world, regardless of the presence of illness (338). See also Gadamer, *The Enigma of Health*; and James Alfred Aho and

Kevin Aho, *Body Matters: A Phenomenology of Sickness, Disease, and Illness* (Lanham, MD: Lexington Books, 2008), 3.

64. Frank, *At the Will of the Body*, 12; emphasis in original.

65. Sidonie Smith and Julia Watson, *Reading Autobiography: A Guide for Interpreting Life Narratives* (Minneapolis,: University of Minnesota Press, 2001), 25.

66. Ibid., 26.

67. Byron J. Good and Mary-Jo DelVecchio Good, "'Fiction' and 'Historicity' in Doctors' Stories," in *Narrative and the Cultural Construction of Illness and Healing*, ed. Cheryl Mattingly and Linda C. Garro (Berkeley: University of California Press, 2000), 50; Kathryn Montgomery Hunter, *Doctors' Stories: The Narrative Structure of Medical Knowledge* (Princeton: Princeton University Press, 1991).

68. Good and DelVecchio Good, "'Fiction' and 'Historicity' in Doctors' Sotries," 51; Hunter, *Doctors' Stories*, xx–xxiii. For Hunter, therapeutic success depends on recognizing that a medical narrative is derived from the patient and that it ultimately must be returned to the patient in a way that is meaningful to that patient in the context of his or her life.

69. Smith and Watson, *Reading Autobiography*, 26.

70. Frank, *At the Will of the Body*, 13.

71. Neither scientific nor phenomenological explanations of the phenomenon of illness will provide us with the whole picture, and we should be suspicious of claims about there being only one correct way of approaching that phenomenon. See Wiener and Ramsey, *Leaving Us to Wonder*, 94.

72. Bishop, *The Anticipatory Corpse*, 294.

73. Frank, *At the Will of the Body*, 10–11.

74. Sometimes a patient's suffering is caused not by an illness, per se, but simply by *being in the world*. Medicine, however, is not particularly well equipped for handling existential suffering, and more often than not, this suffering is either conceived as falling outside (bio)medicine's purview and thus ignored, or attributed to biological or biochemical dysfunction and is thus medicalized and treated pharmacologically. Thus, rather than seeing the anguish that can come from patients being in the world—that what they might need is another to acknowledge their suffering—physicians routinely offer to treat them with psychopharmaceuticals. This is not to say, of course, that patients suffering from debilitating depression or anxiety may not benefit from such treatment. See Aho, "Medicalizing Mental Health."

75. Frank, *The Wounded Storyteller*, 84.

76. Nuland, *How We Die*, 224.

Notes

77. Shapiro, "Walking a Mile in Their Patients' Shoes," 14.

78. Ibid.; see also Scott A. Fields and W. Michael Johnson, "Physician-Patient Communication: Breaking Bad News," *West Virginia Medical Journal* 108, no. 2 (2012): 32–35.

79. Frank, *At the Will of the Body*, 101.

80. Annette C. Baier, "Alternative Offerings to Asclepius?" *Medical Humanities Review* 6, no.1 (1992): 11.

81. See, for example, Quill and Abernethy, "Generalist plus Specialist Palliative Care."

82. Atul Gawande, *Being Mortal: Medicine and What Matters in the End* (New York: Metropolitan Books, 2014), 7.

83. Bishop, *The Anticipatory Corpse*, 17.

84. Camilla Zimmerman and Gary Rodin, "The Denial of Death Thesis: Sociological Critique and Implications for Palliative Care," *Palliative Medicine* 18, no. 2 (2004): 121.

85. Ernest Becker, *The Denial of Death* (New York: Free Press Paperbacks, 1997). Later in his career, Freud dealt extensively with ideas about death and the conflict between Eros and Thanatos.

86. Sam Keen, "Foreword," in Becker, *The Denial of Death*, xii.

87. Becker, *The Denial of Death*, xiii. Becker refers to the search for ways to transcend death as the "hero system."

88. Alice Stewart Trillin, "Of Dragons and Garden Peas: A Cancer Patient Talks to Doctors," *New England Journal of Medicine* 304, no. 12 (1981): 699.

89. Paul Ramsey, *The Patient as Person: Explorations in Medical Ethics* (New Haven: Yale University Press, 1970), 156. There are limitations to Ramsey's argument, given that an overwhelming majority of Americans identified (and still identify) as religious, despite recent declines in religious affiliation; see Pew Research Center, "America's Changing Religious Landscape, May 12, 2015, http://www.pewforum.org/2015/05/12/americas-changing-religious-landscape/. The major point here, however, is that, in the frightening face of death, many people—even those who identify as religious, turn to medicine to palliate their anxiety. As William F. May says in *The Physician's Covenant*, 16: "Latent religious forces are still at work in contemporary medicine, religious forces that shape the perceptions and responses that men and women oppose to the crushing power of disease, suffering, and death."

90. Charles E. Rosenberg, *The Care of Strangers: The Rise of America's Hospital System* (New York: Basic Books, 1987), 9; see also Paul Starr, *The Social Transformation of American Medicine* (New York: Basic Books, 1982).

91. Zimmermann and Rodin, "The Denial of Death Thesis," 125.

92. Howard F. Stein, *American Medicine as Culture* (Boulder: Westview Press, 1990); see also George L. Engel, "Selection of Clinical Material in Psychosomatic Medicine: The Need for a New Physiology," *Psychosomatic Medicine* 16 (1954): 369.

93. Stein, *American Medicine as Culture*, xvi.

94. Nuland, *How We Die*, 258, 224.

95. Herman Feifel, "Death," in *Taboo Topics*, ed. Norman L. Farebrow (New York: Atherton Press, 1963), 11.

96. On the other hand, some physicians assume a "parental role" with terminal patients as a way of sheltering them from the reality of their impending death. See May, *The Physician's Covenant*, 26: see also Aleksandra Ciałkowska-Rysz and Tomasz Dzierżanowski, "Personal Fear of Death Affects the Proper Process of Breaking Bad News," *Archives of Medical Science* 9, no. 1 (2013): 127–131; Fields and Johnson, "Physician-Patient Communication"; Feifel, "Death," 10; and Elisabeth Kübler-Ross, *On Death and Dying* (New York: Macmillan, 1969).

97. Sandra Kocijan Lovko, Rudolf Gregurek, and Dalibor Karlovic, "Stress and Ego-Defense Mechanisms in Medical Staff at Oncology and Physical Medicine Departments," *European Journal of Psychiatry* 21, no. 4 (December 2007): 279–286.

98. Ibid., 285; see also Robert Plutchik, Henry Kellerman, and Hope R. Conte, "A Structural Theory of Ego Defenses and Emotions," in *Emotions in Personality and Psychopathology*, ed. Carroll E. Izard (New York: Plenum Press, 1979), 229–256.

99. Peter Maguire, "Barriers to Psychological Care of the Dying," *British Medical Journal (Clinical Research Ed.)* 291, no. 6510 (1985): 1712.

100. Herman Feifel, Susan Hanson, and Robert Jones, "Physicians Consider Death," in *Proceedings of the 75th Annual Convention of the American Psychological Association* 2 (1967): 201–202. See also Anne C. Kane and John D. Hogan, "Death Anxiety in Physicians: Defensive Style, Medical Specialty, and Exposure to Death," *Omega: Journal of Death and Dying* 16, no. 1 (1985): 11–22.

101. Heidegger, *Being and Time*, 294, 395.

102. Ibid., 234.

103. Ibid., 307; Dahlstrom, *The Heidegger Dictionary*, 52; Iain Thomson, "Death and Demise in *Being and Time*," in *The Cambridge Companion to Heidegger's Being and Time*, ed. Mark A. Wrathall (New York: Cambridge University Press, 2013), 260–290.

104. Thomson, "Death and Demise in *Being and Time*," 264.

105. Ibid. For Heidegger, Dasein does not merely perish, for human existence is not a biological entity. To exist means to interpret and understand the world around us. As such, existence comes to an end through demise or ontological death.

106. Ibid.

107. Heidegger, *Being and Time*, 307.

108. The discussion about death in *Afflicted* might be described as reflecting Heidegger's early philosophy only. In his later philosophy, he begins to equate death "with the sort of world collapse that can befall a cultural epoch, and dying is striving to preserve the culture's understanding of being while being ready to sacrifice it when confronted with anomalous practices that portend the arrival of a new cultural world." See Hubert L. Dreyfus, "Foreword," in Carol J. White, *Time and Death: Heidegger's Analysis of Finitude*, ed. Mark Ralkowski (Aldershot, UK: Ashgate, 2005), xxxi.

109. Thomson, "Death and Demise in *Being and Time*," 275.

110. Gardiner, *Kierkegaard*, 106. As Huntington argues in "Heidegger's Reading of Kierkegaard Revisited," 45, "Heidegger's ontology of being is indebted to the Kierkegaardian notions of *Existenz*, repetition, and ethical identity (authenticity), among other concepts." See also Dahlstrom, *The Heidegger Dictionary*, 111.

111. See Søren Kierkegaard, *The Sickness unto Death*, in *Fear and Trembling and The Sickness unto Death*, trans. Walter Lowrie (Princeton: Princeton University Press, 1968).

112. Ibid., 155; Thomson, "Death and Demise in *Being and Time*," 270.

113. Inwood, *Heidegger*, 35; Heidegger, *Being and Time*, 175. Though *Grundstimmung* is translated as "state-of-mind" in Macquarrie and Robinson's translation, this turn of phrase risks being misunderstood. The phrase inaccurately suggests a kind of conscious cognitive state, rather than one's being disposed toward the world in a way that permeates one's interpretive activity and colors the way one understands one's world.

114. Inwood, *Heidegger*, 35; Heidegger, *Being and Time*, 175, 176.

115. Heidegger, *Being and Time*, 284.

116. Thomson, "Death and Demise in *Being and Time*."

117. Ibid., 280–283.

118. See, for example, David Field, "Palliative Medicine and the Medicalization of Death" *European Journal of Cancer Care* 94, no. 3 (1994): 58–62; Jane Gibbins, Rachel McCoubrie, and Karen Forbes, "Why Are Newly Qualified Doctors Unprepared to Care for Patients at the End of Life?" *Medical Education* 45, no. 4 (2011): 389–399.

119. Because our ontological structure is being-in-the-world, when something like illness, loss, or trauma strikes, it not only affects "us," but it disrupts our ability to make sense of the world as we see it and ourselves in that world.

120. Heidegger, *Being and Time*, 284, 294; emphasis in original.

121. Ibid., 281.

122. Ibid., 175.

123. Ibid.

124. Ibid., 234.

125. Ibid., 165.

126. Aho, "Why Heidegger Is Not an Existentialist," 8.

127. Gardiner, *Kierkegaard*, 91, 114, 110.

128. Kierkegaard, *The Sickness unto Death*, 168. Kierkegaard claims that the highest form of despair belongs to those who are unaware that they are in despair. The condition of despair, according to Kierkegaard, is almost a default position belonging to all human beings—something that lurks beneath and can always return, even for those who have engaged in previous efforts to overcome it. See *Sickness unto Death*, part I, section B, 147–150.

129. Huntington, "Heidegger's Reading of Kierkegaard Revisited," 47.

130. Heidegger, *Being and Time*, 220.

131. Aho, "Why Heidegger Is Not an Existentialist," 7.

132. Huntington, "Heidegger's Reading of Kierkegaard Revisited," 53.

133. Inwood, *Heidegger*, 22.

134. Heidegger, *Being and Time*, 168.

135. Inwood, *Heidegger*, 22.

136. Heidegger, *Being and Time*, 219, 220. As Heidegger says, "'Fallenness' into the 'world' means an absorption into the Being-with-one-another, in so far as the latter is guided by idle talk, curiosity [as opposed to wonder], and ambiguity" (220).

137. Inwood, *Heidegger*, 49.

138. Heidegger, *Being and Time*, 295; emphasis in original.

139. Inwood, *Heidegger*, 62; Heidegger *Being and Time*, 307.

140. Inwood, *Heidegger*, 62.

141. Heidegger, *Being and Time*, 297; emphasis in original.

142. Ibid., 298.

143. Leo Tolstoy, *The Death of Ivan Ilych and Other Stories*, trans. Aylmer Maude and J. D. Duff (New York: Signet Classic 2003), 100.

144. Ibid. After noticing connections between Tolstoy's novella and Heidegger's *Being and Time*, I found that academics have critiqued both Heidegger and Heideggerian

scholars for not emphasizing the debt of inspiration that Heidegger owes to Leo Tolstoy and his work. See William Irwin, "Death by Inauthenticity: Heidegger's Debt to Ivan Il'ich's Fall," *Tolstoy Studies Journal* 25 (2013).

145. Heidegger, *Being and Time*, 223.

146. For an examination of the shortcomings of contemporary medical epistemology, see Montgomery, *How Doctors Think*. For one of the few articles I have found that attempts to uncover the reasons *why* such an epistemology persists, see Shapiro, "Walking a Mile in Their Patients' Shoes."

147. Shapiro, "Walking a Mile in Their Patients' Shoes," 15.

148. Nietzsche, *On the Genealogy of Morals*, third essay, section 23, 147; emphasis in original.

149. Treadway, "Perspective," 1275.

150. Gawande, *Being Mortal*, 3.

151. Ibid.

152. Pauline W. Chen, *Final Exam: A Surgeon's Reflections on Mortality* (New York: Vintage Books, 2008), 205.

153. Ibid.

154. Codes, policies, and procedures that center on "technical performance," for example, serve an "invaluable psychological function," for they help "free the physician from the [perceived] destructive consequences of involvement" with patients. See May, *The Physician's Covenant*, 102.

155. Craig C. Earle, Elyse R. Park, Bonnie Lai, Jane C. Weeks, John Z. Ayanian, and Susan Block, "Identifying Potential Indicators of the Quality of End-of-Life Cancer Care from Administrative Data," *Journal of Clinical Oncology* 21, no. 6 (2003): 1133–1138.

156. Montgomery, *How Doctors Think*, 158, 196.

157. Frank, *At the Will of the Body*, 12.

158. Heidegger, *Being and Time*, 312.

159. Ibid.

160. Anonymous, "I Never Understood the Loss of Empathy."

161. For example, research has shown that chemotherapy may have an anxiety-reducing effect for patients since they feel that they are "actively fighting" the cancer. See Ben Edwards and Valerie Clarke, "The Psychological Impact of a Cancer Diagnosis on Families: The Influence of Family Functioning and Patients' Illness Characteristics on Depression and Anxiety," *Psycho-Oncology* 13, no. 8 (2004): 562–576; see also

John W. Lannaman and Linda M. Harris, "Ending the End-of-Life Communication Impasse: A Dialogic Intervention," in *Cancer, Communication, and Aging*, ed. Lisa Sparks, Dan O'Hair, and Gary Kreps (Cresskill, NJ: Hampton, 2008), 293–320.

162. Lannaman and Harris, "Ending the End-of-Life Communication Impasse," 306.

163. Gadamer, *The Enigma of Health*, 64.

164. Frank, *At the Will of the Body*, 67.

165. Ibid.; emphasis in original.

166. Maguire, "Barriers to Psychological Care," 1711.

167. According to May, *The Physician's Covenant*, 182, 185, some of the prevailing images of the physician are promoted by larger medical institutions. With the result that when an institution holds the image of the physician as a technician as paramount, for example, it elevates a doctor's technical acumen from an instrumental to a final good.

168. Danielle Ofri, "Why Doctors Don't Take Sick Days?," *New York Times*, November 15, 2013, http://www.nytimes.com/2013/11/16/opinion/sunday/why-doctors-dont-take-sick-days.html.

169. Ibid.

170. Heidegger, *Being and Time*, 298.

171. Gadamer, *The Enigma of Health*, 70.

172. Michele A. Carter, "Abiding Loneliness: An Existential Perspective on Loneliness," *Second Opinion* 2000, no. 3: 51.

Chapter 3

1. Indeed, "vocation" is derived from the Latin *vocatio* (stem *vocation-*), meaning "a calling" or "a being called." If we conceive of a career in medicine as a vocation, then it would be natural to assume that medical professionals are called to help, to heal, to care for (compare this to Max Weber's use of "vocation" in note 9 to chapter 1). In the fifteenth century, "vocation" was used to describe a "spiritual calling," a point that resonates with both May in *The Physician's Covenant* and Paul Ramsey in *The Patient as Person*, where Ramsey maintains that God's covenant with humans to offer fidelity and steadfast love should be mirrored in human relationships. The doctor, then, enters into a covenant with the patient, acknowledging the sanctity and dignity of the individual and offering help in the patient's time of need. See Ramsey, *The Patient as Person*, xii.

2. May, *The Physician's Covenant*, 98.

Notes

3. Frank, *At the Will of the Body*, 14.

4. Inwood, *Heidegger*, 62; Heidegger *Being and Time*, 307.

5. See Thomson, "Death and Demise," 268.

6. Gardiner, *Kierkegaard*, 109; see also Kierkegaard, *The Sickness unto Death*, 147. It is easy to view Heidegger's secularized rendition of Kierkegaard's conversation narrative as utterly nihilistic, given that an honest confrontation with death is a confrontation with the "Nothing." For some scholars, "Nothingness" is nothing to despair, for our potential-for-"Nothingness" can bring meaning and intensity to our present being-in-the-world, whereas, for others, the idea of the "Nothing" renders existence utterly meaningless. Still others have argued that Heidegger's emphasis on our desire to evade the facticity of our finitude actually points to his own unspoken "desire to transcend finitude"—a sense that there must be something more than finitude and nothingness. Perhaps what transcends Dasein's everyday being-in-the-world is an authentic being-with—or love—that can transcend the finite. Our existential anxiety, then, is less about our finite being-in-the-world and more about our no longer being able to be with others who bring our life meaning. For more on Heidegger's thinking in this regard, see Judith Wolfe, *Heidegger's Eschatology: Theological Horizons in Martin Heidegger's Early Work* (New York: Oxford University Press, 2015).

7. Heidegger, *Being and Time*, 321, 325.

8. Ibid., 275, 303. Heidegger says, "Inauthenticity is based on the possibility of authenticity" (303).

9. Inwood, *Heidegger*, 71.

10. Heidegger, *Being and Time*, 308.

11. Ibid., 232; emphasis in original.

12. Frank, *At the Will of the Body*, 120.

13. Ibid. In his *New York Times* article of February 2015, Oliver Sacks expresses a similar sentiment as he faces and reflects upon his recent terminal diagnosis: "I feel intensely alive, and I want and hope in the time that remains to deepen my friendships, to say farewell to those I love, to write more, to travel if I have the strength, to achieve new levels of understanding and insight. . . . I feel a sudden clear focus and perspective. There is no time for anything inessential. I must focus on myself, my work, and my friends. I shall no longer look at 'NewsHour' every night. I shall no longer pay any attention to politics or arguments about global warming." See Oliver Sacks, "Oliver Sacks on Learning He Has Terminal Cancer," *New York Times*, February 19, 2015, http://www.nytimes.com/2015/02/19/opinion/oliver-sacks-on-learning-he-has-terminal-cancer.html.

14. Frank, *At the Will of the Body*, 132.

15. Heidegger, *Being and Time*, 376; Heidegger's "Augenblick" is inspired by Kierkegaard's *Øieblik*, which can be traced back to the Greek *kairos*, meaning "time outside (chronological) time." See Koral Ward, *Augenblick: The Concept of the "Decisive Moment" in 19th- and 20th-Century Western Philosophy* (Aldershot, UK: Ashgate, 2008), 3, 12.

16. Heidegger, *Being and Time*, 337, 223.

17. Frank, *At the Will of the Body*, 119.

18. Ibid.

19. Heidegger, *Being and Time*, 265; emphasis in original.

20. Heidegger borrows this notion of "repetition" from Kierkegaard. See Huntington, "Heidegger's Reading of Kierkegaard," 45.

21. Richard P. McQuellon and Michael A. Cowan, "Turning toward Death Together: Conversation in Mortal Time," *American Journal of Hospice & Palliative Care* 17, no. 5 (2000): 314. McQuellon and Cowan conceptualize "death" as the end of one's physical being, a narrower notion of death than the idea of death as world collapse (which can also refer to physical death) used throughout the present work.

22. Heidegger, *Being and Time*, 265.

23. Ibid., 307.

24. Dahlstrom, *The Heidegger Dictionary*, 53.

25. Inwood, *Heidegger*, 61.

26. Jerome Miller, "The Trauma of Evil and the Traumatological Conception of Forgiveness," *Continental Philosophy Review* 42, no. 3 (2009): 409.

27. Dahlstrom, *The Heidegger Dictionary*, 185; Heidegger, *Being and Time*, 343–344.

28. Heidegger, *Being and Time*, 308; emphasis in original.

29. Ibid., 307.

30. Ibid., 311; emphasis in original. But it is important to consider as well the peace and contentment that can come with being absorbed in the everyday, especially for those who are sick. Being ill pulls us out of our typical ways of being, and when we are ill, we have trouble disappearing into the seamlessness of everyday life. The personal knowledge of illness, especially illness that is life threatening, can make one feel "other," even when the othering is not imposed from without. The apparent seamlessness of everyone else's life becomes conspicuous—and perhaps even intolerable—to the ill person. In this way, being wrenched from the "they" can become something undesirable.

31. Though the core idea of "releasement" (*Gelassenheit*) is already present in *Being and Time*—with Heidegger's use of "resoluteness" (*Entschlossenheit*) as "openness"

or "unclosedness," for example—in his later writings, "authenticity" and "resoluteness" become synonymous with "releasement." See, for example, Martin Heidegger, "Conversation on a Country Path about Thinking" and "Memorial Address," both in *Discourse on Thinking*, trans. John M. Anderson and E. Hans Freund (New York: Harper and Row, 1969), 58–90; 43–57.

32. Gadamer, *The Enigma of Health*, 158.

33. Aho, "Medicalizing Mental Health," 252.

34. Heidegger, "Memorial Address," 54.

35. Ibid., 55.

36. Frank, *At the Will of the Body*, 59.

37. In the 1910 Flexner Report, which is still a touchstone for the development of medical curricula in the United States, Abraham Flexner emphasized the need to cultivate "scientific curiosity" among medical students rather than the capacity to engage in rote memorization of scientific and clinical facts. More recently, "curiosity" is noted as an important quality to foster during the development of students' professional identities. See David M. Irby, David M., Molly Cooke, and Bridget C. O'Brien, "Calls for Reform of Medical Education by the Carnegie Foundation for the Advancement of Teaching: 1910 and 2010," *Academic Medicine: Journal of the Association of American Medical Colleges* 85, no. 2 (2010): 220–227. See also H. M. Evans, "Wonder and the Patient," *Journal of Medical Humanities* 36, no. 1 (2014): 47–58.

38. Montgomery, *How Doctors Think*, 37. As Wiener and Ramsey put it in *Leaving Us to Wonder*, 1: "Always, no matter how much or how often we satisfy our never-ending curiosity with facts, something profound remains untouched. That which remains—something far apart from curiosity—is the experience of wonder." In her early work "The Evolution of Medical Uncertainty," *Milbank Memorial Fund Quarterly* 58, no. 1 (1980): 1, 5–6, Renée C. Fox points out that, even though some would like to believe that the "scientific endeavor" of medicine is not subject to the uncertainty and fallibility of some of the "softer" sciences or the humanities, it is actually the case that "uncertainty and death [are] the only certainties" in medical practice and that, "below their medical scientific surface, medical acts and events intersect with the human condition of patients, their relatives, and of the medical professionals themselves—their most profound aspirations, hopes, and fulfillments, their deepest worries, anxieties, and fears"—and are therefore anything but certain.

39. Montgomery, *How Doctors Think*, 36; emphasis added.

40. Kevin Aho, "Guignon on Self-Surrender and Homelessness in Dostoevsky and Heidegger," in *Horizons of Authenticity in Phenomenology, Existentialism, and Moral Psychology*, ed. Hans Pedersen and Megan Altman (Dordrecht: Springer, 2015), 70.

41. Evans, "Wonder and the Patient," 50. Undoubtedly, the terms "mystery" and "wonder" are metaphysically loaded terms. In this context, these terms are meant in both a literal and an epistemological sense (confronting the reality that there are things that we simply cannot "know" for certain) and also in an aesthetic sense (there are moments in medicine, for instance, when we are stunned, even awestruck, by the beauty of the profound complexities of the human body and of the human connection and love that can occur in the midst of tragedy and loss).

42. Frank, *At the Will of the Body*, 62.

43. Shapiro, "Walking a Mile in Their Patients' Shoes," 10.

44. Wiener and Ramsey, *Leaving Us to Wonder*, 99; Friedrich Wilhelm Nietzsche, *Beyond Good and Evil*, trans. Walter Kaufmann (New York: Vintage, 1966), part I, section 10, 16.

45. See Gardiner, *Kierkegaard*, 113.

46. Ibid.

47. Heidegger, *Being and Time*, 344; emphasis in original.

48. Ibid., 155, 233. According to Heidegger, "*Authentic being-one's-Self* does not rest upon an exceptional condition of the subject, a condition that has been detached from the 'they'; it is *rather an existential modification of the 'they'*" (168; emphasis in original).

49. Inwood, *Heidegger*, 35.

50. Dahlstrom, *The Heidegger Dictionary*, 37.

51. Heidegger, *Being and Time*, 396, 158. Heidegger refers to our being-toward *entities* in the world as "concern" (*Besorgen*). He distinguishes this from our care or concern for others (Dasein), which he calls "solicitude" (*Fürsorge*). Our solicitude takes both negative and positive forms. Negative solicitude is a deficient mode, defined by an indifference toward the other, whereas positive solicitude acknowledges the other. Positive solicitude, for its part, can take two forms: inauthentic solicitude, which still acknowledges the other, but *leaps in* for the other, taking over and dominating the other, making decisions for the other rather than letting the other make his or her own decisions; and authentic solicitude, which *leaps ahead* of the other and by helping to reveal the other's possibility for his or her own authenticity, "liberates" the other (158–159).

52. Ibid., 344; see also Aho "Why Heidegger Is Not an Existentialist," 8.

53. Wiener and Ramsey, *Leaving Us to Wonder*, 86.

54. Frank, *At the Will of the Body*, 121. But Frank also warns that, although illness is a unique opportunity for reflection, "this opportunity has its dangers, not the least of which is romanticizing illness. . . . Illness is not a kind of enlightenment" (136).

Notes

55. Heidegger, *Being and Time*, 344.

56. Ibid. Heidegger goes on to say that Dasein can "co-disclose this potentiality in the solicitude which leaps forth and liberates. When Dasein is resolute, it can become the 'conscience' of Others." See note 51.

57. McQuellon and Cowen, "Turning toward Death Together," 312.

58. Ibid., 313. The inverse can also be true: doctors who are themselves resolute and do not turn away from the frightening reality of finitude or death might co-disclose their authenticity to their patients, helping those who are ready to confront their own potential for death or world collapse: "Professionals [and others who care for the patient] can help someone who is dying to wrest life-enhancing meaning and value from a situation in which many can find only despair. They do so primarily by their willingness to engage in authentic conversation with the one who is dying" (ibid., 316); see also Kevin Aho, "Heidegger, Ontological Death, and the Healing Professions," *Medicine, Healthcare and Philosophy* 19, no. 1 (2016): 55–63.

59. Heidegger, *Being and Time*, 344: "Only by authentically Being-their-Selves in resoluteness can people authentically be with one another."

60. Shapiro, "Walking a Mile in Their Patients' Shoes," 15–16.

61. Eleonore Stump, *Wandering in Darkness: Narrative and the Problem of Suffering* (New York: Oxford University Press, 2010), 76.

62. Ibid., 53.

63. Rita Charon, "Narrative Medicine: A Model for Empathy, Reflection, Profession, and Trust," *Journal of the American Medical Association* 286 (2001): 1898, 1899.

64. Ibid., 1899.

65. Heidegger, *Being and Time*, 265.

66. Inwood, *Heidegger*, 73.

67. Dreyfus, "Foreword," xx. Heidegger's position, Inwood tells us in *Heidegger*, 74, is that "there are no objectively correct answers to life's basic problems, nor any decision procedure for discerning them. . . . One's decisions, like one's assertions are always made in a specific situation. What looks good to me in this situation may not look so good to others now or later, or even to myself in a *later* situation" (emphasis in original).

68. Inwood, *Heidegger*, 75. One should note, however, that, for Heidegger, morality and ethics are an ontic endeavor that departs from his fundamental ontology. See Aho, "Why Heidegger Is Not an Existentialist," 14.

69. Heidegger, *Being and Time*, 318.

70. Aho, "Guigon on Self-Surrender," 71. This critique is particularly significant, given Heidegger's involvement with Nazism. Heidegger joined the Nazi Party in 1933, and though a year later he resigned from the rectorship of the University of Freiburg and stopped participating in Nazi Party meetings, he remained a member of the Nazi Party until the end of World War II. The extent of Heidegger's involvement and complicity with Nazism continues to be debated. For more on Heidegger's involvement with the Nazi Party and anti-Semitism and the recent release of the "Black Notebooks," see Paul Hockenos, "Release of Heidegger's 'Black Notebooks' Reignites Debate Over Nazi Ideology," *Chronicle of Higher Education*, February 24, 2014, http://chronicle.com/article/Release-of-Heidegger-s/144897.

71. Michael L. Morgan, *The Cambridge Introduction to Emmanuel Levinas* (New York: Cambridge University Press, 2011), 7.

72. Ibid., 98.

73. Emmanuel Levinas, *Is It Righteous to Be? Interviews with Emmanuel Levinas*, ed. Jill Robbins (Stanford: Stanford University Press, 2001), 62.

74. Bettina Bergo, "Emmanuel Levinas," in *Stanford Encyclopedia of Philosophy*, ed. Edward N. Zalta, Summer 2013, http://plato.stanford.edu/archives/sum2013/entries/levinas/.

75. Morgan, *The Cambridge Introduction to Emmanuel Levinas*, 237–238.

76. Levinas, *Is It Righteous to Be?*, 40.

77. Morgan, *The Cambridge Introduction to Emmanuel Levinas*, 4.

78. Ibid.

79. Ibid., 69.

80. Ibid., 42.

81. Levinas, *Is It Righteous to Be?*, 191.

82. Ibid.

83. Richard M. Zaner, *Conversations on the Edge: Narratives of Ethics and Illness* (Washington, DC: Georgetown University Press, 2004), 33.

84. Ibid.

85. Levinas, *Is It Righteous to Be?*, 48, 1.

86. Morgan, *The Cambridge Introduction to Emmanuel Levinas*, 59.

87. Ibid., 10.

88. Emmanuel Levinas, *Totality and Infinity* (Pittsburgh: Duquesne University Press, 1969), 172.

Notes

89. May, *The Physician's Covenant*, 111, 140–141.

90. Frank, *At the Will of the Body*, 54.

91. Ibid., 104. Though Frank does not explicitly draw on Levinas in *At the Will of the Body*, he does do so in his later work, particularly in *The Renewal of Generosity*.

92. Morgan, *The Cambridge Introduction to Emmanuel Levinas*, 40. In *Being and Time*, 314, Heidegger says, "Calling is a mode of discourse. The call of conscience has the character of an *appeal* to Dasein by calling it to its ownmost potentiality-for-Being-its-Self" (emphasis in original).

93. Levinas, *Is It Righteous to Be?*, 4; Emmanuel Levinas, "Transcendence and Height," in *Emmanuel Levinas: Basic Philosophical Writings*, ed. Adriaan T. Peperzak, Simon Critchley, and Robert Bernasconi (Bloomington: Indiana University Press, 1996), 54.

94. Levinas, "Transcendence and Height," 17.

95. Levinas, *Is It Righteous to Be?*, 2, 3, 5.

96. Ibid., 6, 165.

97. Carter, "Abiding Loneliness," 51.

98. Ibid., 40.

99. Ibid., 41.

100. Zaner, *Conversations on the Edge*, 33.

101. Frank, *The Renewal of Generosity*, 115.

102. Ibid.

103. Ibid., 116.

104. Morgan, *The Cambridge Introduction to Emmanuel Levinas*, 3.

105. Ibid.

106. Margaret Urban Walker, *Moral Understandings: A Feminist Study in Ethics*, 2nd ed. (New York: Oxford University Press, 2007), 16. See also Sherwin, *No Longer Patient*.

107. Walker, *Moral Understanding*, 44, 57–58.

108. Ibid., 112.

109. Ibid.

110. Fredrik Svenaeus, "Hermeneutics of Medicine in the Wake of Gadamer," 416.

111. Ibid., 408, 415.

112. Kurt Mueller-Vollmer, *The Hermeneutics Reader: Texts of the German Tradition from the Enlightenment to the Present* (New York: Continuum, 1985), 256.

113. Acknowledging biases and prejudice is key for Gadamer, for he contends that the Enlightenment demand to overcome all prejudices "will itself prove to be a prejudice, and removing it opens the way to an appropriate understanding of our finitude, which dominates not only our humanity, but also our historical consciousness." See Hans-Georg Gadamer, *Truth and Method*, trans. Donald G. Marshall and Joel Weinsheimer (New York: Bloomsbury Academic, 2004), part II, chapter 4, section 1B, 277.

114. Svenaeus, "Hermeneutics of Medicine in the Wake of Gadamer," 426.

115. Svenaeus, *The Hermeneutics of Medicine*, 158.

116. Hans-Georg Gadamer, "Hermeneutics as Practical Philosophy," in *The Gadamer Reader: A Bouquet of the Later Writings*, trans. and ed. Richard E. Palmer (Evanston: Northwestern University Press, 2007), 240.

117. Svenaeus, "Hermeneutics of Medicine in the Wake of Gadamer," 417.

118. Howard Waitzkin, "A Critical Theory of Medical Discourse: Ideology, Social Control, and the Processing of Social Context in Medical Encounters," *Journal of Health and Social Behavior* 30, no. 2 (1989): 223; see also Carl Edvard Rudebeck, "Grasping the Existential Anatomy: The Role of Bodily Empathy in Clinical Communication," in *Handbook of Phenomenology and Medicine*, ed. S. Kay Toombs (Dordrecht: Kluwer Academic, 2001). In his phenomenological approach to the clinical encounter, Rudebeck argues that Western physicians often become more intrigued by the pathology behind certain symptoms and more preoccupied with determining whether or not the symptoms fall into preconceived categories of disease than they do in attempting to understand how the symptoms might be affecting the patient's life (297). He claims that two immediate risks are associated with physicians assuming this attitude: they may be left with a "shallow" understanding of what their patients present, thus influencing their diagnoses or misdiagnoses, or the patients may be left feeling as if the physicians are uninterested in their particular situation, causing them to question or ignore the physicians' suggested treatment or to seek care elsewhere (297). Thus the physician, according to Rudebeck, must acknowledge and respond to the patient's phenomenological "body experience" in order to gain a richer and more differentiated perception of the symptom presentation. Doing so not only leads to a more informed clinical judgment in terms of diagnosis and treatment, but it also allows the physician to better explain this clinical judgment to the patient in a way that aligns within the patient's own interpretation of his or her symptoms, potentially leading to better outcomes. It should be noted that such hermeneutic approaches to the clinical encounter are informed by the work of George L. Engel, who proposed the "biopsychosocial model" in 1980. See George L. Engel, "The Clinical Application of the Biopsychosocial Model," *American Journal of Psychiatry* 137, no. 5 (1980): 535–544.

119. Mariana Ortega, "'New Mestizas,' '"World" Travelers,' and 'Dasein': Phenomenology and the Multi-Voiced, Multi-Cultural Self," *Hypatia* 16, no. 3 (2001): 4.

120. Ibid., 11.

121. Ibid., 17. Ortega's work is, in part, a response to the work of María Lugones, who argues that the "world" traveler not only traverses different worlds, but is also a *different self* in those worlds. Ortega, however, contends that Lugones's idea of multiple selves fails to account for identity, agency, and responsibility, and offers instead the idea of the multiplicitous self that—despite being complex, ambiguous, and sometimes contradictory—still retains a sense of togetherness. She uses Heidegger's fundamental ontology to make this argument, specifically his ideas about "mineness," our ever-present concern with our own being that stays with us throughout our travels into other worlds. See Maria Lugones, "Playfulness, 'World'-Travelling, and Loving Perception," *Hypatia* 2, no. 2 (1987): 3–19.

122. Daniel F. Davis, "*Phronesis*, Clinical Reasoning, and Pellegrino's Philosophy of Medicine," *Theoretical Medicine* 18, nos. 1–2 (1997): 186.

123. Ibid., 187. For Gadamer, moral understanding and hermeneutic understanding are similar in that one does not simply "apply" some kind of pregiven knowledge to the situation at hand to determine the right action to take. Rather, choosing what is good and right requires making decisions while embedded in the particular hermeneutic situation. See Gadamer, *Truth and Method*, part II, chapter 4, section 2B, 309–319.

124. Pellegrino, "The Internal Morality of Clinical Medicine."

125. Stephen Toulmin, "The Marginal Relevance of Theory to the Humanities," *Common Knowledge* 2, no. 1 (1993): 79.

126. Stephen Toulmin, "The Recovery of Practical Philosophy," *American Scholar* 57, no. 3 (1988): 345–346.

127. Svenaeus, "Hermeneutics of Medicine in the Wake of Gadamer," 409, 418, emphasis in original.

128. McQuellon and Cowen, "Turning toward Death Together," 316.

129. Ronald A. Carson, "The Hyphenated Space: Liminality in the Doctor-Patient Relationship," in *Stories Matter: The Role of Narrative in Medical Ethics*, ed. Rita Charon and Martha Montello (New York: Routledge, 2002), 171–182.

130. As Carson points out in "Education the Moral Imagination," 28, this is not the same as the "Romantic fallacy" that implied it was possible to "get inside another person's skin." Rather, I am referring here to a kind of *knowledge of* what it might be like to suffer in the same way as the patient before me.

131. Ronald A. Carson, "On Metaphorical Concentration: Language and Meaning in Patient-Physician Relations," *Journal of Medicine and Philosophy* 36, no. 4 (2011): 387; emphasis in original.

132. McQuellon and Cowen, "Turning toward Death," 317.

133. Gadamer, *Truth and Method,* part II, chapter 4, section 1A, 271.

134. Merleau-Ponty asserts that alterity is not an either-or concept; we should not assume that in the face of alterity we can never understand the other (as Sartre might argue), nor should we ignore our fundamental difference. Indeed, if we remain open to each other, we might be changed in beneficial and generative ways by the difference the other brings to bear on our encounter with him or her. See Jack Reynolds, "Maurice Merleau-Ponty," *Internet Encyclopedia of Philosophy: A Peer-Reviewed Academic Resource,* 2014, http://www.iep.utm.edu/merleau/.

135. Gadamer, *Truth and Method,* part II, chapter 4, section 1B, 303.

136. Charles Taylor, "The Dialogical Self," in *The Interpretive Turn: Philosophy, Science, Culture,* ed. David R. Hiley, James Bohman, and Richard Shusterman (Ithaca: Cornell University Press, 1991), 307.

137. Ibid.

138. Ibid., 311.

139. Ibid., 314; Frank, *The Renewal of Generosity,* 43.

140. Mikhail Bakhtin, *Problems of Dostoevsky's Poetics* (Minneapolis: University of Minnesota Press, 1984), 59.

141. Gary Saul Morson and Caryl Emerson, *Mikhail Bakhtin: Creation of a Prosaics.* (Stanford: Stanford University Press, 1990), 49.

142. Bakhtin, *Problems of Dostoevsky's Poetics.*

143. Ibid., 287.

144. Ibid.

145. Frank, *The Renewal of Generosity,* 44.

146. Mikhail Bakhtin, *Art and Answerability: Early Philosophical Essays,* ed. Michael Holquist and Vadim Liapunov, trans. Vadim Liapunov (Austin: University of Texas Press, 1990), 35.

147. Frank, *The Renewal of Generosity,* 20.

148. Bishop, *The Anticipatory Corpse,* 311.

149. Ibid., 304.

150. Ibid.

151. Zaner, *Conversations on the Edge,* 34.

152. Louise Arnold and David Thomas Stern, "What Is Medical Professionalism?," in *Measuring Medical Professionalism,* ed. David Thomas Stern (New York: Oxford University Press, 2006), 27.

153. Heidegger, *Being and Time*, 185–186.

154. Frank, *The Wounded Storyteller*, 25.

155. Ibid., 84.

156. Arthur Kleinman, *The Illness Narratives: Suffering, Healing, and the Human Condition* (New York, Basic Books, 1988), xii.

157. Carter, "Abiding Loneliness," 51.

158. As Levinas remarks in *Is It Righteous to Be?*, 53: "I am responsible for the death of the other, I cannot leave him alone to die, even if I cannot stop it. This is how I have always interpreted the 'Thou shalt not kill.' . . . Practically, this goodness, this kindness, this nonindifference to the death of the other is precisely the very perfection of love."

159. May, *The Physician's Covenant*, 103.

160. Ibid., 206.

161. Frank, *At the Will of the Body*, 56.

162. McQuellon and Cowen, "Turning toward Death," 315. In a similar vein in *Being Mortal*, 188, Gawande argues that because "people die only once" and have no previous experience to draw on, they need clinicians who are willing to have hard conversations, to "say what they have seen," and help prepare patients for what is to come.

163. Hilary Putnam, "Levinas and Judaism," in *The Cambridge Companion to Levinas*, ed. Simon Critchley and Robert Bernasconi (Cambridge, UK: Cambridge University Press, 2002), 36.

164. As Carson explains in "On Metaphorical Concentration," 392: "Charles Taylor's expressivist conception of the self, and of language as constitutive of shared meaning and mutual understanding, can be seen to provide an aspirational standard for patient-physician relations that can be steadily striven for and more regularly approximated as a counterforce to prevailing bureaucratized and commercialized conceptions of care."

165. Levinas, Is It Righteous to Be?, 7, 55.

166. Morgan, *The Cambridge Introduction to Emmanuel Levinas*, 74. According to Morgan (110), Levinas asserts that justice puts limits on our responsibility. So, despite the fact that it is our fundamental responsibility to the other that grants the state any legitimacy, it is the law, the state, and justice that limit our responsibilities "by subjecting them to calculation and regimentation," giving us a sense of who we ought to serve, support, stand up to, and so on.

167. Ibid., 241.

168. Ibid., 241–242.

169. Sherwin, *No Longer Patient*, 51.

170. Morgan, *The Cambridge Introduction to Emmanuel Levinas*, 99.

171. McQuellon and Cowen, "Turning toward Death," 318; Chen, *Final Exam*, 207.

172. From the Latin *compassio* (stem *compassion-*)—*com-*, meaning "with" or "together," and *passio* (stem *passion-*), meaning "suffering." See Edmund E. Pellegrino, "The Anatomy of Clinical-Ethical Judgments in Perinatology and Neonatology: A Substantive and Procedural Framework," *Seminars in Perinatology* 1, no. 3 (1987): 208.

173. Martha C. Nussbaum, *Cultivating Humanity: A Classical Defense of Reform in Liberal Education* (Cambridge, MA: Harvard University Press, 1998), 91.

174. Heidegger, *Being and Time*, 186. Because our being is temporal, we continually project ourselves forward into our possibilities—our roles, identities, or projects. This pressing forward into our possibilities (e.g., desires or plans to become a doctor, a mother, a teacher, a criminal) affects who we are now (and how we interpret or reinterpret our past), even if we never actualize the possibilities that we project ourselves into. For more on Heidegger's thinking in this regard, see Iain Thomson, "Heidegger's Perfectionist Philosophy of Education in *Being and Time*," *Continental Philosophy Review* 37, no. 4 (2004): 439–467.

175. Anatole Broyard, "Doctor Talk to Me," *New York Times*, August 26, 1990, http://www.nytimes.com/1990/08/26/magazine/doctor-talk-to-me.html.

176. Tolstoy, *The Death of Ivan Ilych and Other Stories*, 119.

177. Morgan, *The Cambridge Introduction to Emmanuel Levinas*, 240.

Chapter 4

1. Heidegger, "Memorial Address," 47.

2. Frank, *At the Will of the Body*, 21; emphasis added.

3. Shapiro, "Walking a Mile in Their Patients' Shoes," 17.

4. Thomas R. Cole, Nathan S. Carlin, and Ronald A. Carson, *Medical Humanities: An Introduction* (New York: Cambridge University Press, 2014), 16.

5. Sharon Dobie, "Viewpoint: Reflections on a Well-Traveled Path: Self-Awareness, Mindful Practice, and Relationship-Centered Care as Foundations for Medical Education," *Academic Medicine: Journal of the Association of American Medical Colleges* 82, no. 4 (2007): 423. Deborah Cook and Graeme Rocker, for example, describe what they call "vicarious traumatization," arguing that "clinicians who detect physical or psychic pain and other negative symptoms may suffer indirectly, yet deeply.

Vicarious traumatization results from repeated empathic engagement with sadness and loss." See Deborah Cook and Graeme Rocker, "Dying with Dignity in the Intensive Care Unit," *New England Journal of Medicine* 370, no. 26 (2014): 2510.

6. Diane E. Meier, Anthony L. Back, and R. Sean Morrison, "The Inner Life of Physicians and Care of the Seriously Ill," *Journal of the American Medical Association* 286, no. 23 (2001): 3007, 3008. See also Aleksandra Ciałkowska-Rysz and Tomasz Dzierżanowski, "Personal Fear of Death Affects the Proper Process of Breaking Bad News." For more on the complex emotions clinicians experience, see Danielle Ofri, *What Doctors Feel: How Emotions Affect the Practice of Medicine* (Boston: Beacon Press, 2014).

7. Meier, Back, and Morrison, "The Inner Life of Physicians and Care of the Seriously Ill," 3008.

8. Ibid.; see also Pranay Sinha, "Why Do Doctors Commit Suicide?" *NYTimes.com*, September 5, 2014, http://www.nytimes.com/2014/09/05/opinion/why-do-doctors-commit-suicide.html.

9. Eric R Jackson, Tait D. Shanafelt, Omar Hasan, Daniel V. Satele, and Liselotte N. Dyrbye, "Burnout and Alcohol Abuse/Dependence among U.S. Medical Students," *Academic Medicine: Journal of the Association of American Medical Colleges* 90, no. 9 (2016): 1253.

10. Sinhay, "Why Do Doctors Commit Suicide?"

11. Ronald M. Epstein's 1999 article "Mindful Practice" has been highly influential in this area of research. See Ronald M. Epstein, "Mindful Practice," *Journal of the American Medical Association* 282, no. 9 (1999): 833–839. See also Dobie, "Viewpoint"; Delese Wear, Joseph Zarconi, Arno Kumagai, and Kathy Cole-Kelly, "Slow Medical Education," *Academic Medicine: Journal of the Association of American Medical Colleges* 90, no. 3 (2015): 289–293; Arno K. Kumagai, "On the Way to Reflection: A Conversation on a Country Path," *Perspectives in Biology and Medicine* 56, no. 3 (2013): 362–370; Johanna Shapiro, Deborah Kasman, and Audrey Shafer, "Words and Wards: A Model of Reflective Writing and Its Uses in Medical Education," *Journal of Medical Humanities* 27, no. 4 (2006): 231–244.

12. According to Carol P. Tresolini and the Pew Health Professions Commission: "The phrase 'Relationship-Centered Care' captures the importance of the interaction among people as the foundation of any therapeutic or healing activity. Further, relationships are critical to the care provided by nearly all practitioners (regardless of discipline or subspecialty) and a source of satisfaction and positive outcomes for patients and practitioners." See Carol P. Tresolini and the Pew Health Professions Commission, *Health Professions Education and Relationship-Centered Care: Report* (San Francisco: Pew Health Professions Commission: University of California, San Francisco, Center for the Health Professions,1994), 11, available at http://docplayer.net/11036381-Relationship-centered-care.html; see also Dobie, "Viewpoint."

13. Dobie, "Viewpoint," 423. See also Mary Catherine Beach, Thomas Inui, and the Relationship-Centered Care Research Network, "Relationship-Centered Care: A Constructive Reframing," *Journal of General Internal Medicine* 21, suppl. 1 (2006): S3–S8. Relationship-centered care is not unlike narrative approaches to clinical care and clinical ethics. According to Carson, "The Hyphenated Space," 172: "Narrative approaches aim to accommodate just this element of mutuality. Practitioners of narrative ethics share an attentiveness to the experiential dimensions of illness, a conviction that experiences of illness are story-shaped, and a commitment to relationality and reflexivity as preconditions for understanding such experiences."

14. Tait D. Shanafelt, "Enhancing Meaning in Work: A Prescription for Preventing Physician Burnout and Promoting Patient-Centered Care," *Journal of the American Medical Association* 302, no. 12 (2009): 1338–1340.

15. Kumagai, "On the Way to Reflection," 367.

16. Ibid.

17. Dennis H. Novack, Ronald M. Epstein, and Randall H. Paulsen, "Toward Creating Physician-Healers: Fostering Medical Students' Self-Awareness, Personal Growth, and Well-Being," *Academic Medicine: Journal of the Association of American Medical Colleges* 74, no. 5 (1999): 516–517.

18. Shapiro, "Walking a Mile in Their Patients' Shoes," 14.

19. Ibid.

20. Wear et al., "Slow Medical Education," 292.

21. Ibid., 289. This same criticism can be offered in the context of higher education more broadly. According to May, *The Physician's Covenant*, 196: "As the institution that trains the modern professional, the university has done a brilliant job of equipping the professional with technical competence, but it has not always accepted responsibility for nourishing that moral substance and cultivating those virtues that a society has a right to expect in professionals."

22. Arnold and Stern, "What Is Medical Professionalism?," 18.

23. Ibid., 23–27; Jordan Cohen, "Foreword," in *Measuring Medical Professionalism*, ed. Stern, vii.

24. Inui, "A Flag in the Wind," 11.

25. Ramsey, *The Patient as Person*, xvi.

26. Matthew K. Wynia, Maxine A. Papadakis, William M. Sullivan, and Frederic W. Hafferty, "More Than a List of Values and Desired Behaviors: A Foundational Understanding of Medical Professionalism," *Academic Medicine: Journal of the Association of American Medical Colleges* 89, no. 5 (2014): 712–714.

27. Janet Grant, "The Incapacitating Effects of Competence: A Critique," *Advances in Health Sciences Education: Theory and Practice* 4, no. 9 (1999): 271–277. According to Kumagai, although there is no agreement about what exactly we mean by "competencies" in medical education, "several themes are consistent. One: There is an emphasis on the outcomes achieved as a benchmark for progress rather than the underlying learning process itself. Two: Outcomes must be observable. Underlying competence is then inferred from observable actions. Three: Standardization of outcomes and assessments is a priority, as is the generation of 'objective' data. Four: A learner's progression is measured in terms of fulfillment of competencies rather than the time taken to achieve these goals." See Arno K. Kumagai, "From Competencies to Human Interests: Ways of Knowing and Understanding in Medical Education," *Academic Medicine: Journal of the Association of American Medical Colleges* 89, no. 7 (2014): 980.

28. Grant, "The Incapacitating Effects of Competence," 272, 273; Frederic Hafferty, "Measuring Professionalism: A Commentary," in *Measuring Medical Professionalism*, ed. Stern, 283.

29. Grant, "The Incapacitating Effects of Competence," 273.

30. Ibid.

31. Shapiro et al., "Medical Humanities and Their Discontents," 195.

32. See Kinghorn, "Medical Education as Moral Formation"; Coulehan, "Viewpoint."

33. Kinghorn, "Medical Education as Moral Formation," 94.

34. Coulehan, "Viewpoint," 892.

35. Morgan, *The Cambridge Introduction to Emmanuel Levinas*, 78, 112.

36. Kinghorn, "Medical Education as Moral Formation," 89.

37. Ibid.

38. As quoted in Kleinman, *The Illness Narratives*, 216.

39. Hafferty, "Professionalism and the Socialization of Medical Students," 53–54.

40. Ibid., 57; emphasis in original.

41. Arnold and Stern, "What Is Medical Professionalism?," 31.

42. Hafferty, "Professionalism and the Socialization of Medical Students," 54; emphasis in original. As Hafferty so candidly puts it in "Measuring Professionalism," 283: "Ultimately medicine must avoid the self-serving inconsistency of claiming to establish professionalism as an internalized and deep competency while willing to settle for graduates who manifest it only as at a surface phenomenon. . . . A professionalism that is deep must exist at the level of identity. Surface professionalism, on the other hand, is nothing more than doing one's job in a 'professional manner.'"

43. Mark Holden, Era Buck, Mark Clark, Karen Szauter, and Julie Trumble, "Professional Identity Formation in Medical Education: The Convergence of Multiple Domains," *HEC Forum* 24, no. 4 (2012): 245.

44. Ibid., 246.

45. Hafferty, "Professionalism and the Socialization of Medical Students," 60.

46. Inui, "A Flag in the Wind," 27.

47. See Holden et al., "Professional Identity Formation in Medical Education"; Mark D. Holden, Era Buck, John Luk, Frank Ambriz, Eugene V. Boisaubin, Mark A. Clark, et al., "Professional Identity Formation: Creating a Longitudinal Framework through TIME (Transformation in Medical Education)," *Academic Medicine: Journal of the Association of American Medical Colleges* 90, no. 6 (2015): 761–767.

48. Inui, "A Flag in the Wind," 4.

49. See Nancy Sherman, *The Fabric of Character: Aristotle's Theory of Virtue* (Oxford: Oxford University Press, 1991).

50. Judith Andre, "The Medical Humanities as Contributing to Moral Growth and Development," in *Practicing the Medical Humanities: Engaging Physicians and Patients*, ed. Ronald Carson, Chester Burns, and Thomas R. Cole (Hagerstown, MD: University Publishing Group, 2003),44.

51. Ibid., 54; see also Svenaeus, "Hermeneutics of Medicine in the Wake of Gadamer."

52. Alasdair MacIntyre, *After Virtue: A Study in Moral Theory*, 2nd ed. (Notre Dame: University of Notre Dame Press, 1984), 187.

53. Ibid., 191. MacIntyre also suggests that although virtues can be specific to the particular internal goods of a specific practice, one must "accept as necessary to any practice with internal goods and standards of excellence the virtues of justice, courage, and honesty" (191). Without these three virtues, a practice devolves into a mere means of achieving external goods. Accepting these three virtues, as well as accepting the authority of the standards of the particular practice one enters into, MacIntyre claims, works against the idea of moral relativism (191).

54. Ibid., 196.

55. Pellegrino, "The Internal Morality of Clinical Medicine," 565.

56. Ibid., 568.

57. Ibid., 576.

58. May, *The Physician's Covenant*, 209.

59. Kinghorn, "Medical Education as Moral Formation," 87.

Notes

60. I am grateful to the anonymous reviewer who so eloquently pointed this out to me.

61. Svenaeus, "Hermeneutics of Medicine in the Wake of Gadamer," 408; Aristotle, *Nicomachean Ethics* (Oxford: Clarendon Press, 1908), book VI, chapter 3, http://classics.mit.edu/Aristotle/nicomachaen.6.vi.html.

62. Kinghorn, "Medical Education as Moral Formation," 100. For Aristotle, the highest good of all human practice is *eudaimonia*, or human flourishing. Living well and flourishing consists in engaging in activities determined by reason to be in accordance with virtue or excellence. According to Kinghorn, Aristotle considered the practice of medicine during his time to be a form of technē, though whether he was correct to consider it as such has been debated (99).

63. Gadamer, *Truth and Method*, part II, chapter 4, section 2B, 315.

64. Ibid., 318.

65. Sherman, *The Fabric of Character*, 3.

66. Ibid., 5; Aristotle, *Nicomachean Ethics*, book VI, chapter 3.

67. Kinghorn, "Medical Education as Moral Formation," 100. For Aristotle, the way one becomes a good or virtuous clinician is similar to the way one becomes a proficient or skilled one—through habitual practice.

68. Ibid., 101. Aristotle also argues that phronesis is necessary for determining the "golden mean" between two extremes (e.g., courage is the mean between cowardice and temerity) and also for determining what is called for when two virtues or principles conflict (e.g., when is too much honesty detrimental to this particular patient? When does courage teeter on the edge of paternalism?) See Glenn McGee, "*Phronesis* in Clinical Ethics," *Theoretical Medicine* 17, no. 4 (1996): 318.

69. Toulmin, "The Marginal Relevance of Theory to the Humanities," 78.

70. Kinghorn, "Medical Education as Moral Formation," 95.

71. It seems to me that what is clinically salient and what is morally salient are one in the same.

72. Sherman, *The Fabric of Character*, 48.

73. Coulehan, "Viewpoint," 896. Although the factors that affect personal development in medical education are complex and multifarious, according to Cruess and colleagues, among "the most powerful" are role models and mentors. See Richard L. Cruess, Sylvia R. Cruess, J. Donald Boudreau, Linda Snell, and Yvonne Steinert, "A Schematic Representation of the Professional Identity Formation and Socialization of Medical Students and Residents: A Guide for Medical Educators," *Academic Medicine: Journal of the Association of American Medical Colleges* 90, no. 6 (2015): 718–725.

74. Brainard and Brislen,"Viewpoint," 1012.

75. Hafferty, "Professionalism and the Socialization of Medical Students," 61; Brainard and Brislen, "Viewpoint." Portions of this section appear in Piemonte, "Last Laughs: Gallows Humor in Medical Education."

76. Jerald Kay, "Traumatic Deidealization and the Future of Medicine," *Journal of the American Medical Association* 263, no. 4 (1990): 572–573.

77. Ibid., 573.

78. Ibid.

79. David P. Sklar, "Mistreatment of Students and Residents: Why Can't We Just Be Nice?," *Academic Medicine: Journal of the Association of American Medical Colleges* 89, no. 5 (2014): 693–695; see also Brian Mavis, Aron Sousa, Wanda Lipscomb, and Marsha D. Rappley, "Learning about Medical Student Mistreatment from Responses to the Medical School Graduation Questionnaire," *Academic Medicine: Journal of the Association of American Medical Colleges* 89, no. 5 (2014): 705–711.

80. Sklar, "Mistreatment of Students and Residents."

81. Alyssa F. Cook, Vineet M. Arora, Kenneth A. Rasinski, Farr V. Curlin, and John, D. Yoon, "The Prevalence of Medical Student Mistreatment and its Association with Burnout," *Academic Medicine: Journal of the Association of American Medical Colleges* 89, no. 5 (2014): 749–754.

82. William E. Bynum, and Brenessa Lindeman, "Caught in the Middle: A Resident Perspective on Influences from the Learning Environment That Perpetuate Mistreatment." *Academic Medicine: Journal of the Association of American Medical Colleges* 91, no. 3 (2016): 302.

83. Sklar, "Mistreatment of Students and Residents," 694.

84. Geoffrey C. Williams and Edward L. Deci, "The Importance of Supporting Autonomy in Medical Education," *Annals of Internal Medicine* 129, no. 4 (1998): 303–308; Thomas J. Beckman and Mark C. Lee, "Proposal for a Collaborative Approach to Clinical Teaching," *Mayo Clinic Proceedings* 84, no. 4 (2009): 339–344.

85. Beckman and Lee, "Proposal for a Collaborative Approach to Clinical Teaching," 339.

86. Kinghorn, "Medical Education as Moral Formation," 102.

87. For example, at the University of Texas Medical Branch, there are faculty mentors in the "Physician-Healer Track" who provide quality mentorship, encourage mindfulness, and provide students with opportunities for honest reflection. Students also mentioned that they received quality mentorship from some of the faculty scholars in the John P. McGovern Academy of Oslerian Medicine. The problem, however, is that such mentorship is not available to all students but mainly to those enrolled in

the Physician-Healer Track or inducted into the Academy of Oslerian Medicine. For more on the kind of mentorship students receive during medical training, see Delese Wear and Joseph Zarconi, "Can Compassion Be Taught? Let's Ask Our Students," *Journal of General Internal Medicine* 23, no. 7 (2008): 948–953.

88. Carson, "On Metaphorical Concentration," 390.

89. Montgomery, *How Doctors Think*, 166.

90. MacIntyre, *After Virtue*, 187.

91. Ibid., 205.

92. Ibid.

93. Ibid., 204, 205.

94. Robert Coles, "Medical Ethics and Living a Life," *New England Journal of Medicine* 301, no. 8 (1979): 444.

95. Ibid., 445.

96. Robert Kegan, *The Evolving Self: Problem and Process in Human Development* (Cambridge, MA: Harvard University Press, 1982), 248.

97. Ibid., 249.

98. Barnard, "Love and Death," 409.

99. Carter, "Abiding Loneliness," 47.

100. Frank, *The Wounded Storyteller*, 157; Montgomery, *How Doctors Think*, 197.

101. Kumagai, "On the Way to Reflection," 365.

102. Carson, "On Metaphorical Concentration," 389.

103. Frank, *At the Will of the Body*, 14.

104. May, *The Physician's Covenant*, 98.

105. Jack Coulehan and Peter C. Williams, "Vanquishing Virtue: The Impact of Medical Education." *Academic Medicine: Journal of the Association of American Medical Colleges* 76, no. 6 (2001): 600.

106. Ibid.

107. Ibid., 598.

108. Inui, "A Flag in the Wind," 27.

109. Heidegger, *Being and Time*, 159; emphasis in original.

110. Cruess et al., "A Schematic Representation of the Professional Identity Formation and Socialization of Medical Students and Residents," 4.

111. Kumagai, "On the Way to Reflection," 363.

112. Liselotte N. Dyrbye, Matthew R. Thomas, and Tait D. Shanafelt, "Medical Student Distress: Causes, Consequences, and Proposed Solutions," *Mayo Clinic Proceedings* 80, no. 12 (2005): 1614.

113. See, for example, Shapiro et al., "Words and Wards"; Block and Billings, "Learning from the Dying"; Barbara Head, Lori Earnshaw, Ruth Greenberg, Robert Morehead, Mark Pfeifer, and Monica Ann Shaw, "'I Will Never Forget': What We Learned from Medical Student Reflections on a Palliative Care Experience," *Journal of Palliative Medicine* 15, no. 5 (2012): 535–521.

114. Treadway, "Perspective," 1275.

115. Thirusha Naidu and Arno K. Kumagai, "Troubling Muddy Waters: Problematizing Reflective Practice in Global Medical Education," *Academic Medicine: Journal of the Association of American Medical Colleges* 91, no. 3 (2016): 317–321; Alan Bleakley, "From Reflective Practice to Holistic Reflexivity," *Studies in Higher Education* 24, no. 3 (1999): 315–330.

116. Baier, "Alternative Offerings to Aesclepius?," 12; Kumagai, "On the Way to Reflection," 364. For Kumagai and Naidu, reflective practice in medicine involves *reflecting* during or after doing something, *critically reflecting* on the connection of individual identity and the social context, and being *reflexive*—making a connection with human needs and values, being introspective, and analyzing issues of social conditions and injustice. See Arno K. Kumagai and Thirusha Naidu, "Reflection, Dialogue, and the Possibilities of Space," *Academic Medicine: Journal of the Association of American Medical Colleges* 90, no. 3 (2015): 283–288. For more on reflective practice and reflective writing, see Gillie Bolton, *Reflective Practice: Writing and Professional Development*, 3rd ed. (Thousand Oaks, CA: Sage, 2010).

117. Kumagai and Naidu, "Reflection, Dialogue, and the Possibilities of Space," 285.

118. Ibid.

119. Ibid., 286, 287.

120. Wear et al., "Slow Medical Education," 290.

121. Cruess, et al., "A Schematic Representation of the Professional Identity Formation and Socialization of Medical Students and Residents," 4.

122. Shapiro, "Walking a Mile in Their Patients' Shoes," 16.

123. Cruess et al., "A Schematic Representation of the Professional Identity Formation and Socialization of Medical Students and Residents," 3.

124. Ibid., 6. See also Dobie, "Viewpoint," 426; Epstein, "Mindful Practice," 838.

125. Kumagai and Naidu, "Reflection, Dialogue, and the Possibilities of Space"; Wear et al., "Slow Medical Education, 289.

126. Facebook posting by third-year medical student, March 15, 2015; quoted with permission; name withheld to protect his privacy.

127. Inui, "A Flag in the Wind," 19.

128. As Cruess and colleagues point out in "A Schematic Representation of the Professional Identity Formation and Socialization of Medical Students and Residents," 5, the practice of medicine can bring deep joy, though this point is rarely emphasized in medical education or practice.

Chapter 5

1. See Gardiner, *Kierkegaard*, 37.

2. Ibid.

3. Heidegger, "Memorial Address," 46.

4. Pedersen, "Empathy Development in Medical Education," 599.

5. Ibid., 598.

6. Following Heidegger, Iain Thomson argues that the goal of genuine education, is to "bring us full circle back to ourselves, by first turning us away from the world in which we are most immediately immersed and then turning us back to this world in a more reflexive way." See Thomson, "Heidegger's Perfectionist Philosophy of Education in *Being and Time*," 457.

7. Ibid.; see chapter 3, note 51.

8. See Luca Chiapperino and Giovanni Boniolo, "Rethinking Medical Humanities," *Journal of Medical Humanities* 35, no. 4 (2014): 377–387.

9. See Shapiro et al., "Medical Humanities and Their Discontents," 192.

10. Cole, Carlin, and Carson, *Medical Humanities*, 1.

11. See, for example, Therese Jones, Michael Blackie, Rebecca Garden, and Delese Wear, "The Almost Right Word: The Move from Medical to Health Humanities," *Academic Medicine: Journal of the Association of American Medical Colleges* 92, no. 7 (July 2017): 932-935; Paul Crawford, "Health Humanities: We Are Here to Collaborate, Not to Compete," *Guardian*, March 30, 2015, http://www.theguardian.com/higher-education-network/2015/mar/30/health-humanities-here-to-collaborate-not-compete.

12. T. Jones et al., "The Almost Right Word," 3.

13. Ibid.; Lester D. Friedman, "The Precarious Position of the Medical Humanities in the Medical School Curriculum," *Academic Medicine: Journal of the Association of American Medical Colleges* 77, no. 4 (2002): 322.

14. Cole, Carlin, and Carson, *Medical Humanities*, ix. There is debate whether the medical humanities should be considered "multidisciplinary" (different disciplines staying within their own domain and offering varying perspectives), "interdisciplinary" (different disciplines interacting and cooperating with one another to explore questions), or "transdisciplinary" (blending the different disciplines under a model that shares a common language and way of thinking in order to attend to questions in the field). Because so much in the medical humanities is concerned with exploring questions of value, meaning, and being human, from my perspective, an inter- or transdisciplinary approach where experts (including patients and clinicians) work together offers richer insight into such complex questions. For more on the nature of the field, see Chiapperino and Boniolo, "Rethinking Medical Humanities."

15. Cole, Carlin, and Carson, *Medical Humanities*, ix; emphasis in original.

16. Ibid., 2. It is their focus on wisdom and virtue and the belief in the power of literature, poetry, and narrative, and rhetoric—pursuits central to the *studia humanitatis* (studies of humanity)—that unite contemporary medical humanities and Renaissance humanism. The Renaissance humanists of fifteenth-century Europe, particularly the "Father of Humanism," Petrarch (Francesco Petrarca), were disillusioned by the dominant culture's preoccupation with logic and ratiocination; they turned to the ancients and advocated the pedagogy of the studia humanitatis to address the very human problems of their time, including the pervasive sense of incoherence, loss, and contingency in the face of the Black Death. The studia humanitatis emerged in Italy as part of a "cultural revolution" against the largely technical approach to education and the emphasis on pure logic and linguistic analysis in the scholastic theology of the time; the humanists studed classical Latin and the works of the ancients to find inspiration for how to live well in the midst of the cultural and religious crises of their time. See Robert E. Proctor, *Defining the Humanities: How Discovering a Tradition Can Improve Our Schools*, 2nd ed. (Bloomington: Indiana University Press, 1998), xxiv, xxv, 39, 89.

17. See Anne Hudson Jones, "Why Teach Literature and Medicine? Answers from Three Decades," *Journal of Medical Humanities* 34, no. 4 (2013): 415–428.

18. Cole, Carlin, and Carson, *Medical Humanities*, 3.

19. Stephen Toulmin states in "The Marginal Relevance of Theory," 77, that "our nontheoretical (or pretheoretical) experience includes the primary subject matter of the humanities."

20. Jeffrey Bishop, "Rejecting Medical Humanism: Medical Humanities and the Metaphysics of Medicine," *Journal of Medical Humanities* 29, no. 1 (2008): 15–25.

21. Ibid., 21.

22. Ibid., 21, 22.

23. Nancy M. P. King and Ann Folwell Stanford, "Patient Stories, Doctor Stories, and True Stories: A Cautionary Reading," *Literature and Medicine* 11, no. 2 (1992), 186, 189.

24. Anne Hudson Jones, "Reading Patients—Cautions and Concerns," *Literature and Medicine* 13, no. 2 (1994): 190–200.

25. See Sarah Atkinson, Ronan Foley, and Hester Parr, "Introduction: Spatial Perspectives and Medical Humanities," *Journal of Medical Humanities* 36, no. 1 (2014): 1–4.

26. See David S. Jones, Jeremy A. Greene, Jacalyn Duffin, and John Harley Warner, "Making the Case for History in Medical Education," *Journal of the History of Medicine and Allied Sciences* 70, no. 4 (2015): 623–652.

27. See Jonathan M. Metzl and Anna Kirkland, eds., *Against Health: How Health Became the New Morality* (New York: New York University Press, 2010).

28. See Carson, "Engaged Humanities," 325.

29. Carson, "Educating the Moral Imagination," 26.

30. See Evans, "Wonder and the Patient," 50. Related to the moral imagination is what sociologist C. Wright Mills called the "sociological imagination"—the ability to consider the larger social, historical, and economic background of the people we encounter and to shift our particular perspectives from individuals to the larger contexts in which they find themselves. Both of these imaginative capacities are critical to caring for patients. See Wright C. Mills, *The Sociological Imagination* (New York: Oxford University Press, 1959).

31. Carson, "Educating the Moral Imagination," 31.

32. Charon, "Two Hemispheres Unite," 148.

33. Levinas, *Time and the Other*, trans. Richard A. Cohen (Pittsburgh: Duquesne University Press, 1987), 75, 84.

34. Elmore, "A Piece of My Mind," 1526.

35. Ibid.

36. Ibid.

37. Carson, "Educating the Moral Imagination," 26, 28.

38. Gunderman and Kanter, "Perspective," 1161.

39. Ibid. Evans states in "Wonder and the Patient," 51, that he very much believes that "openness to wonder is an educational good that could well be promoted in aspects of the medical curriculum."

40. Carson, "Educating the Moral Imagination," 37.

41. Toulmin, "The Marginal Relevance of Theory," 83.

42. Arthur Frank, *Letting Stories Breathe: A Socio-Narratology* (Chicago: University of Chicago Press, 2010), 4, 47–48.

43. Frank, *The Wounded Storyteller*, 63.

44. Ibid., 146.

45. Ibid., 145.

46. Ibid., 146.

47. Arno K. Kumagai, "Acts of Interpretation: A Philosophical Approach to Using Creative Arts in Medical Education," *Academic Medicine: Journal of the Association of American Medical Colleges* 87, no. 8 (2012): 1139.

48. Frank, *Letting Stories Breathe*, 95.

49. Ibid.

50. Kumagai, "Acts of Interpretation," 1143; Gadamer, *Truth and Method*, 302, 305.

51. Charon, "Narrative Medicine," 1898, 1899.

52. See, for example, Wendy G. Anderson, Jillian E. Williams, James E. Bost, and David Barnard, "Exposure to Death Is Associated with Positive Attitudes and Higher Knowledge about End-of-Life Care in Graduating Medical Students," *Journal of Palliative Medicine* 11, no. 9 (2008): 1227–1233; Gibbins, McCoubrie, and Forbes, "Why Are Newly Qualified Doctors Unprepared to Care for Patients at the End of Life?"

53. Anderson et al., "Exposure to Death Is Associated with Positive Attitudes and Higher Knowledge about End-of-Life," 1228.

54. Delese Wear, "'Face-to-Face with It': Medical Students' Narratives about Their End-of-Life Education," *Academic Medicine: Journal of the Association of American Medical Colleges* 77, no. 4 (2002): 271.

55. Amy M. Sullivan, Matthew D. Lakoma, and Susan D. Block, "The Status of Medical Education in End-of-Life Care: A National Report," *Journal of General Internal Medicine* 18, no. 9 (2003): 685–695.

56. Wear, "'Face-to-Face with It,'" 276.

57. Sullivan, Lakoma, and Block, "The Status of Medical Education in End-of-Life Care," 689.

58. Ibid., 692.

59. Gibbins, McCoubrie, and Forbes, "Why Are Newly Qualified Doctors Unprepared to Care for Patients at the End of Life?," 398.

60. Ibid., 393.

61. Ibid.

62. Ibid., 398.

63. Ibid., 394, 396.

64. Ibid., 394.

65. Ibid.

66. Gail Austin Cooney, "Integrating Curative and Palliative Care: It Can Be Done," *Medscape Education*, May 31, 2005, http://www.medscape.org/viewarticle/505234.

67. Quill and Abernethy, "Generalist Plus Specialist Palliative Care," 1173–1174.

68. See, for example, Head et al., "'I Will Never Forget.'"

69. Heather L. Servaty, Mark J. Krejci, and Bert Hayslip, "Relationships among Death Anxiety, Communication Apprehension with the Dying, and Empathy in Those Seeking Occupations as Nurses and Physicians," *Death Studies* 20, no. 2 (1996): 149–161.

70. David E. Weissman, Susan D. Block, and Linda Blank, Joanna Cain, Ned Cassum, Deborah Danoff, et al., "Recommendations for Incorporating Palliative Care Education into the Acute Care Hospital Setting," *Academic Medicine: Journal of the Association of American Medical Colleges* 74, no. 8 (1999): 874.

71. Head et al., "'I Will Never Forget,'" 535.

72. Ibid., 537.

73. Ibid., 539, 538.

74. See Cynthia M. Williams, Cindy C. Wilson, and Cara H. Olsen, "Dying, Death, and Medical Education: Student Voices," *Journal of Palliative Medicine* 8, no. 2 (2005): 372–381.

75. Head et al., "'I Will Never Forget,'" 539.

76. Charon, "Two Hemispheres Unite," 145.

77. Ibid.

78. Ibid. Charon argues in "Narrative Medicine," 1897, that studying and closely reading literary works can translate into "narrative competence" in the clinic—"the competence that human beings use to absorb, interpret, and respond to stories." Likewise, Anne Hudson Jones, in her foreword to Gillie Bolton, *Reflective Practice: Writing and Professional Development* (Thousand Oaks, CA: Sage, 2010), xii, finds that engaging in reflective writing may also foster one's narrative skills or "narrative competence" in the clinic.

79. Cole, Carlin, and Carson, *Medical Humanities*, 13.

80. Craig M. Klugman and Diana Beckmann-Mendez, "One Thousand Words: Evaluating an Interdisciplinary Art Education Program," *Journal of Nursing Education* 54, no. 4 (2015): 220–223, have found that using "fine arts instructional strategies" with students in nursing and the other healthcare professions can lead to improvement in their observational skills, greater tolerance for ambiguity, and increased interest in interpersonal communication.

81. May, *The Physician's Covenant*, 108.

82. Nussbaum, *Cultivating Humanity*, 111. Nussbaum argues that literature can cultivate what she calls the "narrative imagination."

83. See Martin Heidegger, "The Origins of a Work of Art," in *Poetry, Language, Thought*, trans. Albert Hofstadter (New York: Harper Perennial, 1975), 15–86.

84. Ibid., 60.

85. Kumagai, "On the Way to Reflection," 366.

86. See Gary Saul Morson and Caryl Emerson, *Mikhail Bakhtin: Creation of a Prosaics* (Stanford: Stanford University Press, 1990).

87. Ibid., 27.

88. Frank, *The Wounded Storyteller*, 84, 5; see also Montgomery, *How Doctors Think*, 39–41.

89. Frank, *The Wounded Storyteller*, 7.

90. Anne Hunsaker Hawkins, *Reconstructing Illness: Studies in Pathography* (West Lafayette: Purdue University Press, 1999), 2.

91. Simone de Beauvoir, *A Very Easy Death* (New York: Pantheon, 1985).

92. Ibid., 53.

93. Ibid.

94. Ibid., 78.

95. Ibid., 73.

96. KillerGibsons, "Why I Make Terrible Decisions, or, Poverty Thoughts," *KillerMartinis* (blog), posted October 22, 2013, http://killermartinis.kinja.com/why-i-make-terrible-decisions-or-poverty-thoughts-1450123558. The author of this blog, Linda Tirado, has recently published a book related to this topic. See Linda Tirado, *Hand to Mouth: Living in Bootstrap America* (New York: G. P. Putnam's Sons, 2014).

97. KillerGibsons, "Why I Make Terrible Decisions."

98. Jack Coulehan, "'A Gentle and Humane Temper': Humility in Medicine," *Perspectives in Biology and Medicine* 54, no. 2 (2011): 213.

Notes

99. Rafael Campo, "Iatrogenic," in *Alternative Medicine* (Durham: Duke University Press, 2013), 35. This poem was reprinted here with express permission from the author, who holds copyrights on all poems in the volume.

100. Sherman, *The Fabric of Character*, 44–45.

101. Ibid., 45.

102. Ibid., 48.

103. Amy-Lee Bredlau, "Where Do You Put the Pain?" *Journal of the American Medical Association* 315, no. 10 (2016): 983.

104. A. Jones, "Why Teach Literature and Medicine?," 427.

105. Jane Gallop, "The Ethics of Reading: Close Encounters," *Journal of Curriculum Theorizing* 16, no. 3 (2000): 13.

106. See Ayelet Kuper, "Literature and Medicine: A Problem of Assessment," *Academic Medicine: Journal of the Association of American Medical Colleges* 81, no. 10 (2006): S128–S137.

107. Wear et al., "Slow Medical Education," 291. According to Sharon Dobie, "Viewpoint," 424, the more students and doctors know about themselves, the better able they will be to hear another's narrative.

108. Smith and Watson, *Reading Autobiography*, 45.

109. Shapiro, Kasman, and Shafer, "Words and Wards," 243.

110. Good and DelVecchio Good, "'Fiction' and 'Historicity' in Doctors' Stories," 65.

111. Ibid.

112. See, for example, Shapiro, Kasman, and Shafer, "Words and Wards"; Williams, Wilson, and Olsen, "Dying, Death, and Medical Education"; James W. Pennebaker, *Opening Up: The Healing Power of Expressing Emotions* (New York: Guilford Press, 1997).

113. Shapiro, Kasman, and Shafer, "Words and Wards" 238. See also Hedy S. Wald, David Anthony, Tom A. Hutchinson, Stephen Liben, Mark Smilovitch, and Anthony A. Donato, "Professional Identity Formation in Medical Education for Humanistic, Resilient Physicians: Pedagogic Strategies for Bridging Theory to Practice," *Academic Medicine: Journal of the Association of American Medical Colleges* 90, no. 6 (2015): 753–760.

114. See Sandra Jarvis-Selinger, Daniel D. Pratt, and Glenn Regehr, "Competency Is Not Enough: Integrating Identity Formation into Medical Education Discourse," *Academic Medicine: Journal of the Association of American Medical Colleges* 87, no. 9 (2012): 1185–1190.

115. Kumagai, "Acts of Interpretation," 1142.

116. Shapiro, Kasman, and Shafer, "Words and Wards," 235–236.

117. Ibid., 241.

118. Lloyd Rucker and Johanna Shapiro, "Becoming a Physician: Students' Creative Projects in a Third-Year IM Clerkship," *Academic Medicine: Journal of the Association of American Medical Colleges* 78, no. 4 (2003): 396.

119. Ibid.

120. Shapiro, Kasman, and Shafer, "Words and Wards," 236.

121. Jeffrey P. Gross, Corina D. Mommaerts, David Earl, and Raymond G. De Vries, "Perspective: After a Century of Criticizing Premedical Education, Are We Missing the Point?" *Academic Medicine: Journal of the Association of American Medical Colleges* 83, no. 5 (2008): 519.

122. Ibid.

123. Nathaniel P. Morris, "It's Time to Retire Premed," *Scientific American Blog Network*, posted May 12, 2016, http://blogs.scientificamerican.com/guest-blog/it-s-time-to-retire-premed/.

124. Gunderman and Kanter, "Perspective," 1158.

125. Steven L. Kanter, "Toward a Sound Philosophy of Premedical Education," *Academic Medicine: Journal of the Association of American Medical Colleges* 83, no. 5 (2008): 423.

126. See David A. Gruenewald, "The Best of Both Worlds: A Critical Pedagogy of Place," *Educational Researcher* 32, no. 4 (2003): 3–12; Paulo Freire, *Pedagogy of the Oppressed* (New York: Continuum, 1995; first published in 1970); and Henry A. Giroux, *Teachers as Intellectuals: Toward a Critical Pedagogy of Learning* (South Hadley, MA: Bergin Garvey, 1988).

127. hooks, *Teaching to Transgress*, 8.

128. Ibid., 21.

129. Kenneth Saltman and Alexander Means, "Students as Critical Citizens/Educated Subjects but Not as Commodities/Tested Objects," in *The Sage Guide to Curriculum in Education*, ed. Ming-Fang He, Brain D. Schultz, and William H. Schubert (Thousand Oaks, CA: Sage, 2015), 288, 290.

130. Delese Wear and Joseph Zarconi, "Challenging the Profession: Mentoring for Fearlessness," in *Mentoring in Academic Medicine*, ed. Holly Humphrey (Philadelphia: American College of Physicians Press, 2010), 62.

131. Gross et al., "Perspective," 519.

132. William T. Branch, "Use of Critical Incident Reports in Medical Education." *Journal of General Internal Medicine* 20, no. 11 (2005): 1063–1067. Critical incidences are experiences (positive or negative) that one might identify as influencing one's personal and professional development. Reflecting on them by writing "critical incidence reports," for example, can help draw attention to the process of physician formation, for such reflections "bear witness to the travails and challenges of becoming and being a doctor" (1063). It is also important to note that, although much of a person's character is shaped during childhood and adolescence, the development of practical and moral discernment (phronesis), though marked by spurts and impasses, proceeds continuously, especially when one is confronted with new experiences. See also Sherman, *The Fabric of Character*, 159.

133. LCME (Liaison Committee on Medical Education), "Structures and Functions of a Medical School: Standards for Accreditation of Medical Education Programs Leading to the MD Degree," March 2016, https://med.virginia.edu/ume-curriculum/wp-content/uploads/sites/216/2016/07/2017-18_Functions-and-Structure_2016-03-24.pdf; see also D. Jones et al., "Making the Case for History in Medical Education."

134. Kuper, "Literature and Medicine"; Cheryl J. Erwin, "Development of a Medical Humanities and Ethics Certificate Program in Texas," *Journal of Medical Humanities* 35, no. 4 (2014): 391.

135. See Jakob Ousager and Helle Johannessen, "Humanities in Undergraduate Medical Education: A Literature Review," *Academic Medicine: Journal of the Association of American Medical Colleges* 85, no. 6 (2010): 988–998.

136. See, for example, Antoinette S. Peters, Rachel Greenberger-Rosovsky, Charlotte Crowder, Susan D. Block, and Gordon T. Moore, "Long-Term Outcomes of the New Pathway Program at Harvard Medical School: A Randomized Controlled Trial," *Academic Medicine: Journal of the Association of American Medical Colleges* 75, no. 5 (2000): 470–479; Erwin, "Development of a Medical Humanities and Ethics Certificate Program in Texas"; Miller et al., "Sounding Narrative Medicine"; Rucker and Shapiro, "Becoming a Physician."

137. See Erwin, "Development of a Medical Humanities and Ethics Certificate Program in Texas"; Miller et al., "Sounding Narrative Medicine."

138. Ousager and Johannessen, "Humanities in Undergraduate Medical Education," 988.

139. Ibid., 993.

140. D. Jones et al., "Making the Case for History in Medical Education," 29.

141. Kumagai, "From Competencies to Human Interests," 981.

142. Ibid.

143. Because of the potential for reflective writing to demonstrate identity development, some educators have suggested using portfolios—compilations of (usually written) reflective works that are at least partly selected by students that demonstrate what the students have accomplished or how they have developed over time—in order to assess their growth and formation during medical school. However, it seems unlikely that students will express doubt, worry, fear, or frustration in written works that will be archived and thus "follow" them throughout their medical education. Given the enormous pressures associated with residency applications, it is unlikely that students will view portfolios, which may be read by current faculty and administrators or future residency program directors, as safe spaces for authentic reflection. For more on the use of portfolios in medical education, see Kuper, "Literature and Medicine," S131; Coulehan, "Today's Professionalism"; Carol Carraccio and Robert Englander, "Evaluating Competence Using a Portfolio: A Literature Review and Web-Based Application to the ACGME Competencies," *Teaching and Learning in Medicine* 16, no. 4 (2004): 381–387; Erik Driessen, Jan van Tartwijk, Jan D. Vermunt, and Cees P. M. van der Vleuten, "Use of Portfolios in Early Undergraduate Medical Training," *Medical Teacher* 25, no. 1 (2003): 18–23.

144. In "parallel charts," students are encouraged to write about aspects of patient care that do not fit into the confines of the typical medical chart but that should be considered and written down somewhere. Doing so can help attune students to the hermeneutic situation of the patients they encounter. See Kuper, "Literature and Medicine," S134.

145. Lyuba Konopasek, John Norcini, and Edward Krupat, "Focusing on the Formative: Building an Assessment System Aimed at Student Growth and Development," *Academic Medicine: Journal of the Association of American Medical Colleges* 91, no. 11 (2016): 1492.

146. See Kate Scannell, "Writing for Our Lives: Physician Narratives and Medical Practice," *Annals of Internal Medicine* 137, no. 9 (2002): 779–781.

147. Shapiro et al., "The Medical Humanities and Their Discontents," 193.

148. Ibid.

149. D. Jones et al., "Making the Case for History in Medical Education," 15. For more on the serious problems that arise when so much emphasis is placed on exams like the MCAT and the USMLE and ways we might address this issue, see Peter I. Gliatto, Michael Leitman, and David Muller, "Scylla and Charybdis: The MCAT, USMLE, and Degrees of Freedom in Undergraduate Medical Education," *Academic Medicine: Journal of the Association of American Medical Colleges* 91, no. 11 (2016): 1496–1500.

150. See Meaghan P. Ruddy, Linda Thomas-Hemak, and Lauren Meade, "Practice Transformation: Professional Development Is Personal," *Academic Medicine: Journal of the Association of American Medical Colleges* 91, no. 5 (2016): 624–627.

151. Erwin, "Development of a Medical Humanities and Ethics Certificate Program in Texas," 399.

152. Coulehan and Williams, "Vanquishing Virtue," 602.

153. Shapiro et al., "Medical Humanities and Their Discontents," 196.

154. Heidegger, "Memorial Address," 47.

155. See Howard S. Barrows, "Problem-Based Learning in Medicine and Beyond: A Brief Overview," *New Directions for Teaching and Learning* 1996, no. 68: 3–12.

156. D. Jones et al., "Making the Case for History in Medical Education," 27.

157. Scannell, "Writing for Our Lives," 781.

158. Ibid., 780.

159. Indeed, the humanities can also serve as a flight from authenticity, especially since inauthenticity is, according to Heidegger, our standard, everyday mode of being.

Epilogue

1. Levinas, *Is it Righteous to Be?*, 58.

2. Atul Gawande, as quoted in Melissa Dahl, "Atul Gawande on Making Life Meaningful, All the Way to the End," *Science of Us*, nymag.com. http://nymag.com/scienceofus/2014/10/atul-gawande-on-being-mortal.html.

3. A recent meta-analysis of randomized control trials shows that elements of the patient-clinician relationship—including trust, empathy, genuineness, and warmth—lead to better health outcomes, including pain relief and control of blood pressure. See John M. Kelley, Gordon Kraft-Todd, Lidia Schapira, Joe Kossowsky, and Helen Riess,"The Influence of the Patient-Clinician Relationship on Healthcare Outcomes: A Systematic Review and Meta-Analysis of Randomized Controlled Trials," *PLOS ONE* 9, no. 4 (2014): e94207. See also Suzanne Koven, "The Doctor's New Dilemma," *New England Journal of Medicine* 374, no. 7 (2016): 608–609.

4. Ofri, "Why Doctors Don't Take Sick Days."

Bibliography

AAMC (Association of American Medical Colleges). "What's on the MCAT 2015 Exam?" 2015. https://students-residents.aamc.org/applying-medical-school/article/whats-mcat-exam.

Adorno, Theodor W. *Negative Dialectics*. 2nd ed. Trans. E. B. Ashton. New York: Bloomsbury Academic, 1981.

Aho, James Alfred, and Kevin Aho. *Body Matters: A Phenomenology of Sickness, Disease, and Illness*. Lanham, MD: Lexington Books, 2008.

Aho, Kevin. Guignon on Self-Surrender and Homelessness in Dostoevsky and Heidegger. In *Horizons of Authenticity in Phenomenology, Existentialism, and Moral Psychology*, ed. Hans Pedersen and Megan Altman, 63–74. Dordrecht: Springer, 2015.

Aho, Kevin. Heidegger, Ontological Death, and the Healing Professions. *Medicine, Health Care, and Philosophy* 19, no. 1 (2016): 55–63.

Aho, Kevin. *Heidegger's Neglect of the Body*. New York: State University of New York Press, 2010.

Aho, Kevin. Medicalizing Mental Health: A Phenomenological Alternative. *Journal of Medical Humanities* 29, no. 4 (2008): 243–259.

Aho, Kevin. The Missing Dialogue between Heidegger and Merleau-Ponty: On the Importance of the Zollikon Seminars. *Body & Society* 11, no. 2 (2005): 1–23.

Aho, Kevin. Why Heidegger is not an Existentialist: Interpreting Authenticity and Historicity in *Being and Time*. *Florida Philosophical Review* 3, no. 1 (2003): 5–22.

Anderson, Wendy G., Jillian E. Williams, James E. Bost, and David Barnard. Exposure to Death Is Associated with Positive Attitudes and Higher Knowledge about End-of-Life Care in Graduating Medical Students. *Journal of Palliative Medicine* 11, no. 9 (2008): 1227–1233.

Andre, Judith. The Medical Humanities as Contributing to Moral Growth and Development. In *Practicing the Medical Humanities: Engaging Physicians and Patients*, ed.

Ronald A. Carson, Chester A. Burns and Thomas R. Cole, 39–69. Hagerstown, MD: University Publishing Group, 2003.

Anonymous. "I Never Understood the Loss of Empathy during Medical Training . . . Until Now." *Kevin MD.com* (blog). Posted September 2, 2014. http://www.kevinmd.com/blog/2014/09/never-understood-loss-empathy-medical-training-now.html.

Apesoa-Varano, Ester Carolina, and Charles S. Varano. *Conflicted Health Care: Professionalism and Caring in an Urban Hospital.* Nashville: Vanderbilt University Press, 2014.

Aristotle. *Nicomachean Ethics.* Oxford: Clarendon Press, 1908. http://classics.mit.edu/Aristotle/nicomachaen.6.vi.html.

Armstrong, Paul B. Phenomenology. In *The Johns Hopkins Guide to Literary Theory and Criticism*, ed. Michael Groden and Martin Kreisworth, 562–566. Baltimore: Johns Hopkins University Press, 1994.

Arnold, Louise, and David Thomas Stern. What Is Medical Professionalism? In *Measuring Medical Professionalism*, ed. David Thomas Stern, 17–34. New York: Oxford University Press, 2006.

Atkinson, Sarah, Ronan Foley, and Hester Parr. Introduction: Spatial Perspectives and Medical Humanities. *Journal of Medical Humanities* 36, no. 1 (2014): 1–4.

Baier, Annette C. Alternative Offerings to Asclepius? *Medical Humanities Review* 6, no. 1 (1992): 9–19.

Baile, Walter F., Robert Buckman, Renato Lenzi, Gary Glober, Estela A. Beale, and Andrzej P. Kudelka. SPIKES—A Six-Step Protocol for Delivering Bad News: Application to the Patient with Cancer. *Oncologist* 5, no. 4 (2000): 302–311.

Bakhtin, Mikhail. *Art and Answerability: Early Philosophical Essays.* Ed. Michael Holquist and Vadim Liapunov. Trans. Vadim Liapunov. Austin: University of Texas Press, 1990.

Bakhtin, Mikhail. *Problems of Dostoevsky's Poetics.* Minneapolis: University of Minnesota Press, 1984.

Barnard, David. Love and Death: Existential Dimensions of Physicians' Difficulties with Moral Problems. *Journal of Medicine and Philosophy* 13, no. 4 (1988): 393–409.

Barrows, Howard S. Problem-Based Learning in Medicine and Beyond: A Brief Overview. *New Directions for Teaching and Learning* 1996, no. 68: 3–12.

Bartles, William James. "The Status of Epistemology in the Thought of Martin Heidegger (Knowledge, Art, Phenomenology)." Ph.D. diss., Rice University, 1985.

Beach, Mary Catherine, and Thomas Inui, and the Relationship-Centered Care Research Network. Relationship-Centered Care: A Constructive Reframing. *Journal of General Internal Medicine* 21, suppl. 1 (2006): S3–S8.

Bibliography

Becker, Ernest. *The Denial of Death*. New York: Free Press Paperbacks, 1997.

Beckman, Thomas J., and Mark C. Lee. Proposal for a Collaborative Approach to Clinical Teaching. *Mayo Clinic Proceedings* 84, no. 4 (2009): 339–344.

Bergo, Bettina. "Emmanuel Levinas." *Stanford Encyclopedia of Philosophy*. Ed. Edward N. Zalta. Summer 2013. https://plato.stanford.edu/archives/sum2013/entries/levinas.

Bishop, Jeffrey P. *The Anticipatory Corpse: Medicine, Power, and the Care of the Dying*. Notre Dame: University of Notre Dame Press, 2011.

Bishop, Jeffrey P. Rejecting Medical Humanism: Medical Humanities and the Metaphysics of Medicine. *Journal of Medical Humanities* 29, no. 1 (2008): 15–25.

Bleakley, Alan. From Reflective Practice to Holistic Reflexivity. *Studies in Higher Education* 24, no. 3 (1999): 315–330.

Bleakley, Alan. *Medical Humanities and Medical Education: How the Medical Humanities Can Shape Better Doctors*. New York: Routledge, 2015.

Block, Susan D., and J. Andrew Billings. Learning from the Dying. *New England Journal of Medicine* 353, no. 13 (2005): 1313–1315.

Bolton, Gillie. *Reflective Practice: Writing and Professional Development*. 3rd ed. Thousand Oaks, CA: Sage, 2010.

Brainard, Andrew H., and Heather C. Brislen. Viewpoint: Learning Professionalism; A View from the Trenches. *Academic Medicine: Journal of the Association of American Medical Colleges* 82, no. 11 (2007): 1010–1014.

Branch, William T. Use of Critical Incident Reports in Medical Education. *Journal of General Internal Medicine* 20, no. 11 (2005): 1063–1067.

Bredlau, Amy-Lee. Where Do You Put the Pain? *Journal of the American Medical Association* 315, no. 10 (2016): 983.

Broyard, Anatole. "Doctor Talk to Me." *New York Times*. August 26, 1990. http://www.nytimes.com/1990/08/26/magazine/doctor-talk-to-me.html.

Butler, Sandra, and Barbara Rosenblum. *Cancer in Two Voices*. Duluth: Spinsters Ink, 1996.

Bynum, William E. Why Physicians Need to Be More than Automated Medical Kiosks. *Academic Medicine: Journal of the Association of American Medical Colleges* 89, no. 2 (2014): 212–214.

Bynum, William E., and Brenessa Lindeman. Caught in the Middle: A Resident Perspective on Influences From the Learning Environment That Perpetuate Mistreatment. *Academic Medicine: Journal of the Association of American Medical Colleges* 91, no. 3 (2016): 301–304.

Caan, Woody. A Testing Time for Ethical Standards. *BMJ* 330, no. 7506 (2005): 1510.

Cahn, Peter S. "Seven Dirty Words: Hot-Button Language That Undermines Interprofessional Education and Practice." *Academic Medicine: Journal of the Association of American Medical Colleges* (e-publication online ahead of print, November 1, 2016) http://journals.lww.com/academicmedicine/Abstract/publishahead/Seven_Dirty_Words___Hot_Button_Language_That.98360.aspx.

Campo, Rafael. Iatrogenic. In *Alternative Medicine,*, 35. Durham: Duke University Press, 2013.

Carraccio, Carol, and Robert Englander. Evaluating Competence Using a Portfolio: A Literature Review and Web-Based Application to the ACGME Competencies. *Teaching and Learning in Medicine* 16, no. 4 (2004): 381–387.

Carson, Ronald A. Educating the Moral Imagination. In *Practicing the Medical Humanities: Engaging Physicians and Patients*, ed. Ronald A. Carson, Chester A. Burns and Thomas R. Cole, 25–38. Hagerstown, MD: University Publishing Group, 2003.

Carson, Ronald A. Engaged Humanities: Moral Work in the Precincts of Medicine. *Perspectives in Biology and Medicine* 50, no. 3 (2007): 321–333.

Carson, Ronald A. The Hyphenated Space: Liminality in the Doctor-Patient Relationship. In *Stories Matter: The Role of Narrative in Medical Ethics*, ed. Rita Charon and Martha Montello, 171–182. New York: Routledge, 2002.

Carson, Ronald A. On Metaphorical Concentration: Language and Meaning in Patient-Physician Relations. *Journal of Medicine and Philosophy* 36, no. 4 (2011): 385–393.

Carson, Ronald A., Chester R. Burns, and Thomas R. Cole, eds. *Practicing the Medical Humanities: Engaging Physicians and Patients*. Hagerstown, MD: University Publishing Group, 2003.

Carter, Michele A. Abiding Loneliness: An Existential Perspective on Loneliness. *Second Opinion* 2000, no. 3: 37–54.

Carter, Michele A., and Sally S. Robinson. A Narrative Approach to the Clinical Reasoning Process in Pediatric Intensive Care: The Story of Matthew. *Journal of Medical Humanities* 22, no. 3 (2001): 173–194.

Cassell, Eric J. The Nature of Suffering and the Goals of Medicine. *New England Journal of Medicine* 306, no. 11 (1982): 639–645.

Charon, Rita. Narrative Medicine: A Model for Empathy, Reflection, Profession, and Trust. *Journal of the American Medical Association* 286, no. 15 (2001): 1897–1902.

Charon, Rita. Two Hemispheres Unite: Medical Humanities Become Narrative Medicine. In *Practicing the Medical Humanities: Engaging Physicians and Patients*, ed. Ronald

A. Carson, Chester R. Burns and Thomas R. Cole, 143–156. Hagerstown, MD: University Publishing Group, 2003.

Chen, Pauline W. *Final Exam: A Surgeon's Reflections on Mortality*. New York: Vintage Books, 2008.

Chiapperino, Luca, and Giovanni Boniolo. Rethinking Medical Humanities. *Journal of Medical Humanities* 35, no. 4 (2014): 377–387.

Ciałkowska-Rysz, Aleksandra, and Tomasz Dzierżanowski. Personal Fear of Death Affects the Proper Process of Breaking Bad News. *Archives of Medical Science* no. 4 (2013): 127–131.

Cole, Thomas R., Nathan S. Carlin, and Ronald A. Carson. *Medical Humanities: An Introduction*. New York: Cambridge University Press, 2014.

Cole, Thomas R., and Faith L. Lagay. How the Medical Humanities Can Help Revitalize Humanism and How a Reconfigured Humanism Can Help Nourish the Medical Humanities. In *Practicing the Medical Humanities: Engaging Physicians and Patients*, ed. Ronald A. Carson, Chester R. Burns and Thomas R. Cole, 157–177. Hagerstown, MD: University Publishing Group, 2003.

Coles, Robert. Medical Ethics and Living a Life. *New England Journal of Medicine* 301, no. 8 (1979): 444–446.

Cook, Alyssa F., Vineet M. Arora, Kenneth A. Rasinski, Farr V. Curlin, and John D. Yoon. The Prevalence of Medical Student Mistreatment and its Association with Burnout. *Academic Medicine: Journal of the Association of American Medical Colleges* 89, no. 5 (2014): 749–754.

Cook, Deborah, and Graeme Rocker. Dying with Dignity in the Intensive Care Unit. *New England Journal of Medicine* 370, no. 26 (2014): 2510–2514.

Cooney, Gail Austin. "Integrating Curative and Palliative Care: It Can Be Done." *Medscape Education*. 2005. http://www.medscape.org/viewarticle/505234.

Coulehan, Jack. "A Gentle and Humane Temper": Humility in Medicine. *Perspectives in Biology and Medicine* 54, no. 2 (2011): 206–216.

Coulehan, Jack. Viewpoint: Today's Professionalism: Engaging the Mind but Not the Heart. *Academic Medicine: Journal of the Association of American Medical Colleges* 80, no. 10 (2005): 892–898.

Coulehan, Jack, and Peter C. Williams. Vanquishing Virtue: The Impact of Medical Education. *Academic Medicine: Journal of the Association of American Medical Colleges* 76, no. 6 (2001): 598–605.

Crawford, Paul. "Health Humanities: We Are Here to Collaborate, Not to Compete." *Guardian*. March 30, 2015. https://www.theguardian.com/higher-education-network/2015/mar/30/health-humanities-here-to-collaborate-not-compete.

Cruess, Richard L., Sylvia R. Cruess, J. Donald Boudreau, Linda Snell, and Yvonne Steinert. A Schematic Representation of the Professional Identity Formation and Socialization of Medical Students and Residents: A Guide for Medical Educators. *Academic Medicine: Journal of the Association of Medical Colleges* 90, no. 6 (2015): 718–725.

Dahl, Melissa. "Atul Gawande on Making Life Meaningful, All the Way to the End." *Science of Us*. Nymag.com. October 15, 2014. http://nymag.com/scienceofus/2014/10/atul-gawande-on-being-mortal.html.

Dahlstrom, Daniel O. *The Heidegger Dictionary*. New York: Bloomsbury Academic, 2013.

Daston, Lorraine J., and Peter Galison. *Objectivity*. New York: Zone Books, 2010.

Davis, F. Daniel. *Phronesis*, Clinical Reasoning, and Pellegrino's Philosophy of Medicine. *Theoretical Medicine* 18, nos. 1–2 (1997): 173–195.

de Beauvoir, Simone. *A Very Easy Death*. Trans. Patrick O'Brian. New York: Pantheon, 1985.

Dickinson, George E., and Robert E. Tournier. A Decade Beyond Medical School: A Longitudinal Study of Physicians' Attitudes toward Death and Terminally-Ill Patients. *Social Science & Medicine* 38, no. 10 (1994): 1397–1400.

Dobie, Sharon. Viewpoint: Reflections on a Well-Traveled Path: Self-Awareness, Mindful Practice, and Relationship-Centered Care as Foundations for Medical Education. *Academic Medicine: Journal of the Association of American Medical Colleges* 82, no. 4 (2007): 423–427.

Dreyfus, Hubert L. Foreword. In Carol J. White, *Time and Death: Heidegger's Analysis of Finitude*, ed. Mark Ralkowski, ix–xxxvi. Aldershot, UK: Ashgate, 2005.

Driessen, Erik, Jan van Tartwijk, Jan D. Vermunt, and Cees P. M. van der Vleuten. Use of Portfolios in Early Undergraduate Medical Training. *Medical Teacher* 25, no. 1 (2003): 18–23.

Dyrbye, Liselotte N., Matthew R. Thomas, and Tait D. Shanafelt. Medical Student Distress: Causes, Consequences, and Proposed Solutions. *Mayo Clinic Proceedings* 80, no. 12 (2005): 1613–1622.

Earle, Craig C., Elyse R. Park, Bonnie Lai, Jane C. Weeks, John Z. Ayanian, and Susan Block. Identifying Potential Indicators of the Quality of End-of-Life Cancer Care from Administrative Data. *Journal of Clinical Oncology* 21, no. 6 (2003): 1133–1138.

Edwards, Ben, and Valerie Clark. The Psychological Impact of a Cancer Diagnosis on Families: The Influence of Family Functioning and Patients' Illness Characteristics on Depression and Anxiety. *Psycho-Oncology* 13, no. 8 (2004): 562–576.

Elmore, Shekinah. A Piece of My Mind: The Good Doctor. *Journal of the American Medical Association* 306, no. 14 (2011): 1525–1526.

Engel, George L. The Clinical Application of the Biopsychosocial Model. *American Journal of Psychiatry* 137, no. 5 (1980): 535–544.

Engel, George L. Selection of Clinical Material in Psychosomatic Medicine: The Need for a New Physiology. *Psychosomatic Medicine* 16, no. 5 (1954): 368–372.

Epstein, Ronald M. Mindful Practice. *Journal of the American Medical Association* 282, no. 9 (1999): 833–839.

Erwin, Cheryl J. Development of a Medical Humanities and Ethics Certificate Program in Texas. *Journal of Medical Humanities* 35, no. 4 (2014): 389–403.

Evans, H. M. Wonder and the Patient. *Journal of Medical Humanities* 36, no. 1 (2014): 47–58.

Falcon, Andrea. "Aristotle on Causality." *Stanford Encyclopedia of Philosophy*. Ed Edward N. Zalta. Spring 2015. https://plato.stanford.edu/archives/spr2015/entries/aristotle-causality/.

Feifel, Herman. Death. In *Taboo Topics*, ed. Norman L. Farberow, 8–21. New York: Atherton Press, 1963.

Feifel, Herman, Susan Hanson, and Robert Jones. "Physicians Consider Death." In *Proceedings of the 75th Annual Convention of the American Psychological Association* 2 (1967): 201–202.

Feudtner, Chris, Dimitri A. Christakis, and Nicholas A. Christakis. Do Clinical Clerks Suffer Ethical Erosion? Students' Perceptions of Their Ethical Environment and Personal Development. *Academic Medicine: Journal of the Association of American Medical Colleges* 69, no. 8 (1994): 670–679.

Field, David. Palliative Medicine and the Medicalization of Death. *European Journal of Cancer Care* 94, no. 3 (1994): 58–62.

Fields, Scott A., and W. Michael Johnson. Physician-Patient Communication: Breaking Bad News. *West Virginia Medical Journal* 108, no. 2 (2012): 32–35.

Foucault, Michel. *The Birth of the Clinic: An Archaeology of Medical Perception*. Trans. A. M. Sheridan Smith. New York: Vintage Books, 1975.

Fox, Daniel M. Who We Are: The Political Origins of the Medical Humanities. *Theoretical Medicine* 6, no. 3 (1985): 327–341.

Fox, Renée C. The Evolution of Medical Uncertainty. *Milbank Memorial Fund Quarterly* 58, no. 1 (1980): 1–9.

Frank, Arthur W. *At the Will of the Body: Reflections on Illness*. New York: Houghton Mifflin, 1991.

Frank, Arthur W. *Letting Stories Breathe: A Socio-Narratology*. Chicago: University of Chicago Press, 2010.

Frank, Arthur W. *The Renewal of Generosity: Illness, Medicine, and How to Live*. Chicago: University of Chicago Press, 2004.

Frank, Arthur W. *The Wounded Storyteller: Body, Illness, and Ethics*. Chicago: University of Chicago Press, 1997.

Freire, Paulo. *Pedagogy of the Oppressed*. New York: Continuum, 1995.

Friedman, Lauren F. "IBM's Watson Supercomputer May Soon Be The Best Doctor In The World." *Business Insider*. April 22, 2014. http://www.businessinsider.com/ibms-watson-may-soon-be-the-best-doctor-in-the-world-2014-4.

Friedman, Lester D. The Precarious Position of the Medical Humanities in the Medical School Curriculum. *Academic Medicine: Journal of the Association of American Medical Colleges* 77, no. 4 (2002): 320–322.

Frist, William H., and Martha K. Presley. Training the Next Generation of Doctors in Palliative Care Is the Key to the New Era of Value-Based Care. *Academic Medicine: Journal of the Association of American Medical Colleges* 90, no. 3 (2015): 268–271.

Gadamer, Hans-Georg. *The Enigma of Health: The Art of Healing in a Scientific Age*. Trans. Jason Gaiger and Nicholas Walker. Stanford: Stanford University Press, 1996.

Gadamer, Hans-Georg. Hermeneutics as Practical Philosophy. In *The Gadamer Reader: A Bouquet of the Later Writings*, ed. and trans. Richard E. Palmer, 227–245 Evanston: Northwestern University Press, 2007.

Gadamer, Hans-Georg. *Truth and Method*. 2nd ed. Trans. and ed. Donald G. Marshall and Joel Weinsheimer. New York: Bloomsbury Academic, 2004.

Gallop, Jane. The Ethics of Reading: Close Encounters. *Journal of Curriculum Theorizing* 16, no. 3 (2000): 7–17.

Gardiner, Patrick. *Kierkegaard*. New York: Oxford University Press, 1997.

Gawande, Atul. *Being Mortal: Medicine and What Matters in the End*. New York: Metropolitan Books, 2014.

Gibbins, Jane, Rachel McCoubrie, and Karen Forbes. Why Are Newly Qualified Doctors Unprepared to Care for Patients at the End of Life? *Medical Education* 45, no. 4 (2011): 389–399.

Giroux, Henry A. *Teachers as Intellectuals: Toward a Critical Pedagogy of Learning*. South Hadley, MA: Bergin Garvey, 1988.

Gliatto, Peter, I. Michael Leitman, and David Muller. Scylla and Charybdis: The MCAT, USMLE, and Degrees of Freedom in Undergraduate Medical Education. *Academic Medicine: Journal of the Association of American Medical Colleges* 91, no. 11 (2016): 1498–1500.

Good, Byron J., and Mary-Jo DelVecchio Good. "Fiction" and "Historicity" in Doctors' Stories. In *Narrative and the Cultural Construction of Illness and Healing*, ed. Cheryl Mattingly and Linda C. Garro, 50–69. Berkeley: University of California Press, 2000.

Grant, Janet. The Incapacitating Effects of Competence: A Critique. *Advances in Health Sciences Education: Theory and Practice* 4, no. 3 (1999): 271–277.

Groden, Michael, Martin Kreiswirth, and Imre Szeman, eds. *The Johns Hopkins Guide to Literary Theory and Criticism*. 2nd ed. Baltimore: Johns Hopkins University Press, 2004.

Gross, Jeffrey P., Corina D. Mommaerts, David Earl, and Raymond G. De Vries. Perspective: After a Century of Criticizing Premedical Education, Are We Missing the Point? *Academic Medicine: Journal of the Association of American Medical Colleges* 83, no. 5 (2008): 516–520.

Gruenewald, David A. The Best of Both Worlds: A Critical Pedagogy of Place. *JEducational Researcher* 32, no. 4 (2003): 3–12.

Guignon, Charles B. *Heidegger and the Problem of Knowledge*. Cambridge, MA: Hackett, 1983.

Gunderman, Richard B., and Steven L. Kanter. Perspective: "How to Fix the Premedical Curriculum" Revisited. *Academic Medicine: Journal of the Association of American Medical Colleges* 83, no. 12 (2008): 1158–1161.

Hafferty, Frederic. Measuring Professionalism: A Commentary. In *Measuring Medical Professionalism*, ed. David Stern, 281–306. New York: Oxford University Press, 2006.

Hafferty, Frederic. Professionalism and the Socialization of Medical Students. In *Teaching Medical Professionalism*, ed. Richard L. Cruess, Sylvia R. Cruess, and Yvonne Steinert, 53–70. New York: Cambridge University Press, 2009.

Hawkins, Anne Hunsaker. *Reconstructing Illness: Studies in Pathography*. West Lafayette: Purdue University Press, 1999.

Head, Barbara, Lori Earnshaw, Ruth Greenberg, Robert Morehead, Mark Pfeifer, and Monica Ann Shaw. "I Will Never Forget": What We Learned from Medical Student Reflections on a Palliative Care Experience. *Journal of Palliative Medicine* 15, no. 5 (2012): 535–541.

Heidegger, Martin. *Being and Time*. Trans. John Macquarrie and Edward Robinson. New York: Harper & Row, 1962.

Heidegger, Martin. Conversation on a Country Path about Thinking. In *Discourse on Thinking*, trans. John M. Anderson and E. Hans Freund, 58–90. New York: Harper & Row, 1969.

Heidegger, Martin. *Discourse on Thinking*. Trans. John M. Anderson and E. Hans Freund. New York: Harper & Row, 1969.

Heidegger, Martin. Exposition of the Task of a Preparatory Analysis of Dasein. In *Self and Subjectivity*, ed. Kim Atkins, 117–124. Malden, MA: Blackwell, 2005.

Heidegger, Martin. Memorial Address. In *Discourse on Thinking*, trans. John M. Anderson and E. Hans Freund., 43–57. New York: Harper & Row, 1969.

Heidegger, Martin. The Origins of a Work of Art. In *Poetry, Language, Thought*, trans. Albert Hofstadter., 15–86. New York: Harper Perennial, 1975.

Heidegger, Martin. The Question Concerning Technology. In *The Question Concerning Technology, and Other Essays*, trans. William Lovitt, 3–35. New York: Harper & Row, 1977.

Heidegger, Martin. What Is Metaphysics? In *Existentialism from Dostoevsky to Sartre, Revised and Expanded Edition*, ed. and trans. Walter Kaufmann, 242–279. New York: New American Library, 1975.

Heidegger, Martin. *Zollikon Seminars: Protocols, Conversations, Letters*. Ed. Medard Boss. Trans. Franz Mayr and Richard Askay. Evanston: Northwestern University Press, 2001.

"Hermeneutic Phenomenology." *Phenomenology Online*. 2011. http://www.phenomenologyonline.com/inquiry/orientations-in-phenomenology/hermeneutical-phenomenology/.

Hick, Christian. The Art of Perception: From the Life World to the Medical Gaze and Back Again. *Medicine, Health Care, and Philosophy* 2, no, 2 (1999): 129–140.

Hockenos, Paul. "Release of Heidegger's 'Black Notebooks' Reignites Debate over Nazi Ideology." *Chronicle of Higher Education*, February 24, 2014. http://chronicle.com/article/Release-of-Heidegger-s/144897/.

Hojat, Mohammadreza, Michael J. Vergare, Kaye Maxwell, George Brainard, Steven K. Herrine, Gerald A. Isenberg, et al. The Devil Is in the Third Year: A Longitudinal Study of Erosion of Empathy in Medical School. *Academic Medicine: Journal of the Association of American Medical Colleges* 84, no. 9 (2009): 1182–1191.

Holden, Mark D., Era Buck, Mark Clark, Karen Szauter, and Julie Trumble. Professional Identity Formation in Medical Education: The Convergence of Multiple Domains. *HEC Forum* 24, no. 4 (2012): 245–255.

Holden, Mark D., Era Buck, John Luk, Frank Ambriz, Eugene V. Boisaubin, Mark A. Clark, et al. Professional Identity Formation: Creating a Longitudinal Framework Through TIME (Transformation in Medical Education). *Academic Medicine: Journal of the Association of American Medical Colleges* 90, no. 6 (2015): 761–767.

hooks, bell. *Teaching to Transgress: Education as the Practice of Freedom.* New York: Routledge, 1994.

Hunter, Kathryn Montgomery. *Doctors' Stories: The Narrative Structure of Medical Knowledge.* Princeton: Princeton University Press, 1991.

Huntington, Patricia J. Heidegger's Reading of Kierkegaard Revisited: From Ontological Abstraction to Ethical Concretion. In *Kierkegaard in Post/Modernity,* ed. Martin J. Matuštík and Merold Westphal, 43–65. Bloomington: Indiana University Press, 1995.

Inui, Thomas S. *A Flag in the Wind: Educating for Medical Professionalism.* Washington, DC: Association of American Medical Colleges, 2003.

Inwood, Michael J. *Heidegger.* New York: Oxford University Press, 1997.

Irby, David M., Molly Cooke, and Bridget C. O'Brien. Calls for Reform of Medical Education by the Carnegie Foundation for the Advancement of Teaching: 1910 and 2010. *Academic Medicine: Journal of the Association of American Medcal Colleges* 85, no. 2 (2010): 220–227.

Irwin, William. Death by Inauthenticity: Heidegger's Debt to Ivan Il'ich's Fall. *Tolstoy Studies Journal* 25 (2013): 15–21.

Jackson, Eric R., Tait D. Shanafelt, Omar Hasan, Daniel V. Satele, and Liselotte N. Dyrbye. Burnout and Alcohol Abuse/Dependence among U.S. Medical Students. *Academic Medicine: Journal of the Association of American Medcal Colleges* 91, no. 9 (2016): 1251–1256.

Jansen, Lynn A., and Daniel P. Sulmasy. Proportionality, Terminal Suffering and the Restorative Goals of Medicine. *Theoretical Medicine and Bioethics* 23, nos. 4–5 (2002): 321–337.

Jarvis-Selinger, Sandra, Daniel D. Pratt, and Glenn Regehr. Competency Is Not Enough: Integrating Identity Formation into the Medical Education Discourse. *Academic Medicine: Journal of the Association of American Medical Colleges* 87, no. 9 (2012): 1185–1190.

Jones, Anne Hudson. Foreword. In Gillie Bolton, *Reflective Practice: Writing and Professional Development.* 3rd ed. Thousand Oaks, CA: Sage, 2010.

Jones, Anne Hudson. Reading Patients—Cautions and Concerns. *Literature and Medicine* 13, no. 2 (1994): 190–200.

Jones, Anne Hudson. Why Teach Literature and Medicine? Answers from Three Decades. *Journal of Medical Humanities* 34, no. 4 (2013): 415–428.

Jones, David S., Jeremy A. Greene, Jacalyn Duffin, and John Harley Warner. Making the Case for History in Medical Education. *Journal of the History of Medicine and Allied Sciences* 70, no. 4 (2015): 623–652.

Jones, Therese, Michael Blackie, Rebecca Garden, and Delese Wear. The Almost Right Word: The Move from Medical to Health Humanities. *Academic Medicine: Journal of the Association of American Medical Colleges* 92, no. 7 (July 2017): 932–935. http://journals.lww.com/academicmedicine/Citation/2017/07000/The_Almost_Right_Word___The_Move_From_Medical_to.31.aspx.

Kane, Anne C., and John D. Hogan. Death Anxiety in Physicians: Defensive Style, Medical Specialty, and Exposure to Death. *Omega* 16, no. 1 (1985): 11–22.

Kanter, Steven L. Toward a Sound Philosophy of Premedical Education. *Academic Medicine: Journal of the Association of American Medical Colleges* 83, no. 5 (2008): 423–424.

Kay, Jerald. Traumatic Deidealization and the Future of Medicine. *Journal of the American Medical Association* 263, no. 4 (1990): 572–573.

Keen, Sam. Foreword. In Ernest Becker, *The Denial of Death*, xi–xvi. New York: Free Press Paperbacks, 1997.

Kegan, Robert. *The Evolving Self: Problem and Process in Human Development*. Cambridge, MA: Harvard University Press, 1982.

Kelley, John M., Gordon Kraft-Todd, Lidia Schapira, Joe Kossowsky, and Helen Riess. The Influence of the Patient-Clinician Relationship on Healthcare Outcomes: A Systematic Review and Meta-Analysis of Randomized Controlled Trials. *PLoS One* 9, no. 4 (2014): e94207.

Kierkegaard, Søren. *Concluding Unscientific Postscript to Philosophical Fragments*. Trans. Howard V. Hong and Edna H. Hong. Princeton: Princeton University Press, 1992.

Kierkegaard, Søren. *Fear and Trembling and The Sickness unto Death*. Trans. Walter Lowrie. Princeton: Princeton University Press, 1968.

KillerGibsons. "Why I Make Terrible Decisions, or, Poverty Thoughts." *KillerMartinis* (blog). Posted October 22, 2013. http://killermartinis.kinja.com/why-i-make-terrible-decisions-or-poverty-thoughts-1450123558.

King, Nancy M. P., and Ann Folwell Stanford. Patient Stories, Doctor Stories, and True Stories: A Cautionary Reading. *Literature and Medicine* 11, no. 2 (1992): 185–199.

Kinghorn, Warren A. Medical Education as Moral Formation: An Aristotelian Account of Medical Professionalism. *Perspectives in Biology and Medicine* 53, no. 1 (2010): 87–105.

Kissler, Mark J., Ricardo Nuila Ben Saxton, and Dorene F. Balmer. Professional Formation in the Gross Anatomy Lab and Narrative Medicine: An Exploration. *Academic Medicine: Journal of the Association of American Medical Colleges* 91, no. 6 (2016): 772–777.

Kleinman, Arthur. *The Illness Narratives: Suffering, Healing, and the Human Condition*. New York: Basic Books, 1988.

Klugman, Craig M., and Diana Beckmann-Mendez. One Thousand Words: Evaluating an Interdisciplinary Art Education Program. *Journal of Nursing Education* 54, no. 4 (2015): 220–223.

Komesaroff, Paul. The Many Faces of the Clinic: A Levinasian View. In *Handbook of Phenomenology and Medicine*, ed. S. Kay Toombs, 312–330. Dordrecht: Kluwer Academic, 2001.

Konopasek, Lyuba, John Norcini, and Edward Krupat. Focusing on the Formative: Building an Assessment System Aimed at Student Growth and Development. *Academic Medicine: Journal of the Association of American Medical Colleges* 91, no. 11 (2016): 1492–1497.

Koven, Suzanne. The Doctor's New Dilemma. *New England Journal of Medicine* 374, no. 7 (2016): 608–609.

Kübler-Ross, Elisabeth. *On Death and Dying*. New York: Macmillan, 1969.

Kumagai, Arno K. Acts of Interpretation: A Philosophical Approach to Using Creative Arts in Medical Education. *Academic Medicine: Journal of the Association of American Medical Colleges* 87, no. 8 (2012): 1138–1144.

Kumagai, Arno K. From Competencies to Human Interests: Ways of Knowing and Understanding in Medical Education. *Academic Medicine: Journal of the Association of American Medical Colleges* 89, no. 7 (2014): 978–983.

Kumagai, Arno K. On the Way to Reflection: A Conversation on a Country Path. *Perspectives in Biology and Medicine* 56, no. 3 (2013): 362–370.

Kumagai, Arno K., and Thirusha Naidu. Reflection, Dialogue, and the Possibilities of Space. *Academic Medicine: Journal of the Association of American Medical Colleges* 90, no. 3 (2015): 283–288.

Kuper, Ayelet. Literature and Medicine: A Problem of Assessment. *Academic Medicine: Journal of the Association of American Medical Colleges* 81, no. 10 (2006): S128–S137.

Lannaman, John W., and Linda M. Harris. Ending the End-of-Life Communication Impasse: A Dialogic Intervention. In *Cancer, Communication, and Aging*, ed. Lisa Sparks, Dan O'Hair and Gary Kreps, 293–320. Cresskill, NJ: Hampton, 2008.

Laverty, Susann M. Hermeneutic Phenomenology and Phenomenology: A Comparison of Historical and Methodological Considerations. *International Journal of Qualitative Methods* 2, no. 3 (2003): 21–35.

LCME (Liaison Committee on Medical Education). "Structures and Functions of a Medical School: Standards for Accreditation of Medical Education Programs Leading to the MD Degree." March 2016. https://med.virginia.edu/ume-curriculum/wp-content/uploads/sites/216/2016/07/2017-18_Functions-and-Structure_2016-03-24.pdf.

Levinas, Emmanuel. Ethics as First Philosophy. In *The Levinas Reader*, ed. S. Hand. Oxford: Blackwell, 1989.

Levinas, Emmanuel. *Is It Righteous to Be? Interviews with Emmanuel Levinas*. Ed. Jill Robbins. Stanford: Stanford University Press, 2001.

Levinas, Emmanuel. *Time and the Other*. Trans. Richard A. Cohen. Pittsburgh: Duquesne University Press, 1987.

Levinas, Emmanuel. *Totality and Infinity*. Trans. Alphonse Lingis. Pittsburgh: Duquesne University Press, 1969.

Levinas, Emmanuel. Transcendence and Height. In *Emmanuel Levinas: Basic Philosophical Writings*, ed. Adriaan T. Peperzak, Simon Critchley and Robert Bernasconi, 11–32. Bloomington: Indiana University Press, 1996.

Lovko, Sandra Kocijan, Rudolf Gregurek, and Dalibor Karlovic. Stress and Ego-Defense Mechanisms in Medical Staff at Oncology and Physical Medicine Departments. *European Journal of Psychiatry* 21, no. 4 (2007): 279–286.

Ludmerer, Kenneth. *Time to Heal: American Medical Education from the Turn of the Century to the Era of Managed Care*. New York: Oxford University Press, 2005.

Lugones, María. Playfulness, "World"-Travelling, and Loving Perception. *Hypatia* 2, no. 2 (1987): 3–19.

MacIntyre, Alasdair. *After Virtue: A Study in Moral Theory*. 2nd ed. Notre Dame: University of Notre Dame Press, 1984.

Maguire, Peter. Barriers to Psychological Care of the Dying. *British Medical Journal (Clinical Research Edition)* 291, no. 6510 (1985): 1711–1713.

Malpas, Jeff. "Hans-Georg Gadamer." *Stanford Encyclopedia of Philosophy*. Ed. Edward N. Zalta. Winter 2014. http://plato.stanford.edu/archives/win2014/entries/gadamer/.

Matustík, Martin J., and Merold Westphal, eds. *Kierkegaard in Post/Modernity*. Bloomington: Indiana University Press, 1995.

Mavis, Brian, Aron Sousa, Wanda Lipscomb, and Marsha D. Rappley. Learning about Medical Student Mistreatment from Responses to the Medical School Graduation Questionnaire. *Academic Medicine: Journal of the Association of American Medical Colleges* 89, no. 5 (2014): 705–711.

May, William F. *The Physician's Covenant: Images of the Healer in Medical Ethics*. 2nd ed. Louisville: Westminster John Knox Press, 2000.

McGee, Glenn. *Phronesis* in Clinical Ethics. *Theoretical Medicine* 17, no. 4 (1996): 317–328.

McQuellon, Richard P., and Michael A. Cowan. Turning toward Death Together: Conversation in Mortal Time. *American Journal of Hospice & Palliative Care* 17, no. 5 (2000): 312–318.

Meier, Diane E., Anthony L. Back, and R. Sean Morrison. The Inner Life of Physicians and Care of the Seriously Ill. *Journal of the American Medical Association* 286, no. 23 (2001): 3007–3014.

Merleau-Ponty, Maurice. *Phenomenology of Perception*. Trans. Colin Smith. New York: Routledge, 2002. (Originally published in French in 1945.)

Metzl, Jonathan M., and Anna Kirkland, eds. *Against Health: How Health Became the New Morality*. New York: New York University Press, 2010.

Miller, Eliza, Dorene Balmer, Nellie Hermann, Gillian Graham, and Rita Charon. Sounding Narrative Medicine: Studying Students' Professional Identity Development at Columbia University College of Physicians and Surgeons. *Academic Medicine: Journal of the Association of American Medical Colleges* 89, no. 2 (2014): 335–342.

Miller, Jerome A. The Trauma of Evil and the Traumatological Conception of Forgiveness. *Continental Philosophy Review* 42, no. 3 (2009): 401–419.

Mills, C. Wright. *The Sociological Imagination*. New York: Oxford University Press, 1959.

Montgomery, Kathryn. *How Doctors Think: Clinical Judgment and the Practice of Medicine*. New York: Oxford University Press, 2005.

Moran, Dermot. *Introduction to Phenomenology*. New York: Routledge, 2000.

Morgan, Michael L. *The Cambridge Introduction to Emmanuel Levinas*. New York: Cambridge University Press, 2011.

Morris, Nathaniel P. "It's Time to Retire Premed." *Scientific American Blog Network*. Posted May 12, 2016. http://blogs.scientificamerican.com/guest-blog/it-s-time-to-retire-premed/.

Morson, Gary Saul, and Caryl Emerson. *Mikhail Bakhtin: Creation of a Prosaics*. Stanford: Stanford University Press, 1990.

Mueller-Vollmer, Kurt. *The Hermeneutics Reader: Texts of the German Tradition from the Enlightenment to the Present*. New York: Continuum, 1985.

Naidu, Thirusha, and Arno K. Kumagai. Troubling Muddy Waters: Problematizing Reflective Practice in Global Medical Education. *Academic Medicine: Journal of the Association of American Medical Colleges* 91, no. 3 (2016): 317–321.

Neumann, Melanie, Friedrich Edelhäuser, Diethard Tauschel, Martin R. Fischer, Markus Wirtz, Christiane Woopen, et al. Empathy Decline and Its Reasons: A

Systematic Review of Studies with Medical Students and Residents. *Academic Medicine: Journal of the Association of American Medical Colleges* 86, no. 8 (2011): 996–1009.

Newton, Bruce W., Laurie Barber, James Clardy, Elton Cleveland, and Patricia O'Sullivan. Is There Hardening of the Heart during Medical School? *Academic Medicine: Journal of the Association of American Medical Colleges* 83, no. 3 (2008): 244–249.

Nietzsche, Friedrich Wilhelm. *Beyond Good and Evil*. Trans. Walter Kaufmann. New York: Vintage Books, 1966.

Nietzsche, Friedrich Wilhelm. *The Gay Science*. Trans. Walter Kaufmann. New York: Vintage Books, 1974.

Nietzsche, Friedrich Wilhelm. *On the Genealogy of Morals*. Trans. Walter Kaufmann and R. J. Hollingdale. New York: Vintage Books, 1989.

Novack, Dennis H., Ronald M. Epstein, and Randall H. Paulsen. Toward Creating Physician-Healers: Fostering Medical Students' Self-Awareness, Personal Growth, and Well-Being. *Academic Medicine: Journal of the Association of American Medical Colleges* 74, no. 5 (1999): 516–520.

Nuland, Sherwin B. *How We Die: Reflections on Life's Final Chapter*. New York: Vintage Books, 1995.

Nussbaum, Martha C. *Cultivating Humanity: A Classical Defense of Reform in Liberal Education*. Cambridge, MA: Harvard University Press, 1998.

Ofri, Danielle. *What Doctors Feel: How Emotions Affect the Practice of Medicine*. Boston: Beacon Press, 2014.

Ofri, Danielle. "Why Doctors Don't Take Sick Days." *New York Times*, November 15, 2013. http://www.nytimes.com/2013/11/16/opinion/sunday/why-doctors-dont-take-sick-days.html.

Olthuis, Gert, and Wim Dekkers. Medical Education, Palliative Care and Moral Attitude: Some Objectives and Future Perspectives. *Medical Education* 37, no. 10 (2003): 928–933.

Ortega, Mariana. "New Mestizas," "'World' Travelers," and "Dasein": Phenomenology and the Multi-Voiced, Multi-Cultural Self. *Hypatia* 16, no. 3 (2001): 1–29.

Ousager, Jakob, and Helle Johannessen. Humanities in Undergraduate Medical Education: A Literature Review. *Academic Medicine: Journal of the Association of American Medical Colleges* 85, no. 6 (2010): 988–998.

Peabody, Francis W. The Care of the Patient. *Journal of the American Medical Association* 88, no. 12 (1927): 877–882.

Pedersen, Reidar. Empathy Development in Medical Education—A Critical Review. *Medical Teacher* 32, no. 7 (2010): 593–600.

Pellegrino, Edmund D. The Anatomy of Clinical-Ethical Judgments in Perinatology and Neonatology: A Substantive and Procedural Framework. *Seminars in Perinatology* 11, no. 3 (1987): 202–209.

Pellegrino, Edmund D. The Caring Ethic: The Relation of Physician to Patient. In *Physician and Philosopher: The Philosophical Foundation of Medicine*, ed. Roger J. Bulgar, John P. McGovern and Daniel P. Sulmasy, 166–178. Charlottesville, VA: Carden Jennings, 2001.

Pellegrino, Edmund D. The Internal Morality of Clinical Medicine: A Paradigm for the Ethics of the Helping and Healing Professions. *Journal of Medicine and Philosophy* 26, no. 6 (2001): 559–579.

Pennebaker, James W. *Opening Up: The Healing Power of Expressing Emotions*. New York: Guildford Press, 1997.

Peters, Antoinette S., Rachel Greenberger-Rosovsky, Charlotte Crowder, Susan D. Block, and Gordon T. Moore. Long-Term Outcomes of the New Pathway Program at Harvard Medical School: A Randomized Controlled Trial. *Academic Medicine: Journal of the Association of American Medical Colleges* 75, no. 5 (2000): 470–479.

Pew Research Center. "America's Changing Religious Landscape. http://www.pewforum.org/2015/05/12/americas-changing-religious-landscape/. May 12, 2015.

Piemonte, Nicole M. Last Laughs: Gallows Humor and Medical Education. *Journal of Medical Humanities* 36, no. 4 (2015): 375–390.

Plutchik, Robert, Henry Kellerman, and Hope R. Conte. A Structural Theory of Ego Defenses and Emotions. In *Emotions in Personality and Psychopathology*, ed. Carroll E. Izard, 229–256. New York: Plenum Press, 1979.

Proctor, Robert E. *Defining the Humanities: How Discovering a Tradition Can Improve Our Schools*. 2nd ed. Bloomington: Indiana University Press, 1998.

Putnam, Hilary. Levinas and Judaism. In *The Cambridge Companion to Levinas*, ed. Simon Critchley and Robert Bernasconi, 33–62. New York: Cambridge University Press, 2002.

Quill, Timothy E., and Amy P. Abernethy. Generalist plus Specialist Palliative Care—Creating a More Sustainable Model. *New England Journal of Medicine* 368, no. 13 (2013): 1173–1174.

Ramsey, Paul. *The Patient as Person: Explorations in Medical Ethics*. New Haven: Yale University Press, 1970.

Reynolds, Jack. "Maurice Merleau-Ponty." *Internet Encyclopedia of Philosophy: A Peer-Reviewed Academic Resource*. 2014. http://www.iep.utm.edu/merleau/.

Rojan, Tilottama. Hermeneutics. In *The Johns Hopkins Guide to Literary Theory and Criticism*, ed. Michael Groden and Martin Kreisworth, 375–378. Baltimore: Johns Hopkins University Press, 1994.

Rosenberg, Charles E. *The Care of Strangers: The Rise of America's Hospital System*. New York: Basic Books, 1987.

Rucker, Lloyd, and Johanna Shapiro. Becoming a Physician: Students' Creative Projects in a Third-Year IM Clerkship. *Academic Medicine: Journal of the Association of American Medical Colleges* 78, no. 4 (2003): 391–397.

Ruddy, Meaghan P., Linda Thomas-Hemak, and Lauren Meade. Practice Transformation: Professional Development Is Personal. *Academic Medicine: Journal of the Association of American Medical Colleges* 91, no. 5 (2016): 624–627.

Rudebeck, Carl Edvard. Grasping the Existential Anatomy: The Role of Bodily Empathy in Clinical Communication. In *Handbook of Phenomenology and Medicine*, ed. S. Kay Toombs, 297–316. Dordrecht: Kluwer Academic, 2001.

Sacks, Oliver. "Oliver Sacks on Learning He Has Terminal Cancer." *New York Times*, February 19, 2015. http://www.nytimes.com/2015/02/19/opinion/oliver-sacks-on-learning-he-has-terminal-cancer.html.

Saltman, Kenneth, and Alexander Means. Students as Critical Citizens/Educated Subjects but Not as Commodities/Tested Objects. In *The Sage Guide to Curriculum in Education*, ed. Ming Fang He, Brian D. Schultz, and William H. Schubert, 284–292. Thousand Oaks, CA: Sage, 2015.

Sartre, Jean-Paul. *Being and Nothingness: An Essay in Phenomenological Ontology*. Trans. Hazel E. Barnes. New York: Washington Square Press, 1992.

Scannell, Kate. Writing for Our Lives: Physician Narratives and Medical Practice. *Annals of Internal Medicine* 137, no. 9 (2002): 779–781.

Schön, Donald A. *The Reflective Practitioner: How Professionals Think in Action*. New York: Basic Books, 1983.

Servaty, Heather L., Mark J. Krejci, and Bert Hayslip. Relationships among Death Anxiety, Communication Apprehension with the Dying, and Empathy in Those Seeking Occupations as Nurses and Physicians. *Death Studies* 20, no. 2 (1996): 149–161.

Shanafelt, Tait D. Enhancing Meaning in Work: A Prescription for Preventing Physician Burnout and Promoting Patient-Centered Care. *Journal of the American Medical Association* 302, no. 12 (2009): 1338–1340.

Shapiro, Johanna. Walking a Mile in Their Patients' Shoes: Empathy and Othering in Medical Students' Education. *Philosophy, Ethics, and Humanities in Medicine* 3, item no. 10 (2008). doi:10.1186/1747-5341-3-10.

Shapiro, Johanna, Jack Coulehan, Delese Wear, and Martha Montello. Medical Humanities and Their Discontents: Definitions, Critiques, and Implications. *Academic Medicine: Journal of the Association of American Medical Colleges* 84, no. 2 (2009): 192–198.

Bibliography

Shapiro, Johanna, Deborah Kasman, and Audrey Shafer. Words and Wards: A Model of Reflective Writing and Its Uses in Medical Education. *Journal of Medical Humanities* 27, no. 4 (2006): 231–244.

Sherman, Nancy. *The Fabric of Character: Aristotle's Theory of Virtue*. Oxford: Oxford University Press, 1991.

Sherwin, Susan. *No Longer Patient: Feminist Ethics and Health Care*. Philadelphia: Temple University Press, 1992.

Sinha, Pranay. "Why Do Doctors Commit Suicide?" *NYTimes.com*, September 5, 2014. http://www.nytimes.com/2014/09/05/opinion/why-do-doctors-commit-suicide.html.

Sklar, David P. Mistreatment of Students and Residents: Why Can't We Just Be Nice? *Academic Medicine: Journal of the Association of American Medical Colleges* 89, no. 5 (2014): 693–695.

Smith, David Woodruff. "Phenomenology." *Stanford Encyclopedia of Philosophy*. Ed. Edward N. Zalta. Fall 2011. http://plato.stanford.edu/archives/fall2011/entries/phenomenology/.

Smith, Sidonie, and Julia Watson. *Reading Autobiography: A Guide for Interpreting Life Narratives*. Minneapolis: University of Minnesota Press, 2001.

Sontag, Susan. *Illness as Metaphor and AIDS and Its Metaphors*. New York: Picador USA, 2001. (*Illness as Metaphor* originally published in 1978; *AIDS and Its Metaphors* originally published in 1990.)

Starr, Paul. *The Social Transformation of American Medicine*. New York: Basic Books, 1982.

Stein, Howard F. *American Medicine as Culture*. Boulder: Westview Press, 1990.

Stern, David Thomas, ed. *Measuring Medical Professionalism*. New York: Oxford University Press, 2006.

Stump, Eleonore. *Wandering in Darkness: Narrative and the Problem of Suffering*. New York: Oxford University Press, 2010.

Sullivan, Amy M., Matthew D. Lakoma, and Susan D. Block. The Status of Medical Education in End-of-Life Care: A National Report. *Journal of General Internal Medicine* 18, no. 9 (2003): 685–695.

Svenaeus, Fredrik. *The Hermeneutics of Medicine and the Phenomenology of Health: Steps Towards a Philosophy of Medical Practice*. Dordrecht: Kluwer Academic, 2000.

Svenaeus, Fredrik. Hermeneutics of Medicine in the Wake of Gadamer: The Issue of Phronesis. *Theoretical Medicine and Bioethics* 24, no. 5 (2003): 407–431.

Svenaeus, Fredrik. Illness as Unhomelike Being-in-the-World: Heidegger and the Phenomenology of Medicine. *Medicine, Health Care, and Philosophy* 14, no. 3 (2011): 333–343.

Taylor, Charles. The Dialogical Self. In *The Interpretive Turn: Philosophy, Science, Culture*, ed. David R. Hiley, James Bohman, and Richard Shusterman. Ithaca: Cornell University Press, 1991.

Taylor, Charles. *Philosophical Arguments*. New York: Harvard University Press, 1995.

Taylor, Charles. *Philosophy and the Human Sciences*. vol. 2. Philosophical Papers. New York: Cambridge University Press, 1985.

Thomas, Lewis. Notes of a Biology-Watcher: How to Fix the Premedical Curriculum. *New England Journal of Medicine* 298, no. 21 (1978): 1180–1181.

Thomson, Iain. Death and Demise in Being and Time. In *The Cambridge Companion to Heidegger's Being and Time*, ed. Mark A. Wrathall, 260–290. New York: Cambridge University Press, 2013.

Thomson, Iain. Heidegger's Perfectionist Philosophy of Education in *Being and Time*. *Continental Philosophy Review* 37, no. 4 (2004): 439–467.

Tirado, Linda. *Hand to Mouth: Living in Bootstrap America*. New York: G. P. Putnam's Sons, 2014.

Tolstoy, Leo. *The Death of Ivan Ilych and Other Stories*. Trans. Aylmer Maude and J. D. Duff. New York: Signet Classic, 2003.

Toombs, S. Kay. *The Meaning of Illness: Phenomenological Account of the Different Perspectives of Physician and Patients*. Dordrecht: Kluwer Academic, 1993.

Toombs, S. Kay, ed. *Handbook of Phenomenology and Medicine*. Dordrecht: Kluwer Academic, 2001.

Toulmin, Stephen. The Marginal Relevance of Theory to the Humanities. *Common Knowledge* 2, no. 1 (1993): 75–84.

Toulmin, Stephen. The Recovery of Practical Philosophy. *American Scholar* 57, no. 3 (1988): 337–352.

Treadway, Katharine. Perspective: The Code. *New England Journal of Medicine* 357, no. 13 (2007): 1273–1275.

Tresolini, Carol P., and Pew Health Professions Commission. *Health Professions Education and Relationship-Centered Care: Report*. San Francisco: Pew Health Professions Commission; University of California, San Francisco, Center for the Health Professions, 1994.

Trillin, Alice Stewart. Of Dragons and Garden Peas: A Cancer Patient Talks to Doctors. *New England Journal of Medicine* 304, no. 12 (1981): 699–701.

Bibliography

Waitzkin, Howard. A Critical Theory of Medical Discourse: Ideology, Social Control, and the Processing of Social Context in Medical Encounters. *Journal of Health and Social Behavior* 30, no. 2 (1989): 220–239.

Wald, Hedy S., David Anthony, Tom A. Hutchinson, Stephen Liben, Mark Smilovitch, and Anthony A. Donato. Professional Identity Formation in Medical Education for Humanistic, Resilient Physicians: Pedagogic Strategies for Bridging Theory to Practice. *Academic Medicine: Journal of the Association of American Medical Colleges* 90, no. 6 (2015): 753–760.

Walker, Margaret Urban. *Moral Understandings: A Feminist Study in Ethics*. 2nd ed. New York: Oxford University Press, 2007.

Ward, Koral. *Augenblick: The Concept of the "Decisive Moment" in 19th- and 20th-Century Western Philosophy*. Aldershot, UK: Ashgate, 2008.

Wear, Delese. Face-to-Face with It: Medical Students' Narratives about Their End-of-Life Education. *Academic Medicine: Journal of the Association of American Medical Colleges* 77, no. 4 (2002): 271–277.

Wear, Delese, and Joseph Zarconi. Can Compassion Be Taught? Let's Ask Our Students. *Journal of General Internal Medicine* 23, no. 7 (2008): 948–953.

Wear, Delese, and Joseph Zarconi. Challenging the Profession: Mentoring for Fearlessness. In *Mentoring in Academic Medicine*, ed. Holly Humphrey, 51–66. Philadelphia: American College of Physicians Press, 2010.

Wear, Delese, Joseph Zarconi, Arno Kumagai, and Kathy Cole-Kelly. Slow Medical Education. *Academic Medicine: Journal of the Association of American Medical Colleges* 90, no. 3 (2015): 289–293.

Weber, Max. Science as a Vocation. In *From Max Weber: Essays in Sociology*, ed. and trans. H. H. Gerth and C. Wright Mills, 129–156. New York: Oxford University Press, 1946.

Weissman, David E., Susan D. Block, Linda Blank, Joanna Cain, Ned Cassum, Deborah Danoff, et al. Recommendations for Incorporating Palliative Care Education into the Acute Care Hospital Setting. *Academic Medicine: Journal of the Association of American Medical Colleges* 74, no. 8 (1999): 871–877.

Wiener, Linda, and Ramsey Eric Ramsey. *Leaving Us to Wonder: An Essay On The Questions Science Can't Ask*. Albany: State University of New York Press, 2005.

Williams, Bernard. *Philosophy as a Humanistic Discipline*. Ed. A. W. Moore. Princeton: Princeton University Press, 2008.

Williams, Cynthia M., Cindy C. Wilson, and Cara H. Olsen. Dying, Death, and Medical Education: Student Voices. *Journal of Palliative Medicine* 8, no. 2 (2005): 372–381.

Williams, Geoffrey C., and Edward L. Deci. The Importance of Supporting Autonomy in Medical Education. *Annals of Internal Medicine* 129, no. 4 (1998): 303–308.

Wolfe, Judith. *Heidegger's Eschatology: Theological Horizons in Martin Heidegger's Early Work*. New York: Oxford University Press, 2015.

Wynia, Matthew K., Maxine A. Papadakis, William M. Sullivan, and Frederic W. Hafferty. More Than a List of Values and Desired Behaviors: A Foundational Understanding of Medical Professionalism. *Academic Medicine: Journal of the Association of American Medical Colleges* 89, no. 5 (2014): 712–714.

Zaner, Richard M. *Conversations on the Edge: Narratives of Ethics and Illness*. Washington, DC: Georgetown University Press, 2004.

Zimmerman, Camilla, and Gary Rodin. The Denial of Death Thesis: Sociological Critique and Implications for Palliative Care. *Palliative Medicine* 18, no. 2 (2004): 121–128.

Index

Abstraction, 18, 20
   Kierkegaard and, 29–30, 42, 61, 183n8
Accrediting Council for Graduate Medical Education (ACGME), 156, 157, 169
Agent-narrative suffering, 171n5
Aho, Kevin, 51, 70–71
Algorithms, medical, 25
Alterity, 204n134
   and the other, 80–81
Altruism, 2, 3, 88, 102, 107
Anxiety, 72, 101
   disburdening of (*see under* Reductionistic medicine)
   etymology of the term, 80
   Heidegger and, 47–51, 71, 78
   nature of, 48–49, 54
   related to being-in-the-world, 48–49, 78
   resoluteness and, 68, 69, 72
   and the "they," 51–54
   types of, 51 (*see also* Death anxiety; Existential anxiety; Ontological anxiety)
   vulnerability and, 51, 65, 101, 107
Aristotle, xix, 8
   on medicine, 211n62, 211n67
   on phronesis, 85, 109, 110, 211n68
   on virtue, 107, 211nn67–68
Artificial intelligence (AI). *See* Watson
Arts, 143, 220n80. *See also* Authentic engagement through artistic and narrative representation

Ascetic ideal, 184n9
Assessment. *See also under* Doctors
   formative vs. summative, 158
Attunements, 48–49
Authentic engagement through artistic and narrative representation, 142–144
   doctors' stories, 146–151
   engagement through representation: literature and narrative as an example, 144–146
   making curricular inroads, 155–158
   medical humanities and premedical education, 152–155
   reflecting together, 151–152
Authenticity. *See also* Heidegger, Martin; Inauthenticity; *specific topics*
   Levinas and, 75, 79, 81

Bakhtin, Mikhail, xxviii, 87–90, 92
   dialogism, 87–89
   on novels and other stories, 144
Barnard, David, 117, 171n5
Becker, Ernest, 44–45
Being. *See also* Dasein; *specific topics*
   metaphysics and, 179n74
Being-for-oneself, 77
Being-for-the-other, Levinas on, 77, 79, 80, 87–90, 92, 93

Being-in-the-world, xvii, xxviii, 17, 19, 137, 157, 170
  anxiety and dread related to, 48–49, 78
  Dasein and, 180n94, 186n42, 195n6
  death and the collapse of, 50
  deepening our, 67–68, 97
  Heidegger and, 17, 19, 20, 38, 48, 72, 78, 117, 180n94
  homelikeness, unhomelikeness, and, 38–39, 65, 78, 187n63
  illness and, 32, 37–39, 41, 78, 191n119
  interpretation and, 19, 20
  nature of, 19, 32, 180n94
  Nothingness and, 195n6
  resoluteness and, 72, 75
  suffering and, 32, 97, 188n74
  "they" and inauthentic ways of, 66, 157
  transcending, 195n6
Being-in-the-world-with-others, 158. *See also* Being-with-others-in-the-world
Being-toward-death, 29, 53, 65, 67
Being-toward entities in the world, 198n51
Being-with, 73, 75, 90, 195n6. *See also* Being-with-others
Being-with-one-another, 72, 192n136
Being-with-others, 50–51, 60, 71–75, 94, 163. *See also* Dasein
Being-with-others-in-the-world, 52. *See also* Being-in-the-world-with-others
Being-with-the-other, 87, 90
Billings, Andrew, 13
Biology, applied
  medicine defined as, 9
Biomedical paradigm, 9, 14, 27, 85. *See also* Modernist thinking and modernist biomedical paradigm; *specific topics*

Bishop, Jeffrey P., 22, 23, 32
  on altruism, 88
  on being-in-the-world, 32
  calculative thinking and, xix
  on the coldness of medicine, 41
  on death, 44
  on medical education and training, xix, 8, 22
  on medical humanism, 131, 132
  on the metaphysics of medicine, 8
  on suffering, 8, 32, 88
Bleakley, Alan, xxv
Block, Susan, 13
Bodily perception, 186n42
Body. *See also* Embodiment
  Frank on the breaking down of the, 29, 39, 41, 64
  Heidegger and the, 35–36, 186n42
  lived, 35, 36
  and mind, detachment between, 41 (*see also* Mind–body dualism; Mind–body separation)
  phenomenology and the, 35–37
Bracketing (phenomenology), 17–19, 33–34
  defined, 33
Bredlau, Amy-Lee, 148
Broyard, Anatole, 94, 95
Burnout, 99, 125
Bynum, William E., 20, 21, 113

Cahn, Peter, xvi
Calculative approaches, 55. *See also* Watson
Calculative thinking, xxii. *See also under* Meditative thinking
  and the clinical gaze, 22–27
  Heidegger on, xix–xx, 20, 21, 24, 26, 61, 128, 161
  nature of, xix, 20
Called into becoming, 87–89
Calling(s), 176n9, 194n1. *See also* *specific topics*

Index

medicine as a, 194n1
Call of the other, responding to the, 82–89
Campo, Rafael, 147
Cancer, ix, 37–39, 124, 145, 193n161
Cancer diagnosis, 12, 37–39, 94, 195n13
Cancer in Two Voices (Butler and Rosenblum), 37–38
Capitalism, 98–99, 168
Care
  and concern for others, 198n51
  and cure
    conflation of, 9
    division between, 9–10
Carlin, Nathan S., 98, 130, 143
Carson, Ronald A., xxiv, 63, 98, 135, 203n130
  on the arts, 143
  on Charles Taylor, 205n164
  on doctor characteristics, 98, 134
  on language, communication, and expression, 86
  on listening, 134
  on medical education, 134
  on medical humanities, 130, 134
  on medical practice, 98, 115, 118
  on narrative approaches to clinical care and ethics, 208n13
Carter, Michele, xxi, 79–80
Cartesian dualism, 31, 35. *See also* Mind–body dualism
Cartesian model/Cartesian worldview
  Guignon on, 16, 184n14
  Heidegger and, 16, 17, 21, 25
Cassell, Eric, xvi, 8–9, 27
Causes and causation, types of, 8
Certainty. *See also* Uncertainty
  need for, 27, 55, 61, 63, 71, 159
Charon, Rita, 74, 131, 137, 142, 219n78
Chen, Pauline W., 57, 93
Clinical gaze, 23, 31, 70
  calculative thinking and the, 22–27
  defined, 23

Clinical informatics. *See* Watson
"Closed" scientific way of seeing reality, 23–24
Cognitive frameworks of medical culture, 149
Cole, Thomas R., 98, 130, 143
Coles, Robert, 116
Compassion, 125
  detachment and, 120
  meaning and etymology of the term, 93
  vulnerability and, 93–94
Competencies in medical education, 209n27
Competency frameworks, 103
Computer. *See also* Supercomputer
  as model of thinking, 183n131
Concern, types of, 198n51
Consumers, patients as, 98–99
Conversation(s), 86, 166–167. *See also specific topics*
  nature of, 86
Coping strategies, xxii
Corporeal body, xvi, 36–39
Coulehan, Jack, 104, 111, 120, 147, 160
Courage, virtue of, 210n53
Cowan, Michael A., 67, 73, 86, 91, 196n21, 199n58
Critical incidences and critical incidence reports, 223n132
Curative vs. palliative care, 139. *See also* Palliative care
Cure. *See also under* Care; Healing
  dying/terminal patients and, 9, 10, 43, 57, 59
  goal of, 57
  singleminded telos of, 10
Curiosity, 197nn37–38. *See also* Wonder

Dasein
  being-in-the-world and, 180n94, 186n42, 195n6
  defined, 179n70

Dasein (cont.)
  Heidegger on, 17, 29, 47, 67, 179n70, 180n94, 186n42, 190n105, 198n51, 199n56, 201n92
  nature of, 180n94, 190n105
  resoluteness and, 72, 199nn56
Daston, Lorraine J., 176n25
Davis, F. Daniel, 85
Death (and dying), 47, 91, 95, 191n108. *See also* Dying patients/terminal patients
  as collapse (of identity), 47–51
  conceptions and notions of, 196n21
  dream of defeating or indefinitely deferring, 44–46
  and engagement with the other, 137–142
  existential and scientific realities of, 45
  Heidegger and, 47–50, 53, 67, 190n105, 191n108
  hospital culture and learning about, 139
  Levinas on, 166, 205n158
  meaning of, 74, 129
  medical education and, 138
  medicine and the denial of, 44–47
  nature of, 48, 49
  nothingness and, 195n6
  speaking and having conversations about, 166
  terminology, 47
  and the "they," 51, 53–54, 61, 65
    the "they" and inauthentic understandings of death, 53–54
Death anxiety, 47–50, 140, 189n89
  Heidegger and, 47–51
de Beauvoir, Simone, 145–146
Defense mechanisms, 46. *See also* Denial
Deidealization, 113
"Demise," 47
Denial, 57, 59
  of death, 44–47

Depersonalization in medicine, xvii, xxi, 162
Descartes, René, 16–17
Detachment, 91, 115, 158, 176n22
  causes and development of, xix, xxii, 7, 8, 11, 12–13, 71, 115, 120, 121, 141
  compassion and, 120
  culture of, xviii, 120
  as a default position., 12
  ethic of, 120, 158
  impartiality and, xix, 7
  Katharine Treadway on, 12
  Kierkegaard on, 29
  mitigated by finding meaning in one's work, 100
  Nietzsche and, 55, 184n9
  objectivity and, xi, 6–7, 24, 97–98, 101, 120, 177n25
  from one's body, 41 (*see also* Mind–body dualism)
  science and, xviii, xix, 6, 8, 18, 24, 29, 61, 98
  suffering and, xix, 7, 8, 11, 59, 97–98, 121
  as a symptom, xxii
  from the "they," 198n48
  "they-self" notions about, 59
Dialogism, Mikhail Bakhtin's, 87–89
Dialogue, 85–90, 121–123
  nature of, 87–88
Dickinson, George E., 1
Discursive regimes, 40
Disease, 24. *See also* Illness; *specific topics*
  vs. illness, 39–40
  nature of, 39–40
"dis-ease," 24, 40, 128
"Disease talk" vs. "illness talk," 40, 57
Doctors. *See also specific topics*
  attempting to form "good doctors": the distraction of assessment, 118–125
  humanity, xi, 109

Index

images of, 194n167
qualities valued in, 109, 194n167, 208n21
(re)formation, 125–126
as scientists, xxvi, 5, 7–9, 55–57
as wise persons, 85
Dread, 48. *See also* Anxiety
Dying patients/terminal patients, ix–x. *See also* Death (and dying)
   avoiding and distancing oneself from, 9, 43, 46, 47
   caring for, ix, xxii, 9, 10, 45, 46, 61, 63, 95, 145–146, 199n58 (*see also* Palliative care)
   challenges, difficulties, and anguish experienced in, 43–44, 73, 93, 141–142
   extralinguistic engagement in, 90
   medical education and, xxii, 3, 138–142
   mutual benefits gained from, 74, 93, 136–137, 140–141
   caring for loved ones who are dying, ix–x, 145–146
   cure/curing and, 9, 10, 43, 57, 59
   existential and agent-narrative suffering, 9, 43–44, 171n5 (*see also* Existential suffering)
   healing and, 109
   medical paternalism with, 145, 190n96
   "protecting" students from, 138–141
   talking with them about end-of-life issues and dying, ix, 43–44, 138, 141
   vulnerability and, 44 (*see also* Vulnerability: death and)

Earle, Craig, 57
Ecstatic phenomenon, 36
   defined, 186n44
Education, 135–136. *See also* Medical education; Pedagogy
   etymology of the term, 135
   goals of, 215n6
   Heidegger and, 121, 135, 215n6
   nature of, 135
Efficient causation, 8
Elmore, Sheknah, 12, 13, 134–135
Embodiment, 35
   and the lived experience of illness, 32–33
   the lived body and illness, 35–42
   phenomenology and, 33–37
Emotion, Plutchik's theory of, 46
Empathic imagination, 134–135
Empathy, x, 120, 142, 144. *See also* Witnessing
   cultivating and enhancing, 117, 126, 134, 135, 137, 144, 145, 156
   humility and, 134
   loss of, 58, 120 (*see also* Detachment)
   medical humanities courses and, 5, 14
   medical school, medical training, and, 1–3, 5, 13, 58, 102, 112, 117, 124, 142, 173n20
   modernist beliefs creating barriers to, 173n20
   narratives and, 142, 144
   vs. objectivity, 14, 120, 128
Empathy training, 14
End-of-life care, 57, 89, 138–140. *See also* Dying patients/terminal patients; Palliative care
Enlightenment, 17, 22, 25, 174n35, 183n8, 202n113
Epistemology, 6
   contemporary Western medical
   a closer look at, 5–27
   reasons it persists, 14–15
   Heidegger and, 15–20, 61
   intersection of pedagogy and, 10–13
   looking beyond (and before), xx–xxiii
Epstein, Ronald M., 101
Equilibrium of body, natural, 37
Ethical encounter, 75

Ethics. *See also* Moral imagination; Virtue ethics
  Heidegger on, 75, 199n68
  Kierkegaard and, 52, 183n1, 191n10
  Levinas on, 75–77, 81, 205n166
  narrative approaches to, 208n13
Everydayness
  Heidegger's use of the term, 187n45
  of life, 36, 37, 187n45
Existence (and the existential), 29–30. *See also* Dasein; Heidegger, Martin
  nature of, 190n105
Existential anxiety, xxii, 75, 79, 93, 127–129, 171n4, 195n6. *See also* Ontological-existential anxiety
Existential death, 47
Existential reflection, 100–101, 125
Existential suffering, xvii
  conceptions and scope of the term, 171nn4–5
  dying/terminal patients and, 9, 43–44, 171n5
Expressive-collaborative model, 81
External goods, 108

Face, Levinas's phenomenology of the, 1, 75–81
Faith, 30, 184n9
  leap of, 65
Fearlessness. *See also* Anxiety
  mentoring for, 154–155
Feedback, 158
Feminist approach to ethics, xxiv, 81
Feminist theory, xxiv–xxv, 81
Feminist thinkers, xxiv, 92
Fine arts instructional strategies, 220n80
Flexner Report, 197n37
Formative assessment, 158
Foucault, Michel, 8, 22–23, 40
Fox, Daniel, xvii
Frank, Arthur W., 118, 137
  on alterity, 80
  on breaking down of the body, 29, 39, 41, 64
  on clinical encounters, 97
  on death, 66
  on denial, 59
  on "disease talk" vs. "illness talk," 40–41, 57–58
  on doctors' experiences, 71, 72, 88
  on doctors' personalities, 71
  existential questions and, 57–58
  face-to-face encounters with ill people and, 136–137
  on giving up control, 70
  on illness, 39, 66, 198n54
  Levinas and, 78, 80, 201n91
  on listening, 42–43, 89
  on mind–body connection, 41
  narrative plotlines, restitution narratives, and, 10
  on narratives of illness, 136, 144
  on patient–practitioner relationship, 64
  on patients' experiences, 59, 91, 122
  personal narrative of illness, 43, 66, 67, 145
  recognition and, 78
  on suffering, xxix, 42–44
  on wonder, 70
  The Wounded Storyteller, 9–10

Gadamer, Hans-Georg, 59, 61, 203n123
  hermeneutics and, 34, 82, 203n123
  horizons of meaning and, 82–83, 86, 87, 137
  on illness, 37
  on truth, xxviii
Galison, Peter, 176n25
Gallows humor, xxii, 173n24
Gardiner, Patrick, 72
Gawande, Atul, 43–44, 56, 166, 205n162
Grant, Janet, 103
Gross, Jeffrey P., 152

Index

Ground mood (*Grundstimmung*), 48, 191n113
Grundstimmung, 48
 translations and meanings of the term, 191n113
Guignon, Charles B.
 on Cartesian model and Cartesian tradition, 16, 184n14
 Descartes and, 16–17
 Heidegger and, 16, 21, 24
Gunderman, Richard, 4

Hafferty, Frederic W., 5–6, 105–106, 209n42
Hawkins, Anne Hunsaker, 145
Healer(s), xxvi, 93, 94, 130, 149
 becoming a, 5, 94, 152, 157, 170
 being a, xxiv, 89, 151
 cultivating, 97, 101, 109, 114, 152, 170
 development of, 115, 157
 doctor as, 5, 64, 87, 89, 90
 future, 95, 114, 127, 148, 152, 163, 170
Healing, 83, 91, 157, 162
 components of and preconditions/prerequisites for, 89, 93, 101
  authentic engagement, 128
  love, 168
  responding to the other, 94
  trust, 102, 167
 curing compared with, 10
 curing conflated with, 24, 49, 60
 curing contrasted with, 83, 109
 dying patients and, 109
 medicine and, 166
 nature of, 78, 93
Health, modernist assumption of restoration of, 43
"Health humanities," 129, 130. *See also* Medical humanities
Heidegger, Martin, xix–xx, 15–17, 22, 52, 54, 84, 182n111, 197n31, 199n67
 anxiety and, 47–51, 71, 78
 on being, 16, 17, 19, 179n74
 on being and time, 206n174
 being-in-the-world and, 17, 19, 20, 38, 48, 72, 78, 117, 180n94
 on being-with-the-other, 87
 biases and, 25
 and the body, 35–36, 186n42
 on calculative thinking, xix–xx, 20, 21, 24, 26, 61, 128, 161
 on calling, 201n92
 call to "become what you are," 94
 on care and concern for others, 198n51
 Cartesian thought, Cartesian model, and, 16, 17, 21, 25
 criticisms of, 71, 72, 186n42
 on Dasein, 17, 29, 47, 67, 179n70, 180n94, 186n42, 190n105, 198n51, 199n56, 201n92
 death and, 47–50, 53, 67, 190n105, 191n108
 education and, 121, 135, 215n6
 epistemology and, 15–20, 61
 on ethics, 75, 199n68
 on everydayness, 187n45
 on "fallenness" into the "world," 192n136
 hermeneutics and, 18, 34
 Husserl and, 34
 Iain Thomson and, 215n6
 (in)authenticity and, 51, 52, 64–73, 75, 195n8, 198n48, 225n158
 call to authenticity, 65–70, 75, 78
 on interpretation, 15–20, 34–35, 52–54, 151, 190n105
 Kierkegaard and, 29, 48, 51, 52, 65, 71, 183n1, 191n110, 195n6, 196n15, 196n20
 Mariana Ortega and, 203n121
 medicine and, 20, 21, 25, 26, 35–36, 38, 47, 49, 61
 on meditative thinking, 20, 26, 97, 128, 161
 Merleau-Ponty and, 35–36, 186n42

Heidegger (cont.)
  on metaphysics, 179n74
  Michael Inwood and, 199n67
  on mineness, 203n121
  on mystery, 70
  Nazism and, 200n70
  ontology, 15, 191n10
  phenomenology and, 20, 34, 185n31
  and pressing forward into possibilities, 206n174
  on reflections, 151
  releasement and, 69, 196n31
  resoluteness and, 68, 72, 75, 128, 196n31, 199n56, 199nn58–59
  science and, 15–17, 20, 29, 61
  on technology, 20–22
  and the "they," 51–54
  Tolstoy and, 192n144
  on truth, 18–20, 83
  on works of art, 143
Hermeneutical nature of medicine, 118
Hermeneutic dialogue, 86. *See also* Hermeneutics: dialogue-based
Hermeneutic phenomenology, 35, 185n34. *See also* Hermeneutics: phenomenology and
Hermeneutics
  dialogue-based, 82 (*see also* Hermeneutic dialogue)
  Gadamer and, 34, 82, 203n123
  Heidegger and, 18, 34
  interpretation and, 34, 35, 82, 85, 86, 185n34
  medical, 82, 87
    phronesis and, 85–89
  phenomenology and, 34, 35 (*see also* Hermeneutic phenomenology)
  responding to the call of the other, dialogue, and, 82–89
Hermeneutic understanding and moral understanding, 203n123
Hick, Christopher, 23

Hidden curriculum, xviii–xix, 6, 13, 102, 138, 150, 159
Homelikeness and unhomelikeness, 48
  being-in-the-world and, 65, 78, 187n63
  death anxiety and, 50
  Heidegger and, 38, 78
  illness and, 38–39, 50, 55, 78, 187n63
Homelike state, bringing the patient back to a, 55, 78
Honesty, virtue of, 210n53
hooks, bell, xxiv, 153
Horizons of meaning/horizons of understanding, 83, 84, 143
  closed, 86
  expansion of one's, 125, 137, 142, 143, 147
  fusion/merging of, 82–84, 86, 137, 147
  Gadamer and, 82–83, 86, 87, 137
  malleability and permeability, 86
Hospice and palliative care program at University of Texas Medical Branch (UTMB), 141
Hospice care, 43, 138–140. *See also* Palliative care
Hospitality, 78
Human-centered care. *See* Relationship-centered care
Humanism, 102
  dimensions of, 102
  Renaissance, 216n16
Humanities. *See also* Medical humanities
  etymology of the term, 130
  incorporating humanities into medical education, xvii–xviii
Human sciences and natural sciences, 172n14
Humor, 56
  gallows, xxii, 173n24
Husserl, Edmund, 33–34

"Iatrogenic" (Campo), 147
Identity. *See* Death: as collapse (of identity); Self

Index

Illness. *See also specific topics*
  vs. disease, 39–40
  meanings and interpretations of, 32, 83
  nature of, 39
  romanticizing, 198n54
Illness narratives, 37–39, 144–146, 154. *See also* Narratives
  doctors' stories, 146–151
Illness Narratives, The (Kleinman), xi, 105
"Illness talk" vs. "disease talk," 40, 57
Imagination, 134–136, 142. *See also* Moral imagination
  fostering, 154–156, 170
Impartiality, xix, 6, 7, 58, 81, 101. *See also* Objectivity
  detachment and, xix, 7
Inauthenticity. *See also under* Heidegger, Martin
  Kierkegaard on, 51, 52, 55
  and the "they," 53, 54, 66, 157 (*see also* "They"/"they-self")
Inauthentic understandings of death and dying, 53–54
Inauthentic ways of being-in-the-world, 66, 157
Indirect communication, Socratic ideal of, xxiv
Indirection, teaching by, xxiv
Infantilizing medical students, 113–114
Informatics. *See* Watson
Inquiry, types of, 15
Intellectualization, 46
Internal goods, 108–109
Interpretation, 38–40, 52, 83, 84, 149
  of death, 50, 51, 53, 66
  definitive, 83
  Heidegger on, 15–20, 34–35, 52–54, 151, 190n105
  hermeneutics and, 34, 35, 82, 85, 86, 185n34 (*see also* Hermeneutics)
  of illness, 32, 38–40, 55, 83, 84, 128, 202n118
  language and, 82
  Nietzsche on, 30
  phenomenology and, 34, 35, 185n34
  phronesis and, 85
  renunciation of all, 30
  and the "they," 51–55, 66
  of truth, 16, 19
  of the world, xx, xxiv, 15–20, 35, 38, 52, 69, 72, 135, 136, 190n105
Interpretive horizons, 84. *See also* Horizons of meaning/horizons of understanding
Inui, Thomas, xviii–xix, 102, 106–107
Investigation, modes of, 15
Inwood, Michael J., 199n67
I/Other split, 173n20
Ivanovich, Peter, 53–54

Johannessen, Helle, 156–157
Jones, Anne Hudson, 132
Jones, David, 159
Justice, virtue of, 210n53

Kanter, Steven L., 4, 152–153
Kasman, Deborah, 149
Keen, Sam, 44
Kierkegaard, Søren, xxiv, 51, 52, 61, 71, 127–128
  abstraction and, 29–30, 42, 61, 183n8
  anxiety and, 65
  on despair, 65, 192n128
  on dread, 48
  ethics and, 52, 183n1, 191n10
  on the existential, 29, 30
  Heidegger and, 29, 48, 51, 52, 65, 71, 183n1, 191n110, 195n6, 196n15, 196n20
  on inauthenticity, 51, 52, 55
  on indirect communication, xxiv
  on love, 72

Kierkegaard (cont.)
  Nietzsche and, 30, 55
  on philosophical and theological inquiry, 29, 32, 55
  religion and, 29, 30, 55, 65, 183n8
  as a religious thinker, 183n8
  science and, 29, 30, 32, 55
King, Nancy, 131–132
Kingdom of the sick, 38
Kinghorn, Warren A., 104, 114, 211n62
Kleinman, Arthur, xi, 105
Knowing, purpose of, 8
Knowledge, 8, 17, 23–24
  "hard" vs. "soft," 128
"Knowledge that" vs. "knowledge of," 74
Komesaroff, Paul, 6
Kumagai, Arno K., 100, 117, 127, 144, 151, 157, 209n27, 214n116

Language, 86
  of disease, 40–41
  interpretation and, 82
"Leaping ahead" students, 121, 128, 135, 198n51
"Leaping in" for students, 121, 129, 198n51
Levinas, Emmanuel, 77, 93
  alterity and, 80, 84
  Arthur Frank and, 78, 80, 201n91
  authenticity and, 75, 79, 81
  on being-for-the-other, 77, 79, 80, 87–90, 92, 93
  on death, 166, 205n158
  on ethics, 75–77, 81, 205n166
  on expression, 1, 63
  on hospitality, 78
  on humanity, the human condition, and human nature, 76–80, 87, 92, 95, 165–166
  on interpersonal encounters, 75–81, 89
  on the limits of empathy, 134
  love and, 166, 168, 205n158
  Mikhail Bahktin's dialogism and, 87
  as a moral perfectionist, 91–92
  overview, 76
  phenomenology of the face, 1, 75–81
  religion and, 76
  on responsibility, 76–77, 82, 92, 205n158, 205n166
  on rules, codes, and professionalism, 82, 104, 205n166
  suffering and, 75, 77, 81, 90
  vulnerability and, 77, 79, 80, 89
Liaison Committee on Medical Education (LCME), 156, 157, 160
Life. *See also under* Meaning making
  everydayness of, 36, 37, 187n45
  meaning of, 129
  prolonging life at all costs, 45
Lifeworld, 185n24
Lindeman, Brenessa, 113
Literature. *See also* Narratives
  engagement through, 144–146
Lived body, 35, 36. *See also under* Embodiment
Love, 72, 125, 165–166, 168
Luther, Martin, 16

MacIntyre, Alasdair, 107, 108, 116, 210n53
Maguire, Peter, 46, 59–60
Material and efficient causation, 8
Matuštík, Martin J., 183n8
May, William F., 194n167
  on art, 143
  on healing, 78, 91
  on influence of religion in medicine, 189n89
  on medical education, 12, 64, 119, 175n4, 208n21
  on virtues of doctors, 109
McAffee, Andrew, 25
McQuellon, Richard P., 67, 73, 86, 91, 196n21, 199n58
Meaning, 8, 15, 19, 20, 24, 32–34, 185n34. *See also* Horizons of

Index

meaning/horizons of understanding; Meaning making
  death as the end of all, 44
  of the illness (experience), 8, 25, 32
  of life and death, 129 (*see also under* Death)
  questions of, 24
Meaninglessness, 32, 48, 53, 79, 98, 195n6
Meaning making, xvii, 8, 30, 40
  bringing meaning to one's life, 93, 95, 121, 165, 195n6
  finding meaning in one's work, xii, xxi, 93, 100, 169
  searching and striving for meaning, xvii, xxi, xxiv, xxvi, 62, 79, 117
Meaning-making processes, illness as disturbing/disrupting one's, 39
Medical education. *See also under* Self; *specific topics*
  recent curricular changes, xviii–xx
  values in, 64, 119, 175n4, 208n21
Medical humanism, 131
Medical humanities, 216n14
  criticism of, 131, 156
  and the moral imagination, 133–142
  nature of, 129–163
    authentic engagement through artistic and narrative representation, 142–158
    creating change through relationship, 158–163
    engagement with the other: death and dying as an example, 137–142
  need for evidence of effectiveness of, 156–157
  terminology, 129–130
Medical paradigm. *See* Biomedical paradigm
Medical school. *See also* Medical education
  admission policies and admission process, 2–3

Medical school applicants, 2, 3
  reasons for pursuing medicine as a career, 3–4
Medical students and residents mistreated by mentors, 112–115
Medicine. *See also specific topics*
  definitions and conceptions of, 9, 70
  ethos of, xxii, 6, 10, 43
  functions of, 9
  telos of, x, 10, 85, 108
  as a vocation, 194n1
Meditative thinking
  calculative thinking and, 20–22, 150, 162
  contrasted, xxv, 26, 100, 128, 161
  relations between, xxv, 26, 100, 128, 162
  fostering and cultivating, 128, 129, 150, 155–156, 158
  Heidegger on, 20, 26, 97, 128, 161
  hermeneutical nature of medicine and, 118
  medical education and, 161
  medical humanities and, 129, 155
  nature and scope of, xxv, 26, 128
  reflective writing and, 149–151
  relevance to clinical care, 162
Mentoring for fearlessness, 154–155
Mentors, 158
  behaving badly, 112–118
  virtuous, 111
Merleau-Ponty, Maurice, 35–36, 180n84, 186n42, 204n134
Metaphysics
  Being and, 179n74
  of medicine, 8
Metaquestions, asking, 14–15
Miller, Jerome, 68
Mimetic mode. *See* Reflective (vs. mimetic) mode
Mind–body dualism, 8–9, 31. *See also* Cartesian dualism
Mind–body separation, 23, 35

Mindful practice, 99–100
Mineness, 203n121
Modernist thinking and modernist biomedical paradigm, 10, 43, 87, 101, 123, 173n20
Montgomery, Kathryn, xix, 6, 70
Moral imagination, xxiv, 129, 163, 217n30
  medical humanities and the, 133–142
Morgan, Michael, 93
Mortality, turning away from. *See* Denial: of death; Vulnerability: turning away from
Mystery, 70, 128, 198n41. *See also* Uncertainty

Naidu, Thirusha, 214n116
Narrative approaches, 131
  to clinical care and ethics, 208n13
Narrative competence, 219n78
Narrative imagination, 220n82
"Narrative Medicine" (Charon), 219n78. *See also* Charon, Rita
Narrative medicine movement, 131
Narrative plotlines, 10
Narrative representation, engagement through, 144–146. *See also* Authentic engagement through artistic and narrative representation
Narratives, 40, 116, 151
  incorporating narratives into medical training, 142–143
  types of, 10, 144, 151 (*see also* Illness narratives)
Narrative understanding in medical education, ways to incorporate, 153–154
Neoliberalism, 99, 153
Nietzsche, Friedrich Wilhelm, 183n9
  certainty, uncertainty, and, 30, 55, 71
  detachment and, 55, 184n9
  on interpretation, 30
  Kierkegaard and, 30, 55
  perspectivism, 31, 41
  phenomenology and, 32, 41, 184n18
  on science and truth, 30–31, 55, 184n9, 184n18
No-longer-being-able-to-be-there, 47, 50, 67
No-longer-being-here, potential for, 48
Nonreflective professionalism, 120, 121
Nothingness, 195n6. *See also* Meaninglessness
Novack, Dennis H., 101
Nuland, Sherwin, 10–11
Nussbaum, Martha C., 94, 220n82

Objectification, 22, 24, 40, 61. *See also* Clinical gaze
Objectivity, 6–7, 35, 176n25. *See also* Impartiality
  definitions and meanings of the term, 177n25
  detachment and, xi, 6–7, 24, 97–98, 101, 120, 177n25
  vs. empathy, 14, 120, 128
  history of, 176n25
  taking for granted, 14
Ofri, Daniellle, 61, 168
Omniscient, doctors seen as. *See* Clinical gaze
Ontic inquiry, 15
Ontological anxiety, 44, 47–49, 53, 55, 58, 59
Ontological-existential anxiety, 50, 60. *See also* Existential anxiety
Ontology, xxi, 15
  fundamental, 15, 185n31
  Heidegger on, 15, 185n31
Ortega, Mariana, 84
Other, the
  alterity and, 80–81
  I/Other split, 173n20
  responding to the call of the, 82–89

Index

turning toward, 75–81, 90, 107 (*see also* Face: Levinas's phenomenology of the)
Ousager, Jakob, 156–157

Palliative care, 43, 139, 140. *See also* Dying patients/terminal patients
  vs. curative care, 139
  instruction in, 138–141
Parallel charts, 224n144
Parental role. *See* Paternalism
Paternalism, medical, 131–132
  with dying/terminal patients, 145, 190n96
Patient-centered care, 98–99
  vs. relationship-centered care, 100 (*see also* Relationship-centered care)
Paulsen, Randall H., 101
Pedagogical culture, creating a new, 127, 128
Pedagogy, 137, 156, 157. *See also specific topics*
  intersection of epistemology and, 10–13
Pellegrino, Edmund D., 9, 108–109
Personal and professional, distinction between the, 117
Perspectivism, Nietzsche's dynamic, 31, 41
Phenomenology. *See also* Bracketing
  and the body, 35–37
  defined, 185n31
  and fundamental ontology, 185n31
  Heidegger and, 20, 34, 185n31
  vs. hermeneutic phenomenology, 185n34
  interpretation and, 34, 35, 185n34
  nature of, 33–35
Philosophers, 185n8. *See also specific philosophers*
Phronesis, 85, 211n68
  Aristotle on, 85, 109, 110, 211n68

conceptions of and translations of the term, 85
contrasted with other intellectual virtues, 109
functions, 109, 211n68
hermeneutics and, 85–89
medical humanities as cultivating, 130
mentors and the development of, 85, 111, 112
nature of, 85, 117
vs. professionalism, 117
Physicians. *See* Doctors
Plutchik, Robert, 46
Portfolios, 224n143
Possibilities, pressing forward into, 206n174
Presence and being present with patients, 94, 141. *See also* Witnessing
Problem-based learning (PBL), 161
Professional façade, xix
Professional identity formation, 106–107
Professionalism, 209n42. *See also under* Levinas, Emmanuel
  conceptualizations of, 105
  facets/dimensions of, 106
  mask of, 105
  meaning and scope of the term, 102
  nature of, 117
  vs. phronesis, 117
  use of the term, 102
  virtue ethics and, 107–112
Professionalization movement, medical education and the, 102–112
"Providers," doctors as, 168
Putnam, Hilary, 91–92

Ramsey, Paul, 45, 103, 194n1
Ramsey, Ramsey Eric
  on curiosity, 197n38
  on need for control and certainty, 71
  on Nietzsche, 184n18
  on science, xx, 15, 18

Reductionistic interventions, xxiii
Reductionistic medicine, 132
  disburdening of anxiety and, 54–59
  estrangement from ourselves, 60–62
  patients' own disburdening, 59–60
Reductionistic scientific research, 2
Reductionistic understandings of illness and health, x, 14, 24–26, 41, 55, 145, 159, 169
Reflection, 122. *See also specific topics*
  existential, 100–101, 125
  personal, 122–124, 153
Reflective dialogue, 121–123. *See also* Dialogue
Reflective practice, 214n116
Reflective (vs. mimetic) mode, personal accounts told in the, 150
Relationship-centered care, 100, 101, 207–208nn12–13
Releasement, 69–70
  Heidegger and, 69, 196n31
  resoluteness and, 69, 196n31
Religion, 30, 76
  Kierkegaard and, 29, 30, 55, 65, 183n8
  medicine and, 189n89
Resiliency, 169
Resoluteness, 68
  anxiety and, 68, 69, 72
  authenticity and, 68, 69, 71–73, 75, 79, 128, 197n31, 199nn58–59
  Dasein and, 72, 199nn56
  death and, 68, 69
  Heidegger and, 68, 72, 75, 128, 196n31, 199n56, 199nn58–59
  releasement and, 69, 196n31
Responsibility, 205n166
  of all persons for one another, 76–77
  personal, 146
  practices of, 81
Restitution narrative, 10
Robinson, Sally, xxi
Rounds, grand, 113–115, 119, 120, 140

Routine patterns of medical culture, 149
Rudebeck, Carl Edvard, 202n118

Sacks, Oliver, 195n13
Scannell, Kate, 162
Schön, Donald, 174n35
Science, 23, 176n9. *See also specific topics*
  appeal of, 24–25
  defined, 173n16
  detachment and, xviii, xix, 6, 8, 18, 24, 29, 61, 98
  faith, religion, and, 30
  Heidegger and, 15–17, 20, 29, 61
  Kierkegaard and, 29, 30, 32, 55
  limitations of, 24
  Linda Wiener and Ramsey Eric Ramsey on, xx, 15, 18
  Merleau-Ponty on, 180n84
  Nietzsche on, 30–31, 55, 184n9, 184n18
Science claim, giving up the, xx–xxi
Scientific curiosity, need to cultivate medical students', 197n37
Scientism, 15, 31, 95, 98
  defined, 15, 181n99
Scientists, doctors as, xxvi, 5, 7–9, 55–57
Second-person experience, knowledge gleaned from, 73–74
Self. *See also* Death: as collapse (of identity)
  Charles Taylor on the, 87
  medical education and the cultivation of, 101–102
    attempting to form "good" doctors, 118–125
    physician (re)formation, 125–126
    professionalization movement and, 102–112
    when mentors behave badly, 112–118
  modernist understandings of the, 87
  multiplicitous, 203n121

Index

Self-understanding, hermeneutics and, 18
Shafer, Audrey, 149
Shapiro, Johanna, 73
  on empathy, 173n20
  on intellectual bait and switch, 4–5
  on medical education, 73, 149, 151–152
  on medicine, 43
  on metaquestions, 14–15
  modernist thinking and, 43, 123, 173n20
  on role models, 123
Shared existential loneliness, 79
Shared understanding, 83. *See also* Horizons of meaning/horizons of understanding: fusion/merging of
Sklar, David P., 112–113
Socialization process, medical education as a, 5–6
Sociological imagination, 217n30
Solicitude, 198n51
  positive vs. negative, 198n51
SPIKES (Set the stage, Perception, Inform, Knowledge, Empathy, and Summarize) method, xxii–xxiii
Spiritual calling, 194n1
Stanford, Ann Folwell, 131–132
Stein, Howard, 45–46
Stories, talking in, 40. *See also* Narratives
Stump, Eleonore, 73–74
Suffering. *See also specific topics*
  an authentic response to, 89–90
    asking too much of our doctors, 90–91
    realism vs. idealism, 91–93
    a return back to ourselves, 93–95
  being-in-the-world and, 32, 97, 188n74
  causes of, 188n74
  conceptions of, 188n74
  detachment and, xix, 7, 8, 11, 59, 97–98, 121
  Jeffrey Bishop on, 8, 32, 88
  pedagogy of, 136, 144
  defined, xxix
  types of, xvi–xvii, 9, 171nn4–5, 188n74
  why we turn away from, 42–44 (*see also* Vulnerability: turning away from)
    anxiety and disburdening, 51–54
    Heidegger and death anxiety, 47–51
    medicine and the denial of death, 44–47
Suicide among doctors, 99
Supercomputers, 25–26
Supportive autonomy, 114
Surgeons, 167
Svenaeus, Fredrik., 89
  on health, 39
  on homelikeness and unhomelikeness, 38, 187n63
  on illness, 32, 39–40, 83
  on medical hermeneutics, 82, 85
Symptoms, approaches to, 202n118

Tacit equilibrium. *See* Equilibrium of body
Taken-for-granted assumptions, 33, 37–38, 78, 149. *See also* Objectivity
  of Cartesian inquiry, 17
  of medical epistemology, xx, 10
Taylor, Charles, 17, 18, 87, 89, 183n131, 205n164
Technē, 22, 25, 109, 211n62
Technical rationality, 174n35
Technology, 25–26
  etymology and original meaning of the term, 21–22
  Heidegger on, 20–22
  negative effects on doctor–patient interaction, 20–22
Terminal diagnosis, xxiii, 59, 195n13. *See also* Cancer diagnosis; Dying patients/terminal patients

Theoretical-judicial model, 81
"They"/"they-self," the, 51, 52, 54, 55, 58, 61, 187n45, 196n30
  anxiety and, 51–54
  and calculative thinking, 72
  and the call to authenticity, 65–66, 68
  caring for others as, 58
  death and, 51, 53–54, 61, 65
  defined, 51
  detachment from, 198n48
  failure to distinguish ourselves from, 72
  freeing oneself from, 65, 66, 68
  Heidegger and, 51–54
  interpretation and, 51–55, 66
  resoluteness and, 75
  "they-self" notions about detachment, 59
  "they-self" notions of success, 157
  "they-self" understandings of care, 100
  trappings of, 72
  turning toward, 51
Thomson, Iain, 49, 215, 215n6
Tirado, Linda, 146
Tolstoy, Leo, 53, 95, 192n144
Toombs, S. Kay, 32, 35
Toulmin, Stephen, 136
Tournier, Robert E., 1
Traumatic deidealization, 112
Treadway, Katharine, 12, 56, 122
Trust, 102–103, 167
Truth, 15–20, 23
  Heidegger on, 18–20, 83
  medicine as a permanent, 15
  nature of, 83, 143
  Nietzsche on, 30, 31, 184n9
  quest for, 7

Uncertainty, 55, 70, 71, 109, 159, 197n38, 198n41
  leaving room for, 166
  radical, 70

Understanding. *See* Horizons of meaning/horizons of understanding
University of Texas Medical Branch (UTMB), xxviii
  hospice and palliative care program at, 141
  Physician-Healer Track, 212n87

Vicarious traumatization, 206n5
Virtue ethics, 107–108
  professionalism and, 107–112
Virtue(s), 102, 147, 210n53
  Aristotle on, 107, 211nn67–68
  "functional virtues" in medical practice, 43
Virtuous action in the world, orientation toward, 130
Virtuous person
  development of the virtuous whole person, 116–118
  ideas about being a, 107–108
Vulnerability, 80, 105, 107, 135, 148, 154, 163. *See also specific topics*
  anxiety and, 51, 65, 101, 107
  awareness of and recognizing one's, xii, xxix, 62, 64, 65, 68, 72–73, 79, 101
  calls for, 5
  communicating and expressing, 89, 123, 138
  compassion and, 93–94
  concern, caring, and, 73, 77
  connection, closeness, and, 73, 77
  death and, 44, 50, 63
  etymology and meaning of the term, 147–148
  illness evoking realization of one's, 60
  making meaning in the face of, xxiv
  nature of, 77
  responding to others', xii
  shared (sense of), xxi, 73, 80, 95, 125, 127
  suffering and, 63, 93–94

turning away from, xxi–xxiii, xxvi, 43,
   55, 59, 65, 101, 168 (*see also*
   Suffering: why we turn away from)
witnessing others', 62

Walker, Margaret Urban, 81
Watson (computer), 25–26
Wear, Delese, 154
Weber, Max, 176n9
Weissman, David, 140
Westphal, Merold, 183n8
Whole person
   development of the virtuous, 116–118
   notion of, 116
Wiener, Linda
   on curiosity, 197n38
   on need for control and certainty, 71
   on Nietzsche, 184n18
   on science, xx, 15, 18
Williams, Bernard, 181n99
Williams, Peter, 120, 160
Wisdom, practical. *See* Phronesis
Witnessing, 62, 79, 89–90, 100, 136,
   137, 168
Wonder, 70, 143, 198n41. *See also*
   Curiosity
   openness to, 237n39
"World travelers," 84, 86, 203n121
Wounded storytellers. *See also under*
   Frank, Arthur W.
   narratives of illness told by, 144–145
      (*see also* Illness narratives)

Zaner, Richard M., 77, 80, 88
Zarconi, Joseph, 154

Basic Bioethics

Arthur Caplan, editor

Books Acquired under the Editorship of Glenn McGee and Arthur Caplan

Peter A. Ubel, *Pricing Life: Why It's Time for Health Care Rationing*

Mark G. Kuczewski and Ronald Polansky, eds., *Bioethics: Ancient Themes in Contemporary Issues*

Suzanne Holland, Karen Lebacqz, and Laurie Zoloth, eds., *The Human Embryonic Stem Cell Debate: Science, Ethics, and Public Policy*

Gita Sen, Asha George, and Piroska Östlin, eds., *Engendering International Health: The Challenge of Equity*

Carolyn McLeod, *Self-Trust and Reproductive Autonomy*

Lenny Moss, *What Genes Can't Do*

Jonathan D. Moreno, ed., *In the Wake of Terror: Medicine and Morality in a Time of Crisis*

Glenn McGee, ed., *Pragmatic Bioethics*, 2nd edition

Timothy F. Murphy, *Case Studies in Biomedical Research Ethics*

Mark A. Rothstein, ed., *Genetics and Life Insurance: Medical Underwriting and Social Policy*

Kenneth A. Richman, *Ethics and the Metaphysics of Medicine: Reflections on Health and Beneficence*

David Lazer, ed., *DNA and the Criminal Justice System: The Technology of Justice*

Harold W. Baillie and Timothy K. Casey, eds., *Is Human Nature Obsolete? Genetics, Bioengineering, and the Future of the Human Condition*

Robert H. Blank and Janna C. Merrick, eds., *End-of-Life Decision Making: A Cross-National Study*

Norman L. Cantor, *Making Medical Decisions for the Profoundly Mentally Disabled*

Margrit Shildrick and Roxanne Mykitiuk, eds., *Ethics of the Body: Post-Conventional Challenges*

Alfred I. Tauber, *Patient Autonomy and the Ethics of Responsibility*

David H. Brendel, *Healing Psychiatry:Bridging the Science/Humanism Divide*

Jonathan Baron, *Against Bioethics*

Michael L. Gross, *Bioethics and Armed Conflict: Moral Dilemmas of Medicine and War*

Karen F. Greif and Jon F. Merz, *Current Controversies in the Biological Sciences: Case Studies of Policy Challenges from New Technologies*

Deborah Blizzard, *Looking Within: A Sociocultural Examination of Fetoscopy*

Ronald Cole-Turner, ed., *Design and Destiny: Jewish and Christian Perspectives on Human Germline Modification*

Holly Fernandez Lynch, *Conflicts of Conscience in Health Care: An Institutional Compromise*

Mark A. Bedau and Emily C. Parke, eds., *The Ethics of Protocells: Moral and Social Implications of Creating Life in the Laboratory*

Jonathan D. Moreno and Sam Berger, eds., *Progress in Bioethics: Science, Policy, and Politics*

Eric Racine, *Pragmatic Neuroethics: Improving Understanding and Treatment of the Mind-Brain*

Martha J. Farah, ed., *Neuroethics: An Introduction with Readings*

Jeremy R. Garrett, ed., *The Ethics of Animal Research: Exploring the Controversy*

Books Acquired under the Editorship of Arthur Caplan

Sheila Jasanoff, ed., *Reframing Rights: Bioconstitutionalism in the Genetic Age*

Christine Overall, *Why Have Children? The Ethical Debate*

Yechiel Michael Barilan, *Human Dignity, Human Rights, and Responsibility: The New Language of Global Bioethics and Bio-Law*

Tom Koch, *Thieves of Virtue: When Bioethics Stole Medicine*

Timothy F. Murphy, *Ethics, Sexual Orientation, and Choices about Children*

Daniel Callahan, *In Search of the Good: A Life in Bioethics*

Robert Blank, *Intervention in the Brain: Politics, Policy, and Ethics*

Gregory E. Kaebnick and Thomas H. Murray, eds., *Synthetic Biology and Morality: Artificial Life and the Bounds of Nature*

Dominic A. Sisti, Arthur L. Caplan, and Hila Rimon-Greenspan, eds., *Applied Ethics in Mental Health Care: An Interdisciplinary Reader*

Barbara K. Redman, *Research Misconduct Policy in Biomedicine: Beyond the Bad-Apple Approach*

Russell Blackford, *Humanity Enhanced: Genetic Choice and the Challenge for Liberal Democracies*

Nicholas Agar, *Truly Human Enhancement: A Philosophical Defense of Limits*

Bruno Perreau, *The Politics of Adoption: Gender and the Making of French Citizenship*

Carl Schneider, *The Censor's Hand: The Misregulation of Human-Subject Research*

Lydia S. Dugdale, ed., *Dying in the Twenty-First Century: Towards a New Ethical Framework for the Art of Dying Well*

John D. Lantos and Diane S. Lauderdale, *Preterm Babies, Fetal Patients, and Childbearing Choices*

Harris Wiseman, *The Myth of the Moral Brain*

Arthur L. Caplan and Jason Schwartz, eds., *Vaccine Ethics and Policy: An Introduction with Readings*

Tom Koch, *Ethics in Everyday Places: Mapping Moral Stress, Distress, and Injury*

Nicole Piemonte, *Afflicted: How Vulnerability Can Heal Medical Education and Practice*